Autoimmune Diseases in Domestic Animals

Autoimmune Diseases in Domestic Animals

Ian R. Tizard, BVMS, PhD, ACVM (Hons), DSc (Hons)
University Distinguished Professor Emeritus
Department of Veterinary Pathobiology
Texas A&M University
College Station
Texas

ELSEVIER

Elsevier
3251 Riverport Lane
St. Louis, Missouri 63043

AUTOIMMUNE DISEASES IN DOMESTIC ANIMALS   ISBN: 978-0-323-84813-8

Senior Content Strategist: Jennifer Catando
Senior Content Development Manager: Somodatta Roy Choudhary
Senior Content Development Specialist: Shilpa Kumar
Publishing Services Manager: Shereen Jameel
Project Manager: Vishnu T Jiji
Design Direction: Ryan Cook

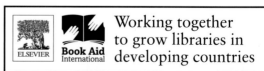

Working together to grow libraries in developing countries

www.elsevier.com • www.bookaid.org

Printed in India

Last digit is the print number: 9   8   7   6   5   4   3   2   1

To Claire

ACKNOWLEDGMENTS

As always, my professional colleagues have proven to be incredibly generous in sharing material with me. The team of pathologists at Texas A&M University have proven to be an inestimable source of high-quality material for the illustrations. These include Drs. Dominique Wiener, Karen Russell, Brian Porter, Roy Pool, Mark Johnson, and Aline Rodrigues Hoffman. I must also single out Dr. Robert Kennis of Auburn University for permitting me to use many of his excellent clinical illustrations. Drs. Unity Jeffery, Erin Scott, and Nick Jeffery also provided invaluable assistance in correcting selected chapters. Nevertheless, I take full credit for all the mistakes in the text. Finally, as always, I must thank my wonderful wife, Claire, for her help and support.

College Station, Texas
May 2021

Veterinary immunology is growing in significance. Once a minor subdiscipline of microbiology, it has established itself as a discipline central to the practice of scientific veterinary medicine. Its growing importance in animal health is reflected in the explosive growth of information regarding infection, immunity, and immunologic diseases in domestic animals. This growth has meant that veterinary immunology can no longer be adequately covered by a single broad-based textbook. Several clinically important subdisciplines such as vaccinology, allergic diseases, and autoimmune diseases have emerged. There is a need for advanced texts that can assist not only students but also practitioners seeking to expand their knowledge and practice their profession based on the most recent scientific information.

This text, the third in this series on advanced immunology, is primarily about autoimmune diseases of animals. It has been written for three main reasons: The first is to draw together the latest information on their causes, pathogenesis, and treatment for the interested veterinarian, comparative immunologist, and veterinary student. Only by connecting peer-reviewed scientific reports from many diverse diseases is it possible to form a coherent picture of current information on the autoimmune-autoinflammatory disease spectrum. The second reason is to seek to resolve confusion regarding the relationships between autoimmunity and other immune-mediated diseases, especially misinformation circulating on the web. The final and by no means least important reason is because the prevalence and the importance of autoimmune diseases are increasing in both humans and their animals.

Because of their significance, research into autoimmune diseases continues apace. This research focuses almost exclusively on the human diseases, and enormous strides have been made in our understanding of their complexity, pathogenesis, and treatment. Large numbers of peer-reviewed papers on autoimmune and rheumatoid diseases are published annually. Unfortunately, the same cannot be said for our domestic species, especially companion animals. Fortunately, it has proved possible to apply many of the findings from human primates to other mammals. For example, it is inevitable that the highly successful monoclonal antibody therapies used in humans will eventually be applied to dogs and cats. But veterinarians need to be prepared to use them appropriately. Issues are sure to arise if there is confusion or misunderstanding regarding disease causation and pathogenesis.

At their simplest, autoimmune diseases result from a loss of immune tolerance that results in adaptive immune responses being targeted at normal body components. However, few autoimmune diseases are that simple. Indeed, much of the evidence relating to autoimmune diseases in the domestic species is circumstantial. This evidence includes specific breed-related susceptibility in dogs, clear immune mediation as evidenced by an infiltration of affected tissues with lymphocytes, an obvious similarity to a proven autoimmune disease in humans, and perhaps most importantly a positive therapeutic response to immunosuppressive and antiinflammatory drug treatment. Even within these guidelines there are many animal diseases that remain difficult to diagnose and classify. Many are unquestionably immune mediated but not necessarily autoimmune.

The immune system not only consists of adaptive immune responses but also encompasses innate immunity, especially inflammation. The term *autoinflammatory diseases* has been coined to describe those diseases where uncontrolled inflammation also causes tissue destruction and disease. Inflammation is also a response to disturbances in adaptive immunity. Thus immune-mediated inflammatory diseases are key components of the autoinflammatory spectrum. They overlap conventional autoimmunity in many ways. Some diseases are primarily autoinflammatory while others are almost exclusively autoimmune in nature. They all form a part of an immune-inflammatory continuum.

Domestic mammals, especially companion animals, do not have a shortage of diseases in which chronic inflammation, with or without autoimmunity, is a key component. Many such diseases result from the overproduction of inflammatory cytokines. It is also clear that for many diseases, especially those mediated by hypersensitivity responses, a distinction must be drawn between primary diseases that appear to occur spontaneously and are currently of unknown etiology and secondary diseases in which the immune-mediated responses are clearly triggered by infections, drugs, or neoplasia. Rather than draw an arbitrary line between the two, these secondary immune-mediated diseases are discussed herein as appropriate.

Another reason for publishing at this time is the growing evidence that these diseases are increasing in prevalence. Recent studies have confirmed the impression that the prevalence of many autoimmune diseases is steadily increasing in humans. For example, the prevalence of anti-nuclear antibodies in the North American population has risen from 11% in 1988-1991 to 12% in 1999-2994 to 16% in 2011-2012. In Alberta, Canada, the prevalence of systemic lupus erythematosus increased from 48 cases per 100,000 in 2000 to 90 per 100,000 in 2015. Other human autoimmune diseases that have steadily increased in prevalence include celiac disease, type 1 diabetes mellitus, and myasthenia gravis. The reasons for this appear to be associated with a Western lifestyle and dietary factors that have altered our commensal microbiota. Unfortunately, there is very little comparable data available for domestic animal species. Nevertheless, there is evidence that the prevalence of autoimmunity in companion animals is also increasing.

Part of my motivation in writing this text also derived from an effort to correct the misinformation spread over the Internet regarding these diseases. There has been a tendency to oversimplify these problems and lump all immune-mediated diseases in a single category, rather than recognizing their diversity and their many differences in causation, pathogenesis, treatment, and significance. As described earlier, there exists, in the minds of many, confusion regarding the precise nature of autoimmune diseases and their relationship to the broader universe of immune-mediated and inflammatory diseases.

In drawing together the material for this text, decisions have had to be made as to what to include and exclude. There are overlaps between the different categories of immune-mediated diseases. Thus, broadly speaking, hypersensitivity and allergic diseases, while critically important in veterinary medicine, form a discrete entity that is best considered on its own. The sharp-eyed reader will, however, note a certain overlap between some of the contents of this text and my previous one on hypersensitivity diseases. For example, milk allergy in dairy cattle is both an allergic disease and an autoimmune disease and warrants inclusion in both. Other overlapping topics include type III hypersensitivity diseases where some autoimmune diseases cause damage by generating immune complexes. Some, such as the vasculitides, may also be triggered by autoimmunity as well as other sources of immune complexes and so require overlapping coverage. However, I do believe that these diseases are best considered as part of this package of autoimmune and inflammatory diseases.

The reader will note that this is primarily a text about canine diseases. Besides the obvious predominance of dogs in companion animal practice, dogs represent uniquely important models of immune diseases. The incredible phenotypic heterogeneity of dogs and their complex genomics ensure that there are enormous variations in disease prevalence and clinical manifestations among breeds. Cats and horses tie for a distant second place, whereas livestock species rarely show up in lists of autoimmune diseases. This is unfortunate, since livestock undoubtedly represent a potential source of much useful information on pathogenesis and immunopathology. Perhaps this text will encourage livestock veterinarians to look out for novel immune-mediated diseases in their species of interest.

Another issue that I have encountered when writing this text is the fact that some animal autoimmune diseases are very rare indeed. This raises the question of how much space to allocate to them. This has been especially difficult for diseases that are both common and important in humans but very rare or trivial in domestic species. The reader may find oneself in disagreement with me in the emphasis or lack of it placed on certain individual rare diseases, but this is a book about diseases of animals and I have sought to minimize coverage of human diseases except when directly relevant to the domestic mammals.

TABLE OF CONTENTS

ACAID	Anterior chamber-associated immune deviation	FoxP3	Forkhead box P3
AChR	Acetylcholine receptor	GBS	Gullain-Barré syndrome
ACPA	Anticitrullinated protein antibodies	GM-CSF	Granulocyte/monocyte colony-stimulating factor
ADCC	Antibody-dependent cellular cytotoxicity	GWAS	Genome-wide association study
AhR	Aryl hydrocarbon receptor	HMGB-1	High mobility group box (protein)-1
AIRE	Autoimmune regulator	HSC	Hematopoietic stem cell
APRIL	Activation and proliferation-induced ligand	HSP	Heat-shock protein
		IBD	Inflammatory bowel disease
APS1	Autoimmune polyglandular syndrome-1	IDDM	Insulin-dependent diabetes mellitus
BAFF	B-cell activating factor	IDO	Indoleamine 2,3-dioxygenase
BCR	B-cell (antigen) receptor		
CCL/CXCL	Chemokines of different structures	IFN	Interferon
		IL	Interleukin
CCR/CXCR	Chemokine receptors	ILC	Innate lymphoid cell
CpG	Paired cytosine-guanosine nucleotides (DNA)	ITP	Immune-mediated thrombocytopenia
CRP	C-reactive protein	IVIG	Intravenous immunoglobulin
CSF	Cerebrospinal fluid	MDSC	Myeloid-derived suppressor cells
CSK	Chronic superficial keratitis		
CTLA-4	Cytotoxic T-lymphocyte–associated antigen 4	MHC	Major histocompatibility complex
DAMP	Damage-associated molecular pattern	MS	Multiple sclerosis
		NET	Neutrophil extracellular trap
DC	Dendritic cell	NK	Natural killer (cell)
DIC	Disseminated intravascular coagulation	NOD	Nonobese diabetic (mice)
EAE	Experimental autoimmune encephalomyelitis	NOD	Nucleotide oligomerization domain (pattern recognition receptors)
EAN	Experimental autoimmune neuritis	NK cells	Natural killer cells
		NKT cells	Natural killer T cells
ELISA	Enzyme-linked immunosorbent assay	PAF	Platelet-activating factor
FcR	Fc (immunoglobulin) receptor	PAMP	Pathogen-associated molecular pattern
		PD-1	Programed cell death 1
FeLV	Feline leukemia virus	PGE	Promiscuous gene expression
FIV	Feline immunodeficiency virus	PRR	Pattern recognition receptor

RA	Rheumatoid arthritis	T1DM	Type 1 diabetes mellitus
RANKL	Receptor activator of nuclear factor kappa-B ligand	TCR	T-cell (antigen) receptor
ROS	Reactive oxygen species	TGFβ	Transforming growth factor-β
SCAR	Severe cutaneous adverse reaction	Th1	Type 1 helper T cell
		Th2	Type 2 helper T cell
SCFA	Short-chain fatty acid	Th17	Type 17 helper T cell
SJS	Stevens-Johnson syndrome	TLR	Toll-like receptor
SLE	Systemic lupus erythematosus	TNF	Tumor necrosis factor
		TRAIL	Tumor necrosis factor-related apoptosis-inducing ligand
SNP	Single nucleotide polymorphisms		
SP	Substance P (a neuropeptide)	Treg	Regulatory T cell
		VEGF	Vascular endothelial growth factor
SRMA	Steroid-responsive meningitis-arteritis		

Basic Immunology: A Review

The function of the immune system is to detect, attack, and destroy harmful invading microorganisms. It is highly effective at this and readily prevents invasion by most potential pathogens. When a microbe invades the body, the first critical step is to recognize its presence. An animal's survival depends on the ability of its immune system to differentiate between a normal body component and an invading foreign organism. Once the invader has been identified as foreign, it is destroyed rapidly, efficiently, and completely. However, molecules identified as normal body components and healthy cells are usually ignored. This distinction is regulated by multiple checks and balances so that tolerance to healthy cells is usually maintained. Under some circumstances, however, the system breaks down, and on occasion a misdirected immune response—an autoimmune response—can cause sufficient damage that can result in disease and death.

Although autoimmune diseases have been considered uncommon, it is estimated that worldwide they affect about 4.5% of the population, including 2.7% of men and 6.4% of women. In the United States and United Kingdom, autoimmune diseases are among the top 10 leading causes of death in women up to age 65 years. The most common of these diseases are lymphocytic thyroiditis and rheumatoid arthritis, with a prevalence of 791 and 860 cases per 100,000, respectively. In domestic animals, autoimmune thyroiditis and autoimmune skin diseases are probably of greatest significance. About 100 autoimmune diseases have been identified in humans and a somewhat smaller number in domestic animals. They therefore cause significant morbidity suffering and mortality. They can be subdivided somewhat arbitrarily into those organ-specific diseases that attack a single organ such as the thyroid, intestine, brain, or muscle. Others are systemic diseases such as systemic lupus erythematosus that attack many different organs. These diseases can be mediated by the innate immune system and/or by the adaptive immune system, including both antibody- and cell-mediated responses.

Innate Immunity

The immune system consists of two distinct subsystems: the innate system and the adaptive system. The innate immune system generates a reflexive, immediate response to microbial invasion (Fig. 1.1). Upon recognizing that the body is under attack, by sensing the presence of foreign molecular patterns, either microbial molecules or molecules released from damaged cells, the process

1

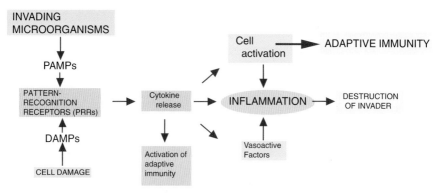

Fig. 1.1 **A** simplified view of the innate immune system. Note that in addition to triggering inflammation, innate responses begin the activation of adaptive immune responses. *DAMPs,* Damage-associated molecular patterns; *PAMPs,* pathogen-associated molecular patterns.

of inflammation is triggered. (Tissue damage and cell breakage release molecules formally called damage-associated molecular patterns [DAMPs]; pathogens are covered with and release their own characteristic molecules called pathogen-associated molecular patterns [PAMPs]. There is a growing tendency to refer to DAMPs as alarmins given their role in triggering immune responses.) DAMPs and PAMPs bind to innate sensors (invariant pattern-recognition receptors), and these in turn cause sentinel cells to release a mixture of proinflammatory proteins called cytokines. The resulting inflammation concentrates protective leukocytes such as neutrophils and antimicrobial proteins such as complement at the sites of invasion. As a result, the invaders are usually destroyed. Inflammation is, however, an uncomfortable process that is often accompanied by some tissue damage. Cells are killed, enzymes leak into tissues, and pain neurons are activated. Under most conditions, though, any residual damage is repaired by the healing process, and affected tissues return to normal. Innate immune responses do not, however, improve with experience. They are not a long-term solution to the body's defensive needs. For this, the body requires an adaptive immune response.

It is also clear that innate immune responses are required to initiate adaptive immune responses. This is well seen in vaccination where adjuvants are employed to trigger a mild inflammatory response that serves to promote a very strong adaptive response to the vaccine antigens. This will also be seen later in this book, where there are many examples of an innate immune response—inflammation—serving as a trigger for the subsequent development of an autoimmune adaptive response. The flood of cytokines generated by innate immune responses provides the essential stimuli needed to trigger adaptive responses. Thus they activate antigen-presenting cells so that antigens are efficiently processed and presented to the adaptive system. The mixture of inflammatory cytokines can, depending on their composition, also provide the signals that determine the nature of the subsequent adaptive response.

The animal body may sometimes lose control of these inflammatory processes. Regulatory pathways may not work properly, and as a result animals may undergo excessive uncontrolled inflammation. Thus autoinflammatory diseases can occur and may cause significant suffering or even death. Likewise, it is believed that dysregulated production of some inflammatory cytokines can initiate many autoimmune diseases. They are discussed in Chapter 14.

Adaptive Immunity

While innate immunity is essential, its limitations mean that a much more potent but less intrusive system is required for survival. This is the role of the adaptive immune system. Unlike innate immunity, adaptive responses detect and respond to specific foreign molecules (i.e., antigens). One reason for its complexity is the need for fail-safe devices to ensure that the body's defensive cells, the lymphocytes, will only attack invading bacteria, viruses, or parasites and will ignore antigens originating in normal, healthy tissues. As might be anticipated, many different regulatory pathways control these lymphocyte functions and serve to minimize the chances of a misunderstanding that results in damaging autoimmunity. Thus a key feature of the adaptive immune system is its ability to ignore normal body components. This ability is called immunologic tolerance. If tolerance is incomplete or fails, then the adaptive immune system may misidentify normal body components and attack them as if they were foreign. This process is termed autoimmunity, and the consequences may be life-threatening.

Lymphocytes mediate adaptive immunity. The two major populations of lymphocytes are B cells and T cells. While both originate in the bone marrow, B cells are antibody-producing cells that also mature in the bone marrow. Immature T cells leave the bone marrow early and develop in the thymus. They mediate the adaptive immune response by interacting with antigen-presenting cells. The key characteristic of both T and B cells is they possess cell surface receptors that bind diverse foreign antigens. Unlike the invariant cell receptors of the innate immune system, T- and B-cell receptors are generated randomly by a process that ensures an animal almost always possesses some lymphocytes capable of binding and responding to the diverse and enormous universe of foreign molecules (called antigenic determinants or epitopes) provided by the world of potential pathogens. Each T and B cell expresses thousands of identical antigen receptors so that each lymphocyte will only respond to a single antigen. Adaptive immune responses occur when foreign antigens are bound by their specific receptors on T or B cells and as a result stimulate these cells to respond and attack the invaders.

Adaptive immune responses proceed in four steps (Fig. 1.2). These are:

Step 1: Foreign antigens are captured and processed so their epitopes can bind lymphocyte receptors in the correct manner.

Step 2: Antigen-processing cells activate helper T cells that then permit the immune response to proceed.

Step 3: Antigen plus helper T cells together cause the activation of B cells and/or T cells. The B cells make antibodies, the T cells mount cell-mediated responses, and both responses eventually eliminate the invaders.

Step 4: As a consequence of the adaptive immune responses, large populations of B and T memory cells are generated. These are, in effect, stored for future use.

STEP 1: ANTIGEN CAPTURE AND PROCESSING

The triggering of adaptive immunity requires the activation of antigen-presenting cells. The most important of these are called dendritic cells (DCs). DCs are activated by a mixture of cytokines, together with PAMPs and DAMPs acting through pattern-recognition receptors generated during the initial innate response. The activated DCs capture and process antigens derived from invading pathogens. DCs have a small cell body with many long cytoplasmic processes (dendrites) extending from their surface. These dendrites promote antigen capture and maximize the area of contact when they encounter lymphocytes. DCs reside in the tissues where they form interlacing networks optimized to trap invaders. They are especially prominent in lymph nodes and under the skin and mucosal surfaces where invading organisms are most likely to be encountered.

Exogenous Antigens

When considering the body's defenses, the diversity of pathogens encountered in everyday life must be taken into account. The two most important of these are bacteria and viruses. Effective defense against these agents requires two very different strategies. Thus when bacteria

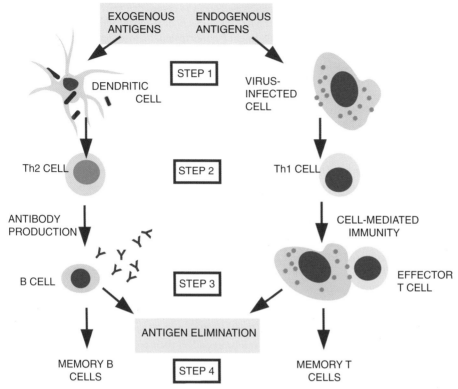

Fig. 1.2 The four major steps of the adaptive immune response. These apply to both the antibody response against exogenous antigens such as bacteria and the T-cell–mediated response against endogenous antigens such as viruses. *Th1,* T helper type 1; *Th2,* T helper type 2.

invade tissues, they multiply in the extracellular environment or in the bloodstream. Conversely, viruses are intracellular pathogens that can only grow inside cells. Viruses only leave one cell in order to invade another. Invading microbes therefore fall into two categories. One, typified by most bacteria, invade tissues and extracellular fluid. These invaders mainly grow outside cells and are classified as exogenous antigens.

Exogenous antigens are first captured and killed by DCs, then processed, and finally presented to helper T cells. When DCs capture foreign antigens and receive danger signals such as DAMPs from tissue damage or PAMPs from infection, as well as the cytokine mixture released by inflammatory cells, they become activated. The activated DCs migrate toward the source of the antigen and capture the invaders by phagocytosis. When they ingest bacteria, they can usually kill them. The ingested bacterial proteins are not, however, totally destroyed. Some peptides remain intact. These surviving peptides are bound to specialized receptors called major histocompatibility complex (MHC) class II molecules. Once a peptide binds to a MHC molecule, the peptide-MHC complex is transported to the DC surface. On arrival on the cell surface, the complex is made available for inspection by any passing T cells (Fig. 1.3). The T cells examine the DCs for the presence of the MHC-peptide complexes. As pointed out earlier, T cells each express thousands of identical antigen receptors (T-cell receptors [TCRs]) on their surface. These TCRs can only recognize peptides attached to MHC molecules. They cannot recognize or respond to the peptides alone. These helper T cells are also characterized by possessing a cell surface molecule called CD4 that binds strongly to MHC class II molecules.

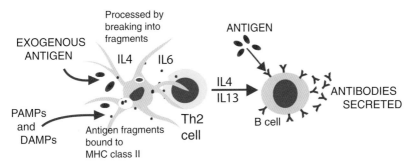

Fig. 1.3 Dendritic cells capture and process antigens, bind the resulting peptides to major histocompatibility complex *(MHC)* molecules, and present them to helper T *(Th2)* cells. If the helper cell receptors can bind the presented MHC–peptide complex, they in turn will permit the B cells to respond to the antigen and produce large quantities of antibodies. Dendritic cells produce cytokines such as interleukin-4 *(IL4)* and IL6 that activate Th2 cells. Th2 cells, in turn, produce other cytokines such as IL4 and IL13 that activate the B cells. *DAMPs,* Damage-associated molecular patterns; *PAMPs,* pathogen-associated molecular patterns.

If a CD4$^+$ T cell happens to possess antigen receptors that can bind one of these MHC-peptide complexes, signals will be exchanged between the DC and the T cell. As a result, the T cell will be activated so that it divides and differentiates. Migrating DCs can also carry their MHC-bound peptides to nearby lymph nodes, where they can be presented to even more helper T cells. Given the number of these T cells, the processed peptides will probably encounter at least a few T cells that can recognize and respond to their antigenic peptides.

MHC class II molecules can bind some but not all of the peptides created during antigen processing, so they effectively select those antigen peptides that are to be presented to the T cells. The response to antigens is thus controlled in large part by an animal's set of MHC genes. It is not surprising, therefore, that MHC genes regulate immune responses and play a major role in controlling both immunity and, by extension, the development of autoimmune diseases (see Chapter 4).

Endogenous Antigens

Antibodies cannot enter cells and as a result cannot attack intracellular viruses. The adaptive immune system therefore must employ a different technique: It simply identifies and destroys any virus-infected cells it encounters. This response is mediated by another T-cell population consisting of cytotoxic T cells. When cytotoxic T cells come into contact with an infected target cell, they transmit a signal triggering cell suicide—apoptosis. When the target cell dies, so too do any viruses hiding within.

Viral or endogenous antigens are processed by the cells in which they are produced. Immune responses against endogenous antigens are therefore directed at the detection and destruction of any cells producing abnormal or foreign proteins. Once they enter a cell, viruses take over its protein-synthesizing machinery and use it to make new viruses. While this is happening, the infected cells recycle a sample of any viral proteins they produce. These proteins are broken up into short peptides and transported to newly formed MHC class I molecules. If they fit the MHC peptide-binding site, the peptides will bind. Once loaded onto the MHC molecule, the MHC-peptide complex is carried to the cell surface and displayed to any passing T cells. T cells can therefore identify a virus-infected cell by detecting any viral proteins expressed on its surface. If a cytotoxic T cell encounters an antigen-MHC complex that can bind to its TCR, providing the helper T cells agree, it will kill the virus-infected cell. These cytotoxic T cells are characterized by expressing a cell surface molecule called CD8 on their surface. CD8 binds strongly to MHC class I molecules.

STEP 2: HELPER T-CELL ACTIVATION

The two antigen-responsive lymphocyte populations, the B cells and the cytotoxic (CD8+) T cells, cannot respond fully to foreign antigens unless they first receive permission from helper (CD4+) T cells. This is a built-in control mechanism to ensure that damaging immune responses to normal components do not occur. Helper T-cell activation is a tightly regulated process that ensures it is only triggered when needed and promptly terminated once the threat has passed.

Helper T cells are found in follicles and germinal centers within lymph nodes. Each helper T cell is covered by approximately 30,000 identical antigen receptors. Antigen binding to these receptors will signal to the cell. This signal will turn on the genes for some cytokines and cell surface molecules, and the cell will begin to divide.

The binding of a MHC-peptide complex to a TCR is usually insufficient by itself to trigger a helper T-cell response. Helper T cells must receive additional signals. A second signal comes from the prolonged strong contact between the DC and the T cells and is mediated by cell surface adhesion molecules. A third set of signals determines the direction in which naïve helper T cells will develop and the precise form the resulting immune response will take. These third signals are provided by the mixture of cytokines secreted by the DCs. For example, some antigens trigger DCs to secrete interleukin-12 (IL12). The IL12 acts on undifferentiated helper T cells (Th0), causing them to develop into type 1 helper (Th1) cells that stimulate cytotoxic T cells. Other antigens are processed in such a way that they cause the DCs to secrete a cytokine mixture containing IL4 and IL6. These cytokines act on Th0 cells to cause them to differentiate into type 2 helper (Th2 cells) that will stimulate B cells to produce antibodies.

It is now usual to refer to adaptive immune responses that rely primarily on cell-mediated immunity as type 1 immune responses. Conversely, those adaptive responses that rely primarily on antibody-mediated immunity are classified as type 2 responses.

DCs that stimulate type 1 responses are called DC1 cells. Those that stimulate type 2 responses are called DC2 cells. A third type of response is mediated by helper T cells that secreted the cytokine IL17. These are called Th17 cells. They trigger type 17 responses and play an important role in promoting inflammation and autoimmune disease.

It is important to point out at this stage that while CD4+ helper T cells have been classified into discrete subtypes based on the cytokine mixture they secrete, this is an oversimplification. Studies on these T cells in vivo have indicated that these phenotypes form a continuum. Single precursor cells may give rise to distinctly different helper cell types, and these T cells can readily switch phenotypes as a result of exposure to a different cytokine mixture.

STEP 3: B- AND T-CELL RESPONSES

The division of the adaptive immune system into type 1 and type 2 responses is based on the need to recognize two distinctly different categories of foreign invaders: exogenous and endogenous. Unlike T cells that can only respond to processed peptides, B cells can respond to antigens in their native form. As a result, antibodies produced by a type 2 response will bind to bacteria, free virus particles, and parasites and so promote their destruction. Antibodies provide the first line of defense against viruses. However, once a virus succeeds in entering a cell, then antibodies will no longer work, and a type 1 response mediated by cytotoxic T cells is required to kill the infected cell, release cytokines that inhibit microbial growth, or prevent viral survival within cells.

B-Cell Responses

B cells are so called because they mature in the *bone* marrow in mammals and in the *bursa* of Fabricius in birds. B cells produce antibodies and are primarily responsible for immunity to bacteria.

Th2 cells are required for B-cell activation, antibody production, and immune memory. B cells can also capture and process antigens, present them to helper T cells, and then receive costimulation from the same T cells. B cells thus play two roles: They respond to native antigen by making antibodies while at the same time, they themselves can act as antigen-presenting cells. Th2 cells manipulate these B-cell responses by secreting a mixture of cytokines as well as through interacting receptor pairs. One important receptor pair consists of CD40, found on the T-cell surface, and its ligand, CD40L, found on B cells. When these two molecules bind, the helper T cell sends a strong stimulatory signal that promotes the B-cell response. In some autoimmune diseases, such as systemic lupus erythematosus and rheumatoid arthritis, this pathway may be overactive. Conversely, blocking the CD40 pathway may reduce the severity of these diseases.

B-cell activation by Th2 cells occurs mainly within lymph nodes. When a B cell encounters an antigen that binds to its receptors (B-cell receptors [BCRs]), it will, with appropriate costimulation, respond by upregulating its receptor genes, increasing their production, and secreting the receptors into body fluids where they are called antibodies. Each B cell is covered with about 200,000 to 500,000 identical antigen receptors. Antibodies are simply BCRs released into body fluids; they are all members of the family of proteins called immunoglobulins. The most important of these are immunoglobulin M (IgM) produced during a primary immune response, IgG that constitutes the bulk of the antibodies found within the body, IgA produced on body surfaces, and IgE that mediates allergic disease. Depending on the species, IgG consists of several different subclasses that play slightly different roles in immunity and autoimmunity.

Although the binding of an antigen to a BCR is an essential first step, this is usually insufficient by itself to activate B cells. Complete activation of a B cell also requires costimulatory signals from helper T cells and their cytokines. When helper T cells "help" B cells, they start the process that leads to B-cell division and development into antibody-secreting cells. As B cells respond to antigen, some become specialized antibody-producing factories. These specialized cells are called plasma cells and despite their name, they are mainly found in lymphoid organs.

When appropriately stimulated and costimulated, B cells divide. This division is asymmetric so that one daughter cell gets lots of antigen while the other daughter cell gets much less. The cell that gets lots of antigen then differentiates into antibody-producing plasma cells. The cell that gets less antigen continues the cycle of dividing and mutating and eventually generates memory cells (Stage 4). The B cells destined to become plasma cells develop a rough endoplasmic reticulum, increase their rate of antibody synthesis, and secrete enormous quantities of immunoglobulins.

A key feature of BCRs is the progressive increase in binding strength between antibodies and their antigens that occurs over time. This increase takes place within germinal centers in lymph nodes and the spleen. B cells stimulated by antigen migrate to the germinal centers, where they proliferate. The B cells divide every 6 to 8 hours so that within just a few days, a single B cell may develop into a clone of several thousand cells. During this phase of rapid cell division, the BCR variable region genes (encoding the antigen-binding sites) mutate on average once per division. This repeated random mutation ensures that progeny B cells have BCRs whose antigen-binding sites differ slightly from those in their parent cell. As the B cells are dividing, they are presented with antigen by DCs. Because of these random mutations, some of the new BCRs will bind the antigen with greater affinity while others will bind it with less. A process of selection then occurs. If the mutation has resulted in greater receptor affinity for the antigen, this will stimulate more B-cell proliferation. If the affinity has dropped, however, then B-cell proliferation and survival are correspondingly reduced. Thus cycles of somatic mutation and selection result in a progressive strengthening in antigen binding, a process called affinity maturation. The high-affinity, antigen-selected B cells eventually leave the germinal center to form either plasma cells or memory B cells. In contrast, those B cells with receptors that have reduced antigen binding will die. Thus the antibodies synthesized by B cells at the beginning of an immune response progressively increase their affinity for antigen and hence their effectiveness as the response proceeds. It is important to note, however, that this random mutation may also generate antibodies that happen to bind to normal body components. In other words, it may trigger an autoimmune response.

THE COMPLEMENT SYSTEM

Antibodies by themselves do not kill invaders or destroy cells. They rely on phagocytic cells such as macrophages or neutrophils to do the killing for them. They also use a set of lethal proteins called the complement system. The complement system consists of over 50 proteins found in serum, on cell surfaces, and even within cells. They work through several distinct pathways. The classical complement pathway, for example, involves serum proteins that are activated by antibodies and thus work in association with adaptive immune response to kill invading microbes. It also plays an important role in tissue destruction in autoimmune diseases. The classical pathway is triggered when antibodies bind to a cell or microorganism. This binding triggers a conformational change that activates the first complement component, C1. IgG is much less efficient than IgM in activating the classical pathway. This is relevant to the pathogenesis of autoimmune hemolytic anemia (see Chapter 11). Sequential activation of complement components eventually generates multiprotein complexes that punch holes in the surface of the microbe or a target cell. When sufficient complexes form on a target, it will be killed by osmotic lysis. Recent studies have also shown that the complement system works within cells. This so-called complosome appears to play an important role in apoptosis and the destruction of intracellular pathogens.

Just as important as direct complement-mediated lysis are the potent inflammatory effects of two small peptides, C3a and C5a, generated during complement activation. C3a and C5a can degranulate mast cells and stimulate platelets to release histamine and serotonin. As a result, they trigger inflammation. C5a is also a powerful attractant for neutrophils and macrophages. It increases vascular permeability, causes lysosomal enzyme release from neutrophils, and regulates some T-cell responses. As a result, complement activation within tissues plays a key role in inflammatory diseases such as systemic lupus erythematosus and rheumatoid arthritis.

T-Cell Responses

T cells are so called because they develop within the *thymus. They have multiple functions. Helper T cells, as described earlier, regulate immune responses by helping to trigger both T- and B-cell responses. These in turn activate cytotoxic (or effector) T cells whose task is to kill virus-infected target cells. Activation of other T-cell populations such as Th17 cells triggers yet more inflammation. Regulatory T cells (Tregs), as their name suggests, have an opposite effect. They serve to control immune responses, especially those that may be inappropriate or damaging. When autoimmune diseases develop, they are often a result of problems occurring in the production and development of Tregs.

CYTOTOXIC T-CELL RESPONSES

In general, organisms such as viruses that enter the cell cytosol or nucleus are killed by cytotoxic T cells, whereas organisms such as intracellular bacteria or parasites that enter endosomes are destroyed by T-cell–activated macrophages. Abnormal cells (or cells perceived as abnormal) are generally destroyed by T-cell–mediated cytotoxicity.

The first step in triggering a cell-mediated response is the activation of antigen-specific cytotoxic $CD8^+$ T cells. Like the antibody response, this involves the interactions of three cell types: antigen-presenting DCs, $CD4^+$ helper T cells, and $CD8^+$ T cells. These $CD8^+$ cells can only be activated when they receive stimuli from both $CD4^+$ helper cells and DCs. The helper T cell first interacts with the antigen-presenting DC through its TCR as well as CD40 and its ligand

CD40L. This activates the DCs, upregulates their expression of MHC class I, and stimulates their production of IL12. The activated DC then binds tightly and presents its antigen to the CD8$^+$ T cell. For complete activation, CD8$^+$ T cells need to receive two additional signals. The first is IL12 from activated DCs. The second comes from IL2 and interferon-gamma (IFNγ) produced by the helper T cells. Only when all three signals are received will the CD8$^+$ T cells respond fully. Binding of 100 to 1000 antigen-MHC complexes is required to trigger cytokine production and T-cell clonal expansion.

Once fully activated, the CD8$^+$ T cells begin to divide, and their numbers grow rapidly. Their progeny leave lymphoid organs and seek out infected cells by themselves. Indeed, most lymphocytes found in the bloodstream and lymphatics are T cells out hunting for potential targets. (B cells are largely content to remain in lymphoid organs and wait for the antigen to come to them.) When T cells recognize an antigen expressed on another cell, they will attack and kill their target.

Cytotoxic T cells recognize any peptide-MHC complexes displayed on the surface of an infected cell by means of their antigen receptors. For example, when a virus infects a cell, cytotoxic T cells will detect the viral peptides on the cell surface. The T cell then uses its CD8 to bind to the MHC class I molecules on the infected cell. Once the two cells are tightly linked and their receptors interact, the signals are exchanged, and as a result the T cell will attack and kill the virus-infected cell.

Very few peptide-MHC complexes on a target cell are required to trigger a T-cell attack. Thus T-cell binding to a single peptide-MHC complex may be sufficient to trigger target cell killing. Cytotoxic T cells need to be highly sensitive to viral peptides so they can kill any infected cells they encounter as rapidly and as effectively as possible. Within seconds after encountering a cytotoxic T cell, the organelles and the nucleus of the target begin to show apoptotic changes, and the target cell is dead in less than 10 minutes. The cytotoxic T cell can then disengage and move on to attack and kill other targets. In addition, several cytotoxic cells may join in killing a single target.

Cytotoxic T cells kill their targets through the secretion of toxic molecules called perforins and granzymes. The perforin pathway effectively injects granzymes into the target cells through pores constructed from perforins. Perforins may also release granzymes from target cell endosomes. The granzymes then activate the natural apoptotic pathways in the target.

There is a second apoptotic pathway that kills cells by signaling through a death receptor called Fas. While the perforin pathway is primarily used to destroy virus-infected cells, the Fas pathway is used mainly by regulatory T cells to kill other unwanted, surplus T cells. Both pathways can contribute to tissue damage and cell destruction in autoimmune diseases.

OTHER CYTOTOXIC MECHANISMS

T-cell–mediated cytotoxicity is not the only way by which the immune system can destroy abnormal cells. For example, cells that have receptors for antibodies on their surface may bind to target cells or bacteria by means of these bound antibodies and then kill them. These cytotoxic cells may include monocytes, eosinophils, neutrophils, B cells, and natural killer (NK) cells. The mechanism of this antibody-dependent cell-mediated cytotoxicity (ADCC) is unclear. However, neutrophils and eosinophils probably release lethal oxidants and toxic granule contents. ADCC is slower and less efficient than direct T-cell–mediated cytotoxicity, taking 6 to 18 hours to occur.

Whether a macrophage participates in ADCC depends on its antibody receptors and its degree of activation. Macrophage-activating cytokines such as IFNγ or granulocyte-macrophage colony-stimulating factor (GM-CSF) promote ADCC. Macrophages may also destroy target cells in an antibody-independent process. For example, when they ingest bacteria or parasites, activated macrophages release nitric oxide, proteases, and tumor necrosis factor-alpha (TNFα). The nitric oxide can kill nearby bacteria and cells, whereas the TNFα is cytotoxic for some tumor cells. These activated macrophages are classified as M1 cells. Macrophages can also change their phenotype to become M2 cells. M2 cells suppress inflammation and promote wound healing.

TH17 CELLS

As naïve Th cells differentiate into different lineages, Th17 cells differentiate under the influence of a cytokine mixture containing IL23, transforming growth factor-beta (TGFβ), and IL6. Th17 cells are very flexible in that if the cytokine mixture changes, they can readily differentiate into other helper cell types. There are few Th17 cells in the circulation. Th17 cells are primarily located under the skin and mucosal surfaces, where they regulate inflammation, tolerance, and tissue repair. Th17 cells are also able to shift their phenotype. Under the influence of the skin or intestinal microbiota as well as their cytokine environment, they can acquire different phenotypes. Thus they can acquire features of Th1, Th2, or even Tregs. Growing evidence suggests there are two major subsets of Th17 cells: Specifically, they are classical Th17 cells and proinflammatory Th17.1 cells activated by IL1β. Classical immunoregulatory Th17 cells are important in host defense against pathogens. Th17-deficient patients suffer from bacterial and fungal infections of the lung and skin. Proinflammatory Th17 cells, in contrast, play important roles in many autoimmune diseases. Th17 numbers are increased in many autoimmune diseases, including systemic lupus erythematosus, rheumatoid arthritis, multiple sclerosis, inflammatory bowel disease, and Sjögren syndrome.

Typically, Th17 cells release members of the IL17 family of cytokines, all of which cause inflammation by upregulating gene expression and triggering the release of proinflammatory cytokines, chemokines, antibacterial peptides, and matrix metalloproteases from target cells such as keratinocytes and fibroblasts. As a result, this attracts large numbers of cells such as neutrophils to an inflammatory site and contributes to the pathogenesis of many immune-mediated inflammatory diseases such as encephalitis, rheumatoid arthritis, and inflammatory bowel disease.

REGULATORY T CELLS

A critically important population of T cells are those that regulate immune responses. They are especially important in terminating T-cell responses once viruses have been eliminated, but they also prevent unwanted immune responses such as autoimmune responses. They ensure that the adaptive immune responses are appropriate to the magnitude of the threat. Thus Tregs play an essential role in preventing autoimmunity and many allergic diseases. They are discussed in detail in the next chapter.

Sources of Additional Information

Tizard IR. *Veterinary Immunology: An Introduction.* 10th ed. St Louis: Elsevier; 2017.

CHAPTER 2

Immunologic Tolerance

The function of the immune system is to detect, attack, and destroy any microorganisms (bacteria, viruses, or parasites) that invade the body. Once a microbe invades, it must be identified as foreign; thus the success of the immune system depends on its ability to differentiate between normal body components and invading foreign organisms. Once the invader is identified as foreign, it is destroyed as rapidly and completely as possible; however, molecules identified as normal body components are usually ignored. This distinction is not absolute, and on occasion a misdirected immune response can cause damage, disease, and death.

Tolerance

B and T cells possess receptors for foreign antigens. When appropriately activated by these foreign antigens, they respond by generating protective type 1 and type 2 immune responses and attack the invaders. If perchance the T or B cells express antigen receptors that can bind normal body cells or tissues, then they may attack these as well and so cause autoimmune disease. This is normally prevented by the development of immune tolerance. Tolerance is the name given to the state in which the cells of the adaptive immune system cannot respond to a specific antigen. Tolerance is primarily directed against self-antigens from normal tissues. If tolerance fails, then autoimmunity develops.

Tolerance develops because most immature T and B cells that express receptors for self-antigens are killed within the thymus or the bone marrow before they can develop into functional cells. This killing results in central tolerance. In addition, just to be safe, regulatory pathways also operate after cells leave the thymus and prevent any surviving self-reactive T or B

11

cells from responding when they encounter a self-antigen. These regulatory pathways therefore promote peripheral tolerance. If tolerance is lost, self-reactive T and B cells can develop and cause disease. Maintenance of central and peripheral tolerance is essential to the prevention of autoimmunity.

THE CLONAL SELECTION THEORY

In the late 1800s as our understanding of immunity developed, it became apparent that some mechanism must exist by which the immune system could recognize foreign invaders while at the same time ignoring normal body components. The German immunologist Paul Ehrlich expressed this basic principle by suggesting that the body had a *horror autotoxicus,* a Latin term meaning "an aversion to autotoxicity." For many years thereafter, it was believed that autotoxicity (renamed autoimmunity) simply could not occur; however, accumulated evidence eventually made the concept of an absolute ban on autoimmunity untenable.

In 1945 Dr. Ray Owen, while working in Wisconsin, observed in some pregnant cows carrying twin calves that the blood vessels in their two placentas commonly joined together. As a result, the calves' blood intermingled freely, and circulating bone marrow stem cells from one calf colonized the other. Consequently, each calf was born with a mixture of blood cells, some of its own and some from its twin. In dizygotic (nonidentical) twins, these animals are called chimeras. The "foreign" blood cells are not destroyed by the recipient but persist indefinitely. This is in marked contrast to the response that would occur if cells from the twin calf were transfused after birth. They would be rapidly destroyed by the recipient's immune system.

In 1949, two Australian immunologists, Frank MacFarlane Burnet and Frank Fenner, wrote *The Production of Antibodies,* in which they explained Owen's results by suggesting that chimeras could only develop because each calf was exposed to the foreign cells early in fetal life at a time when its lymphocytes become tolerant upon encountering self-antigens. They suggested that immune tolerance was not innate but established during fetal and early postnatal development.

Burnet continued to work on these ideas over the next several years, and in 1957 published his clonal selection theory. In this theory, Burnet suggested that the ability to respond to antigens was conferred by antigen-specific receptors on the surface of lymphocytes and that each lymphocyte expressed only one sort of antigen receptor. Burnet explained that the adaptive immune response resulted from the proliferation of lymphocytes responding to antigen binding to their receptors (Fig. 2.1). Thus the antigen effectively selects the cell with appropriate receptors. This binding then

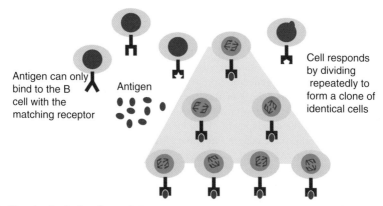

Fig. 2.1 The clonal selection theory. Only when an antigen matches the receptors on a B or T cell will a lymphocyte be triggered to respond. It will divide repeatedly to form a clone of identical lymphocytes that participate in the immune response.

causes the cell to multiply, resulting in the development of a clone of cells that produce identical targeted antibodies.

The clonal selection theory was rapidly accepted by the scientific community. Burnet and Peter Medawar subsequently expanded the theory to explain immunologic tolerance to normal body components. They suggested that only those lymphocytes that cannot recognize and respond to normal body components (self-antigens) are permitted to survive beyond the embryonic stage. Cells that respond to self-antigens before reaching maturity are eliminated. In 1953 Medawar went on to demonstrate this experimentally by injecting foreign white cells into neonatal mice and showed that rather than mounting an antibody response, the mice developed tolerance to the foreign cells. The clonal selection theory has now been shown to be correct in all its essential features. Burnet and Medawar shared the Nobel Prize in medicine in 1960.

Central Tolerance

Since the genes that encode the antigen-binding receptor proteins in both T and B cells are randomly translated and transcribed during cell development, it is clear that the initial production of lymphocytes expressing self-reactive receptors cannot be prevented. Cells do not control these amino acid sequences and hence the binding specificity of their randomly generated receptors. As a result, when first generated, as many as half of the immature lymphocytes may possess receptors that can bind normal body components. If autoimmunity is to be avoided, these self-reactive lymphocytes must be eliminated or at a minimum, actively suppressed.

Immune tolerance is generated in two distinct steps classified as central and peripheral tolerance. To generate central tolerance, immature lymphocytes with self-reactive receptors developing within the "central" lymphoid organs such as the thymus or bone marrow are either killed or forced to alter their receptor specificity. This eliminates most but not all self-reactive T cells. This process occurs within the thymus for T cells and in the bone marrow for B cells. Given, however, the central role played by helper T (Th) cells in initiating adaptive immunity, establishment of central tolerance in the T-cell population is the most critical process.

CD4+ and CD8+ T-cell precursors are derived from lymphoid stem cells in the bone marrow. From the marrow, they migrate to the thymus. On arrival in the thymic cortex, they continue to develop and begin to express random antigen receptors. These immature T cells are then exposed to diverse antigenic peptide–major histocompatibility complexes (MHC) by cortical thymic epithelial cells (cTECs). Two different fates await them. If they have failed to develop a functional antigen receptor and so cannot respond to any presented antigen, they will die. In fact, they receive signals instructing them to commit suicide (apoptosis). On the other hand, if their receptors are functional and can bind to MHC-peptide complexes, then they are permitted to survive (Fig. 2.2). If they make the cut, the developing lymphocytes then begin to divide and differentiate. As they differentiate, the lymphocytes lose either CD4 or CD8 from their surface. In effect, this is a career choice. CD4+ cells become Th cells, and CD8+ cells become cytotoxic T cells.

The developing T cells next migrate from the cortex into the thymic medulla and undergo their second selection step. Here they encounter populations of medullary thymic epithelial cells (mTECs), fibroblasts, and dendritic cells (DCs). These cells present the T cells with a vast and diverse array of MHC-bound self-antigens. If their antigen receptors bind any of these self-antigens with high affinity, then the developing lymphocytes will undergo forced apoptosis, a process called negative selection. The T-cell receptor (TCR) signals to the T cell and triggers the production of BIM, a proapoptotic protein. BIM neutralizes antiapoptotic proteins such as Bcl-2, and as a result the T cell dies. Some cells that respond weakly to self-antigens may otherwise differentiate into regulatory T (Treg) cells.

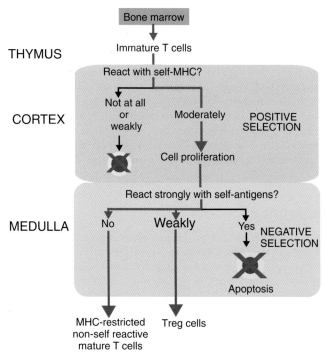

Fig. 2.2 The mechanisms of central T-cell tolerance. Within the thymic cortex, cells with faulty antigen receptors are destroyed, and cells with functional receptors are permitted to survive and multiply. They then move to the thymic medulla, where they are presented with a broad diversity of self-antigens. Strongly reactive T cells are killed. Unreactive T cells are permitted to survive and emigrate. Weakly reactive T cells become regulatory T cells. *MHC,* Major histocompatibility complex; *Treg cell,* regulatory T cell.

THE AUTOIMMUNE REGULATOR

Differentiated cells such as liver, skin, or kidney cells normally express only a limited number of tissue-specific protein genes (i.e., only the ones they need to survive and function). On the other hand, mTECs are unique. To establish and maintain central tolerance, mTECs collectively express thousands of protein coding genes. As a result, they present developing T cells with an enormous library of tissue-specific proteins (Fig. 2.3). Thymic epithelial cells and DCs located within the thymic medulla use a unique protein called the autoimmune regulator (AIRE). AIRE is a protein of 56 KDa that binds to chromatin and regulates gene transcription in such a way that a huge diversity of self-proteins is expressed by a single mTEC. AIRE is not a conventional transcription factor since it does not itself bind directly to DNA. AIRE binds to histones in the chromatin near target genes, and by activating RNA polymerases, it promotes promiscuous gene transcription. As a result, AIRE acts as a superenhancer and mediates the expression of thousands of different proteins that are normally restricted to other body tissues and cell types. This results in a specialized thymic display of the body's repertoire of self-antigens. The half-life of AIRE-positive mTECs is about 12 to 14 days. As a result, every 2 weeks or so a new pool of mTECs is generated, thus presenting developing T cells with a constant supply of diverse self-antigens. B cells that enter the thymus also employ AIRE to express multiple self-antigens and so contribute to the selection process.

It is estimated that a normal mouse genome encodes about 24,000 different proteins. Thymic medullary epithelial cells collectively express about 15,000 of these proteins. They undergo this

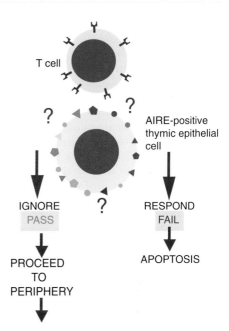

Fig. 2.3 Thymic medullary epithelial cells using the autoimmune regulator *(AIRE)* will produce small quantities of many different self-antigens. If the antigen receptors of a developing T cell bind one of these self-antigens and the T cell responds strongly, then it will be triggered to undergo apoptosis. If it ignores these antigens, then it will be allowed to proceed.

promiscuous gene expression under the influence of AIRE and other transcriptional regulators. Individual mTECs each express a subset (1%–3%) of these proteins, and they still maintain their identity. In effect, therefore, mTECs can collectively present the developing T cells with most of the normal proteins that they are liable to encounter when they leave the thymus and circulate through the body. In this way, the mTECs ensure that self-reactive T cells are exposed to many normal tissue antigens, and as a result most self-reactive cells are eliminated before they are released into the body. Mutations in the AIRE gene in humans result in patients developing a severe disease syndrome called autoimmune polyendocrine syndrome 1 (see Fig. 6.4).

In addition to AIRE, a second transcription factor called Fezf 2 (forebrain-expressed zinc finger 2) also promotes the expression of hundreds of self-antigens on mTECs. These are different from the antigens transcribed by AIRE.

As a result of these selection processes, the T cells that eventually leave the thymus have been purged of dangerous, self-reactive cells. Negative selection is not however foolproof, and some self-reactive T cells can sneak through. In effect, negative selection "prunes" the T-cell repertoire, but it does not completely eradicate self-reactive T cells. It has been calculated that it eliminates only about 60% of self-reactive T cells. Nevertheless, it is also estimated that only 1% to 3% of the immature T cells that enter the thymus survive both positive and negative selection and eventually escape into the periphery. The others are recycled. Once the selected mature, single positive T cells leave the thymus they colonize peripheral lymphoid tissues.

CENTRAL B-CELL TOLERANCE

B lymphocyte synthesis of B-cell receptors (BCRs) that can bind self-antigens is an unavoidable consequence of antibody diversification in the bone marrow. As a result, 55% to 75% of early immature B cells are autoreactive. Unlike the TCR repertoire, BCR/antibody diversity is generated in two phases. The first phase involves gene rearrangement or gene conversion in the bone marrow. This generates a great diversity of different antibody variable regions that form the antigen binding sites. The second phase involves random somatic mutation of these variable region genes within the germinal centers in secondary lymphoid organs. As a result of these random processes, B cells have multiple opportunities to generate receptors that can bind self-antigens. Suppression of these B cells must begin at an early stage in an animal's development. This suppression occurs in the bone marrow and the gastrointestinal tract.

Self-reactive immature B cells in the bone marrow and the intestine can be eliminated once they have rearranged their V-region genes and are committed to express complete immunoglobulin M (IgM) molecules. When these immature cells encounter and bind antigen, the BCR transmits a signal that arrests cell development and triggers apoptosis. This requires exposure to very small amounts of self-antigens. An immature B-cell population can be rendered tolerant by exposure to one-millionth of the dose of an antigen required to make mature B cells tolerant. Immature B cells may also undergo receptor editing, as described later. If receptor editing fails to generate a functional, nonself-reactive B cell, the cell will die. Like T cells, the selection process is not perfect, and some self-reactive B cells can also evade central tolerance induction.

The importance of early B-cell tolerance induction in the gastrointestinal tract stems from the presence of the gut microbiota. Thus microbial antigens produced by these intestinal commensals can trigger B-cell tolerance and so protect themselves against aggressive immunologic attack. Should this tolerance break down in later life, inflammatory bowel disease may result.

Another mechanism by which central tolerance can break down has recently been described in mice. A mouse herpesvirus, roseolovirus, selectively kills thymic medullary epithelial cells in neonatal mice. It reduces thymic expression of AIRE and tissue restricted antigens. As a result, the mice produce a wide array of autoantibodies and develop a severe autoimmune gastritis.

Peripheral Tolerance

The thymus reaches its greatest size and functional activity in early life prior to puberty, thus central tolerance is the predominant control process in the young. Subsequently, as thymic functionality declines, T-cell replenishment occurs in the secondary lymphoid organs, and peripheral tolerance becomes the dominant regulatory process.

While the thymus acts as an efficient filter to remove self-reactive T cells, it is not perfect. Central tolerance does not completely eliminate self-reactive T cells. There are several reasons for this. For example, many self-antigens are made later in life and are not expressed by mTECs controlled by AIRE. Innocuous or microbial antigens may enter the body later in life and trigger autoantibody formation as a result of cross-reactivity. Thus, while central tolerance is critical, it is not sufficient to totally prevent autoimmunity. Peripheral tolerance is required to eliminate or suppress any persistent self-reactive T cells. This peripheral tolerance is mediated by four distinct suppressive mechanisms. These are (1) a failure of lymphocytes to be completely stimulated by self-antigens, resulting in an unreactive state known as anergy, (2) the production of regulatory and inhibitory molecules, (3) active suppression of responsive cells by Treg cells, and (4) changes in antigen binding specificity as a result of receptor editing.

As indicated earlier, central tolerance of B cells is also incomplete. The surviving self-reactive B cells must therefore be eliminated or suppressed by a succession of tolerance-inducing mechanisms. Thus active suppression, receptor editing, and anergy induction also occur after B cells are released into the periphery.

PERIPHERAL T-CELL TOLERANCE

Once released from the thymus, naïve T cells circulate through secondary lymphoid organs until they recognize antigen presented to them by antigen-presenting cells. Once activated, they differentiate into different functional lineages. This activation process provides other opportunities to detect and suppress any cells that react with normal body components.

Anergy

In Chapter 1 it was described how Th cells require multiple costimulatory signals if they are to respond optimally to antigen presented by DCs. If they do not receive the correct signals in the correct amounts and in the correct order, instead of turning on, T cells are turned off. This is known as anergy, a form of peripheral tolerance. It results in the prolonged, antigen-specific suppression of T-cell functions. Once induced, this anergy can be long lasting but is reversible and eventually fades unless reinforced by ongoing exposure to the antigen. Anergy is therefore triggered when T-cell antigen receptors bind antigen in the absence of effective costimulation.

Binding to the TCR by an antigen in the absence of costimulation by molecules such as CD40 activates the TCR tyrosine kinases and phospholipases and raises its intracellular Ca2+. This results in enhanced production of the protein IκB that normally inhibits the NF-κB pathway (Box 2.1; Fig. 2.4). If, as a result of a lack of costimulation, the amount of NF-κB generated is insufficient to activate a T cell, its functions will be suppressed and tolerance results (Fig. 2.5).

Insufficient NF-κB will also prevent a T cell from making cytokines, especially interleukin-2 (IL2). Anergic Th type 1 (Th1) cells produce less than 3% of normal IL2 levels as well as much less interferon-gamma (IFNγ) and tumor necrosis factor-alpha (TNFα). Triggering of TCRs normally requires prolonged interactions with antigen-presenting cells. Anergy induction, on the other hand, is characterized by relatively short interactive episodes. Thus a key difference between Th cell activation and anergy may simply be the duration of their encounter with the presenting cells.

Recent emigrants from the thymus are most susceptible to developing anergy, especially in the absence of inflammation. Anergic CD4+ cells may also convert into Treg cells and suppress autoimmunity. Very high doses of an antigen can induce a form of clonal anergy called immune paralysis. The high doses of the antigen probably bypass antigen-presenting cells, reach the helper cell TCRs directly, and even in the presence of costimulation, trigger T-cell exhaustion and apoptosis.

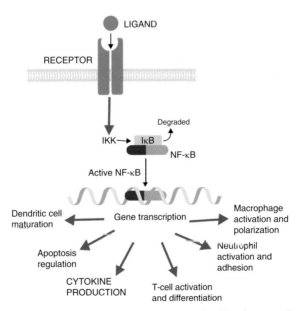

Fig. 2.4 The canonic NF-κB pathway. This signaling pathway can be driven by many diverse signals. These include pathogen-associated molecular patterns binding to toll-like receptors, antigens binding to T-cell receptors, and many different cytokines, including interferon-gamma, interleukin-17, and tumor necrosis factor-beta. A related pathway is used by CD40. The activated NF-κB binds to DNA and regulates gene transcription.

BOX 2.1 ■ The Importance of NF-κB

The cells of the immune system are activated through signals originating in cell surface receptors. These signals influence cell functions through three major transduction pathways. Each pathway is named after its key transduction factor. These are nuclear factor-AT (NF-AT), activator protein-1 (AP-1), and nuclear factor-kappa B (NF-κB). The NF-κB pathway is by far the most important. NF-κBs are a family of dimeric proteins that act as fast-acting transcription factors and play a central role in transducing signals generated by cell surface receptors on the cells of the immune system. As such, they are essential in triggering activation, proliferation, and differentiation that result in inflammatory and adaptive immune responses to antigens and harmful stimuli. They regulate cytokine production as well as cell survival. As key mediators in controlling immunity, NF-κBs play an important role in the development of autoimmunity. Their name is derived from their initial discovery when one was shown to drive immunoglobulin kappa chain production in B cells.

NF-κB1 is a heterodimer consisting of Rel and p50 proteins found in almost all cell types. When not active, it is present in the cytosol, bound to a member of a family of inhibitory proteins, IκBs. The IκB molecule normally masks the NF-κB1 nuclear localization signals. Activation involves removal of IκB by rapid phosphorylation, ubiquitination, and proteolytic degradation. Many different signals can act through cellular receptors to activate NF-κB, including cytokines, damage-associated molecular patterns (DAMPs) and pathogen-associated molecular patterns (PAMPs), DNA damage, oxidative and physical stress, and antigen signaling through B- and T-cell receptors. NF-κB1 is activated by the canonic pathway driven by antigens, PAMPs and DAMPs, or cytokines such as tumor necrosis factor-alpha and interleukin-1-beta (see Fig. 2.4). A second noncanonic pathway activates NF-κB2 and is triggered by cell development molecules, including lymphotoxin b, BAFF, RANKL, and CD40. There is also a third, atypical pathway driven by cell stress. When a cell such as a lymphocyte is activated by the canonic pathway, the extracellular signals activate an enzyme complex consisting of IκB kinases (IKK) plus a regulatory protein called NEMO. These kinases in turn phosphorylate IκB, causing it to separate from the NF-κB1 and eventually be degraded in the proteasome. The NF-κB1 freed from this constraint can translocate to the nucleus, where it binds and activates response elements on the DNA, recruits coactivators and RNA polymerase, and begins the process of transcribing and translating protein genes. The noncanonic pathway activates an NF-κB–inducing kinase (NIK). NF-κB2 is then activated by processing of RelB. This pathway appears to control the production of homeostatic cytokines.

Among the important triggers of the NF-κB pathways are CD40 that activates both pathways and thus is a potent stimulator of adaptive immunity. Conversely, the checkpoint inhibitor, cytotoxic T-lymphocyte–associated antigen 4, inhibits NF-κB activation and so suppresses adoptive immunity.

Dysregulation of NF-κB signaling has been linked to many inflammatory and autoimmune diseases. These include rheumatoid arthritis, inflammatory bowel disease, and multiple sclerosis. It appears that six codons in the Rel gene determine the nature of the cell response to NF-κB signaling by controlling the expression of immune response genes. Inappropriate immune responses such as those in autoimmunity may result from confusing signals generated by defective codon usage. Suppression of the NF-κB pathway is mediated by glucocorticosteroids, the most important drugs used in the treatment of autoimmune diseases of animals.

Adelaja A, Taylor B, Sheu KM, et al. Six distinct NFkB signaling codons convey discrete information to distinguish stimuli and enable appropriate macrophage responses. *Immunity*. 2021. doi:10.1016/j.immuniu.2021.04.011.

Liu T, Zhang L, Joo D, et al. NF-kB signaling in inflammation. *Signal Transduct Target Ther.* 2017. doi:10.1038/sigtrans.2017.25.

PERIPHERAL B-CELL TOLERANCE

As with T cells, self-reactive B cells can leak through the central tolerance screening process. It has been estimated that, after processing within the bone marrow, about 20% of the B cells released into the body are still self-reactive. In general, these cells tend to produce low affinity IgM antibodies and as a result cannot cause disease. Nevertheless, they must still be regulated. Peripheral

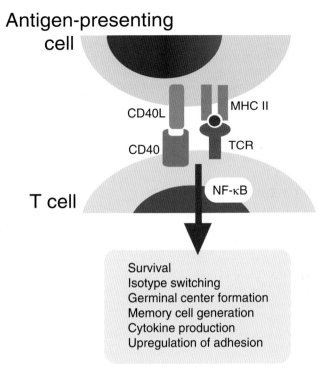

Antigen-presenting cell

CD40L
MHC II
CD40
TCR
NF-κB

T cell

Survival
Isotype switching
Germinal center formation
Memory cell generation
Cytokine production
Upregulation of adhesion

Fig. 2.5 The critical role of the CD40-CD40L system in mediating the normal development of helper T cell responses. In the absence of CD40 signaling the T cell, will undergo apoptosis rather than division, resulting in anergy. Excessive CD40 activity plays an important role in their pathogenesis of some autoimmune diseases. *MHC*, Major histocompatibility complex; *TCR*, T-cell receptor.

B-cell tolerance is induced by multiple mechanisms, including anergy, exhaustion, and apoptosis, as well as inhibition of BCR signaling.

Because BCRs undergo random somatic mutation within germinal centers, self-reactive B cells can develop in secondary lymphoid organs. Three mechanisms remove these autoreactive B cells. First, they may die as a result of high-affinity interactions with self-antigens. Self-antigens are present in large amounts and do not go away. B cells subjected to repeated, exhaustive, antigenic stimulation by persistent self-antigens are driven to differentiate into short-lived plasma cells. If all these B cells develop into such plasma cells, no memory B cells will remain to respond to antigen, and tolerance will result. In effect, they are driven to an early death. Secondly, as they respond to antigens, B-cell antigen receptors continue to be edited as a result of mutation and selection; thus they may no longer bind self-antigens. Finally, if these B cells escape into the body and bind self antigens, they will undergo anergy. Perhaps up to 50% of newly emerged B cells undergo anergy, and it is estimated that 5% to 7% of circulating B cells are in an anergic state. These anergic cells have a half-life of ~5 days compared to 13 to 22 weeks for follicular B cells. These cells cannot make autoantibodies if other members of the team such as antigen-presenting cells and Th cells are absent or if Treg cells are active.

BCR signaling alone is insufficient to promote cell division and trigger effective cell growth pathways such as those mediated by NF-κB; however, the cell's apoptosis pathways remain intact. Anergic B cells show impaired proliferation and antibody secretion. They are not, however, deleted immediately, and some may survive to serve as a reservoir that can eventually be reactivated by inflammation.

Anergy is not a foolproof method of preventing self-reactivity. Even in the absence of T-cell help, B cells may be activated by pathogen-associated molecular patterns (PAMPs) such as bacterial lipopolysaccharide (LPS), flagellins, or bacterial DNA acting through toll-like receptors (TLRs). Bacterial LPS or double-stranded RNA binding to TLRs may provide the B cell with sufficient stimulation to trigger a response. B cells may also be activated by either cross-reacting epitopes or foreign carrier molecules stimulating nontolerant Th cells. B cells are difficult to maintain in an anergic state and will reactivate rapidly unless steps are taken to maintain anergy. Self-reactive B cells must also bind to a critical threshold of self-antigen to be made tolerant. This results in selective silencing of high-affinity B cells. Presumably the failure of low-affinity antiself B cells to become tolerant poses little threat of autoimmune disease because the low-affinity antibodies cannot cause tissue destruction.

DURATION OF TOLERANCE

The duration of tolerance depends on antigen persistence and on the ability of the bone marrow to generate fresh T or B cells. Once an antigen is completely eliminated, tolerance fades. If, however, the antigen is persistent, such as occurs with an animal's own self-antigens, tolerance also persists. In the continued presence of an antigen, newly formed antigen-sensitive cells will undergo anergy or apoptosis as soon as their receptors bind self-antigen. By reconstituting lethally irradiated mice with T or B cells derived from normal or tolerant donors, anergy can be shown to occur in both T- and B-cell populations. However, their susceptibility to peripheral tolerance differs. In mice, for example, T cells can be made anergic rapidly and easily within 24 hours and remain in that state for more than 100 days. In contrast, mouse B cells develop anergy in about 10 days and may return to normal within 50 days.

Regulatory Cells

Although much immune regulation is passive in that self-reactive lymphocytes are eliminated by central tolerance, regulatory cells in peripheral tissues also actively monitor and regulate the immune system. Cells with regulatory functions include T cells, B cells, DCs, and natural suppressor (NS) cells.

REGULATORY T CELLS

Treg cells play a critical role in controlling the immune system. This includes ensuring that immune responses are of an appropriate magnitude and that they are terminated when no longer needed. Tregs are also tasked with maintaining the balance between peripheral tolerance and immunity. This means that they act to prevent autoimmune responses, but they also serve to control immune responses to commensal microorganisms. In their absence, multiorgan autoimmune disease or uncontrolled inflammation results. Treg cells are heterogeneous, and each subpopulation has its own biologic characteristics. Some directly suppress effector T cells, whereas others secrete suppressive cytokines. Some Tregs develop naturally during animal development, whereas others are induced by inflammation, microbial products, or cytokine exposure. Thymic Treg (tTreg) cells originate in the thymus, whereas peripheral Treg (pTreg) cells are produced following antigenic stimulation within secondary lymphoid organs, especially in the intestine.

The main source of tTreg cells is the thymus. tTreg cells possess antigen receptors that have a greater affinity for self-peptide–MHC complexes than do conventional T cells. Thus AIRE promotes deletion of high-affinity autoreactive T cells; however, intermediate affinity self-reactive T cells are not killed. During the negative selection process in the thymic medulla, a subset of self-reactive T cells upregulates a transcription factor called Forkhead box P3 (FoxP3) and develops into tTreg cells. They then emigrate to peripheral tissues, both lymphoid and nonlymphoid, and promote peripheral tolerance. Tregs are also generated in peripheral tissues, especially if they encounter antigens in the presence of IL10 and transforming growth factor-beta (TGFβ). The Treg repertoire may also be expanded by reactions with antigens from the commensal microbiota (Chapter 5). Conversely, interferons produced by activated Th1 cells profoundly suppress Treg cell function.

Under normal conditions, the immune system acts through Treg cells to suppress autoimmunity. However, if Tregs are deficient as a result of a failure to develop, chronic suppression by type 1 interferons, or a functional deficiency, then autoimmune diseases can develop. For example, Treg numbers and their functions are reduced in type 1 diabetes mellitus, systemic lupus erythematosus, myasthenia gravis, and rheumatoid arthritis.

Treg cells are typical lymphocytes that express CD4 and CD25 (the alpha chain of the IL2 receptor). All activated T cells express CD25, but Treg cells are the only ones that express it when naïve. Their most characteristic feature, however, is their use of the specialized transcription factor FoxP3. FoxP3 is a transcriptional regulator that controls Treg functions by inducing transcription of the genes for cytotoxic T-lymphocyte–associated antigen 4 (CTLA-4), TGFβ, and IL10. Mice that fail to make functional FoxP3 develop a lethal lupus-like syndrome (Chapter 22).

Because of the need to prevent an inappropriate attack on the commensal microbiota, the intestine is a major site of pTreg development, and specialized intestinal DCs promote this development through pathways that use a combination of TGFβ and retinoic acid, a metabolite of vitamin A. The retinoic acid is generated by the microbiota and is required for normal T-cell function. Changes in the microbiota may therefore reduce pTreg production. Intestinal pTreg cells may also develop from naïve T cells in response to antigen and costimulation by IL2 and TGFβ. These signals induce the production of FoxP3. Once generated, pTregs spread throughout the body. They account for about 5% of circulating T cells and 10% of lymph node T cells in the dog.

Treg cells suppress the response of Th cells to antigens and prevent inappropriate T-cell activation in the absence of an antigen. Treg cells can also suppress CD4+ and CD8+ T-cell responses by pathways independent of IL10 and TGFβ. For example, they shorten the interaction time between T cells and antigen-presenting cells and so prevent T-cell activation. Oral administration of an antigen may selectively induce pTreg cells. Treg cells from the mesenteric lymph nodes of orally tolerant animals account in large part for tolerance to food antigens. The term *infectious tolerance* is applied to a situation when FoxP3+ Tregs act to convert conventional Th cells into pTregs by secreting the suppressive cytokines TGFβ, IL10, and IL35.

In addition to naturally occurring Tregs and induced Tregs, other minor Treg cell populations include IL10-producing T cells and TGFβ-producing Th cells. Collectively these, with tTregs and pTregs, regulate self-recognition and peripheral tolerance. The pTregs may become especially important in older individuals after thymic involution is complete and the importance of central tolerance is reduced.

Tregs suppress immune responses through multiple pathways. However, these can be divided into those that require direct cell–cell contact and those mediated by secreted soluble factors (Fig. 2.6).

Contact-Dependent Regulation

Given their key role in terminating an immune response once invaders have been eliminated, Treg cells mediate the off switch. They do this by directly contacting and suppressing effector T cells. The delivery of these inhibitory signals can be mediated by binding of membrane-bound suppressive cytokines such as TGFβ or by reverse signaling through inhibitory receptors such as CTLA-4 (described later). Tregs may also kill effector T cells by releasing toxic granzymes or other apoptosis-inducing molecules. Some Tregs can also cause suppression by releasing extracellular vesicles. These vesicles act through microRNA-induced gene silencing, the activities of their

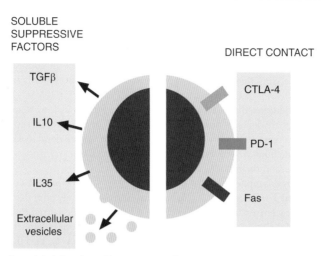

Fig. 2.6 Treg cells and their functions. They can turn off immune responses by two general mechanisms. Thus they may secrete suppressive cytokines or other immunosuppressive molecules and extracellular vesicles, or they can contact their targets directly and transmit suppressive signals through inhibitory cell surface receptors. *CTLA-4*, Cytotoxic T-lymphocyte–associated antigen 4; *IL*, interleukin; *PD-1*, programmed death 1; *TGF*, transforming growth factor.

surface proteins, and the transmission of suppressive enzymes. Presumably they contain suppressive factors packaged within the vesicles.

Tregs express cell surface molecules that can regulate and effectively suppress both T- and B-cell responses. A deficiency of any of these may result in the development of excessive T-cell responses, inflammation, and autoimmunity. These inhibitory checkpoint molecules are key to maintaining control of T-cell–mediated immunity. In effect, they serve to balance protective immunity and immunopathology. Two of the most important checkpoint inhibitors are CTLA-4 and programmed death 1 (PD-1). Both suppress T-cell function. They act at different stages in the immune response. CTLA-4 regulates T-cell proliferation early in the response, especially within lymph nodes. PD-1, in contrast, suppresses T-cell responses later in the response and acts primarily within peripheral tissues.

The CTLA-4 Pathway. In the course of a normal immune response, when effector T cells are activated by antigen and helper cells, they express a cell surface receptor called CD28. This CD28 binds two alternative ligands: either CD80 on antigen-presenting cells (DCs, macrophages, and activated B cells) or CD86 on B cells. This CD28 binding initially stimulates the T-cell response. It promotes T-cell proliferation and increases T-cell survival and the production of cytokines such as IL2. Once it has achieved sufficiency, however, the T cell has to be turned off. To do this, the T cell produces a new surface receptor called CTLA-4. CTLA-4 also binds to CD80 or CD86 and directly competes with CD28, thus blocking its stimulatory signal. In addition, CTLA-4 delivers inhibitory signals to the T cell (Fig. 2.7). When T-cell CTLA-4 binds to CD80 on antigen-presenting cells, it inhibits the key T-cell–activating pathway mediated through the NF-κB transcription factors (see Box 2.1).

Only activated T cells express CTLA-4. Once a T cell is activated by antigen binding, the newly synthesized CTLA-4 is transported to the cell surface. The greater the T-cell activation, the more CTLA-4 is expressed. In effect, therefore, the relative amount of CD28-CD80 binding versus CTLA-4–CD80 binding determines whether the T cell will undergo activation or become anergic. These T-cell responses are not rapid. It takes 48 to 72 hours after T cells are first activated

Fig. 2.7 When an antigen-presenting cell and a helper T cell interact, the peptide-MHC complex on the antigen-presenting cell *(APC)* binds the T-cell receptor *(TCR)*. However, two other pathways mediated by CTLA-4 and PD-1 interfere with TCR signaling. CTLA-4 blocks the stimulatory signal from CD80/86. PD-1 blocks TCR signaling. Collectively, they suppress T-cell responses and hence control peripheral tolerance. *CTLA-4,* Cytotoxic T-lymphocyte–associated antigen 4; *MHC,* major histocompatibility complex; *PD-1,* programmed death 1.

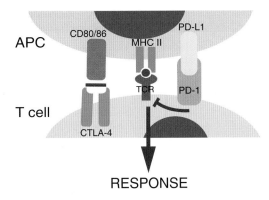

before they begin to express CTLA-4. Because CTLA-4 binds CD80 and CD86 with a higher affinity than CD28, the inhibitory effect of CTLA-4 eventually predominates, and the T-cell response is turned off. CTLA-4 expression is critical for the development of peripheral tolerance.

Unlike effector T cells, Tregs constitutively express CTLA-4, and this contributes to their suppressor functions. In fact, much of the suppressive effect of CTLA-4 is mediated through Tregs. A loss of CTLA-4 expression by Tregs results in autoimmunity (Box 2.2). Defects in CTLA-4 expression have been detected in patients with systemic lupus erythematosus and rheumatoid arthritis. It is also of relevance to note that some dogs with autoimmune diseases make autoantibodies directed against CTLA-4. These could potentially block its functions and promote autoimmunity (see Box 16.2).

The PD-1/PD-L Pathway. A second T-cell checkpoint inhibitor is called PD-1. PD-1 is a transmembrane glycoprotein expressed on activated T cells, Treg cells, and B cells, among others. It is expressed following antigen-mediated T-cell activation, and its levels decrease once the antigen has gone. If the antigen persists, as in normal tissues (or in cancer), PD-1 levels remain high. PD-1 serves as a natural inhibitor of overenthusiastic T cell responses and so contributes to the generation of self-tolerance.

PD-1 has two ligands (PD-L1 and PD-L2). One ligand, PD-L1, is expressed on many cell types, including T and B cells, thymocytes, DCs, macrophages, and stem cells as well as on nonlymphoid cells within immunologically privileged organs such as the eye, placenta, and testes. Importantly, it is also expressed on some tumor cells. The second ligand, PD-L2, is expressed only on macrophages and DCs. The expressions of PL-L1 and PD-L2 are both stimulated by inflammation. For example, inflammatory cytokines such as the interferons and TNFα induce PD-L1 expression on T cells, B cells, endothelial cells, and epithelial cells.

When PD-1 ligands on target cells bind to PD-1 on T cells, they send inhibitory signals to the T cell. These signals inhibit its cytokine synthesis, proliferation, and cytotoxicity. Thus if an effector T cell binds to a target cell expressing PD-1 ligand, this will inhibit the T-cell response. The PD-1 acts by preventing protein phosphorylation in the TCR signaling pathway, thus terminating TCR signaling and blocking T-cell activation. As a result, it reduces T effector functions and keeps them within a desirable physiologic range. Conversely, Treg cell differentiation, maintenance, and function are enhanced by PD-1.

Both PD-1 and PD-L1 are expressed by thymocytes and regulate thymocyte development, and so contribute to central tolerance. PD-1 also contributes to peripheral tolerance through several mechanisms. First, in the presence of TGFβ at inflammatory sites or within immune-privileged organs such as the eye, it promotes the development of Tregs. Second, PD-1 directly inhibits any self-reactive T cells that happen to develop in the periphery. It basically keeps the

---

BOX 2.2 ■ CTLA-4 and Canine Diabetes Mellitus

Lest the reader think that cytotoxic T-lymphocyte–associated antigen 4 (CTLA-4) is not relevant to animal autoimmune diseases, it should be pointed out that canine autoimmune diabetes mellitus is associated with polymorphisms in the promoter region of the CTLA-4 gene. Several dog breeds, such as Samoyeds and Cairn Terriers, are predisposed to developing diabetes mellitus. This is probably an autoimmune disease associated with the production of antibodies against pancreatic islet beta cells. Analysis has shown that some single nucleotide polymorphisms (SNPs) in the promoter region of the CTLA-4 gene are associated with this increased susceptibility. The single nucleotide changes result in a change in the amino acid sequence of this protein. Of the 15 SNPs detected, 9 were shown to be associated with diabetes susceptibility in dogs.

Short AD, Saleh NM, Catchpole B, et al. CTLA4 promoter polymorphisms are associated with canine diabetes mellitus. *Tissue Antigens.* 2010;75:242-252.

---

threshold of T-cell activation high to prevent autoimmunity. PD-1 has been shown to play a key role in preventing the development of type 1 diabetes mellitus, autoimmune encephalomyelitis, rheumatoid arthritis, autoimmune hepatitis, myasthenia gravis, autoimmune uveitis, Sjögren syndrome, systemic sclerosis, psoriasis, vitiligo, systemic lupus, myocarditis, ankylosing spondylitis, and inflammatory bowel diseases. Conversely, PD-1 deficiency in mice results in the development of a lupuslike disease.

While CTLA-4 and PG-1 have similar suppressive effects, their timing, location, and mechanisms are different. Thus CTLA-4 is restricted to T cells, whereas PD-1 is found on activated T and B cells. CTLA-4 acts during T-cell priming. PD-1 acts during the effector phase, especially in peripheral tissues. The ligands for CTLA-4 are restricted to antigen-presenting cells in lymph nodes and the spleen. The ligands for PD-1 are more widely expressed on a variety of immune and nonimmune cell types and can be readily induced. Thus CTLA-4 primarily acts at sites of T-cell priming in which CD28 costimulation is involved. In contrast, PD-1 mainly acts in inflamed peripheral tissues.

Monoclonal antibodies called checkpoint inhibitors can block both these inhibitory proteins and so inactivate them. For example, in many cancer patients, T-cell functions are suppressed by the tumor cells. Administration of monoclonal antibodies against CTLA-4 (ipilimumab), PD-1 (pembrolizumab, nivolumab), or PD-L1 (atezolizumab) will reverse this suppression, activate the T cells, and so permit cancer cell destruction. Monoclonal checkpoint inhibitors have achieved remarkable success in the treatment of many cancers. A combination of anti–PD-1 and anti–CTLA-4 appears to be exceptionally effective in permitting T-cell cytotoxicity to proceed and results in long-term cancer remissions. Unfortunately one of the most important adverse effects of blocking CTLA-4 and PD-1 by these monoclonal antibodies is the development of uncontrolled autoimmune disease.

Contact-Independent Processes

Both CTLA-4 and PD-1 require direct cell-cell contact to suppress T-cell functions. A second set of inhibitory pathways, mediated by secreted cytokines, is used predominantly by pTreg cells. These suppressive cytokines include IL10, IL35, and TGFβ, in addition to indoleamine 2,3-dioxygenase (IDO).

IL10. IL10 is a regulatory cytokine that inhibits both innate and adaptive immune responses (Fig. 2.8). It is a protein of about 178 amino acids produced by macrophages and DCs in response to microbial products. It is also produced by many T-cell subsets, especially Treg cells, but also includes some populations of Th cells in response to high antigen doses. It is produced in especially large amounts by Th1 cells in response to TGFβ.

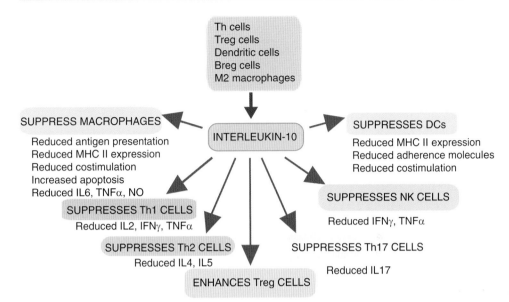

Fig. 2.8 The many suppressive pathways mediated by interleukin-10. These play a key role in maintaining peripheral tolerance and hence preventing the development of autoimmunity. *Breg*, Regulatory B cell; *DC*, dendritic cell; *IL*, interleukin; *IFN*, interferon; *MHC*, major histocompatibility complex; *NK*, natural killer cell; *NO*, nitric oxide; *Th*, helper T cell; *TNFα*, tumor necrosis factor-alpha; *Treg*, regulatory T cell.

IL10 downregulates MHC class II and costimulatory molecule expression on DCs and macrophages and hence impairs antigen presentation. IL10 or IL10-treated DCs can induce a long-lasting, antigen-specific anergic state when T cells are activated in its presence. IL10 inhibits the synthesis of the Th1 cytokines, IL1, IFNγ, and TNFα, and the Th2 cytokines IL4 and IL5. Thus it can suppress both Th1 and Th2 responses. IL10 also inhibits the production of IL5, IL8, IL12, granulocyte-macrophage colony-stimulating factor (GM-CSF), and granulocyte CSF (G-CSF). It also downregulates the production of IFNγ and TNFα by natural killer cells.

IL35. Primarily produced by FoxP3⁺ Treg cells, this cytokine inhibits the activation and differentiation of naïve CD4⁺ Th cells. It promotes their differentiation into CD4⁺ FoxP3⁻ regulatory cells. It also suppresses the production of proinflammatory Th17 cells. A related cytokine, IL37, has similar effects.

TGFβ. TGFβ consists of three glycoproteins (TGFβ1, TGFβ2, and TGFβ3). TGFs are produced by platelets, activated macrophages, neutrophils, B cells, and T cells and act on T and B cells, DCs, macrophages, neutrophils, and fibroblasts. TGFβ is required for the induction and maintenance of FoxP3⁺ Tregs. Membrane-bound TGFβ may also be responsible for some Treg functions (Fig. 2.9). Microbial metabolites such as retinoic acid enhance the tolerogenic properties of TGFβ.

TGFβ regulates macrophage activities. It can enhance phagocytosis by blood monocytes. On the other hand, it suppresses the respiratory burst and nitric oxide production and blocks monocyte differentiation and the cytotoxic effects of activated macrophages. TGFβ is required for optimal DC development and regulates the interaction between follicular DCs and B cells. TGFβ inhibits T- and B-cell proliferation and stimulates their apoptosis. Apoptotic T cells release TGFβ, contributing to the suppressive environment. TGFβ influences the differentiation of Th subsets. It tends to promote Th1 responses and the production of IL2 in naïve T cells, but it also antagonizes

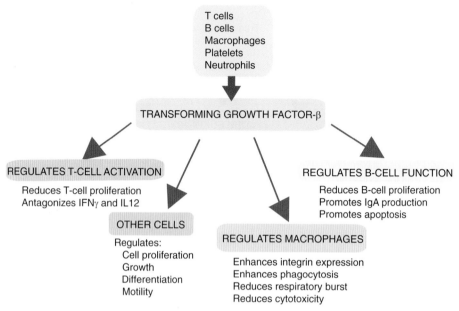

Fig. 2.9 The many suppressive pathways mediated by transforming growth factor-beta. Like interleukin-10, it plays a key role in maintaining peripheral tolerance and the prevention of autoimmunity. *IFN,* Interferon; *IgA,* immunoglobulin A; *IL,* interleukin.

the effects of IFNγ and IL12 on memory cells. It also controls the development and differentiation of B cells, inhibiting their proliferation, inducing apoptosis, and regulating IgA production. IL10 enhances the response of activated T cells to TGFβ by modulating TGF receptor expression. The critical importance of TGFβ1 in controlling lymphocytes can be seen in a mouse knockout model where inactivation of the TGFβ1 genes results in a massive lymphocyte and macrophage infiltration of many organs, development of a progressive wasting syndrome, and death.

IDO. Many regulatory cells, including Tregs, plasmacytoid dendritic cells (pDCs), and some macrophages, produce IDO. This enzyme catalyzes the oxidative degradation of the amino acid tryptophan, resulting in its local depletion. Tryptophan is required for T-cell function so that in its absence T cells undergo cell cycle arrest and apoptosis. IDO therefore inhibits T-cell activation, proliferation, and survival, and promotes peripheral tolerance. Th1 cells appear to be more sensitive to tryptophan depletion than are Th2 cells. Treg cells can induce IDO expression in pDCs. In other situations, IDO production by pDCs is required to confer suppressive functions on Tregs. For example, in experimental autoimmune encephalitis, IDO from pDCs activates Tregs to reduce disease severity. Likewise, IDO plays an important role in maintaining tolerance to testicular antigens. IDO activity has also been documented in suppressing T-cell responses to tumors and as a negative regulator of autoimmune diseases such as rheumatoid arthritis and orchitis, as well as in some allergies.

OTHER REGULATORY CELLS

Regulatory Dendritic Cells

The primary function of DCs is to capture and process foreign antigens for presentation to T cells. However, they also play an important role in maintaining peripheral tolerance by regulating T-cell responses. It has generally been accepted that immature DCs promote tolerance, while the main function of mature DCs is to promote immunogenicity. This is probably an oversimplification, and their functions probably also depend on external signals. These signals depend on their state of maturity, on cellular costimulation, on the presence or absence of inflammatory cytokines, and on their tissue location. Some of these signals can generate tolerogenic DCs. These tolerogenic DCs play an important role in establishing central tolerance within the thymus as well as maintaining peripheral tolerance. Low-affinity self-reactive T cells that leave the thymus must continue to be suppressed in the periphery. This suppression is the function of Treg cells, but the production of Treg cells is in turn controlled by regulatory DCs.

DCs can induce T-cell tolerance either by direct contact or by producing suppressive cytokines and IDO. Contact suppression includes PD-1 signaling or even Fas-mediated apoptosis. For example, TGFβ and IL10 from regulatory DCs promote the differentiation of Treg cells.

In general, if proteins are captured by immature DCs in the absence of inflammation, they trigger tolerance. The DCs silence responding T cells or cause the T cells to differentiate into Treg cells. Likewise, DCs can take up antigens from apoptotic cells, present them to T cells, and under the influence of molecules such as CTLA-4 and PD-1, cause them to undergo clonal anergy or differentiate into Tregs. However, DCs eventually mature, especially in the presence of PAMPs and damage-associated molecular patterns (DAMPs). Once they grow up, they increase their expression of MHC class II and acquire the ability to activate naïve T cells.

The tissue environment also plays a role in determining DC functions, Thus DCs located on body surfaces such as the intestinal mucosa play an important role in maintaining immune tolerance to food antigens and commensal bacteria. This suppressive function is likely triggered by signals transmitted through their pattern-recognition receptors.

Regulatory B Cells

Tolerogenic DCs can also interact with B cells to generate regulatory B (Breg) cells. These Breg cells secrete high levels of IL10, IL35, and TGFβ. As a result, they can suppress the functions of Th17, Th1, and effector T cells; trigger clonal anergy; and promote the differentiation of Treg cells. They may also induce tolerogenic DCs in a tolerogenic feedback loop.

Natural Suppressor Cells

NS cells are large, granular innate lymphocytes that produce cytokines with Treg-inducing activity. They suppress B- and T-cell proliferation as well as immunoglobulin production. NS cells are found normally in the adult bone marrow and the neonatal spleen.

Myeloid-Derived Suppressor Cells

Myeloid-derived suppressor cells (MDSCs) are a heterogeneous group of immature myeloid cells that eventually develop into macrophages, granulocytes, or DCs. When activated, however, these stem cells can also suppress T-cell functions. MDSCs suppress cytotoxic T-cell responses by cell–cell contact through PD-1 or by secreting soluble immunosuppressive mediators such as arginase, IL10, TGFβ, reactive oxygen species, nitric oxide, and peroxynitrite. Peroxynitrite causes nitrate addition to TCRs and thus inactivates them. MDSCs also produce arginase that impairs T-cell function by reducing expression of CD3z, a key component of the TCR. Some MDSCs promote the production of Treg cells. Collectively, therefore, these cells effectively promote tolerance. They accumulate in some autoimmune diseases, such as in rheumatoid arthritis, but their role is unclear.

Sources of Additional Information

Bigley TM, Yang Y, Kang L-I, Saenz JB, et al. Disruption of thymic central tolerance by infection with murine roseolovirus induces autoimmune gastritis. *J Exp Med.* 2022; doi:10.1084/jem.20211403.

Bluestone JA, Anderson M. Tolerance in the age of immunotherapy. *N Engl J Med.* 2020;383:1156–1166.

Boros P, Ochando J, Zeher M. Myeloid derived suppressor cells and autoimmunity. *Human Immunol.* 2016;77:631–636.

Buchbinder EJ, Desai A. CTLA-4 and PD-1 pathways: similarities, differences and implications for their inhibition. *Am J Clin Oncol.* 2016;39:98–106.

Burnet FM. A modification of Jerne's theory on antibody production using the concept of clonal selection. *Aust J Science.* 1957;20:67–69.

ElTanbouly MA, Noelle RJ. Rethinking peripheral T cell tolerance: checkpoints across a T cell's journey. *Nat Rev Immunol.* 2021;21:257–267.

Francisco LM, Sage PT, Sharpe AH. The PD-1 pathway in tolerance and autoimmunity. *Immunol Rev.* 2010;236:219–242.

Jennette JC, Falk RJ. The rise and fall of horror autotoxicus and forbidden clones. *Kidney Int.* 2010;78:533–535.

Khatlani TS, Ma Z, Okuda M, et al. Autoantibodies against T-cell costimulatory molecules are produced in canine autoimmune diseases. *J Immunother.* 2003;26:12–20.

Lippens C, Irla FV, Dubrot J, et al. IDO-orchestrated crosstalk between pDCs and Tregs inhibits autoimmunity. *J Autoimmune.* 2016. doi:10.1016/j.jaut.2016.07.004.

Passos GA, Speck-Hernandez CA, Assis F, et al. Update on Aire and thymic negative selection. *Immunology.* 2017;153:10–20.

Proekt I, Miller CN, Lionakis MS, et al. Insights into immune tolerance from AIRE deficiency. *Curr Opin Immunol.* 2017;49:71–78.

Rojas C, Campos-Mora M, Carcamo I, et al. T regulatory cells-derived extracellular vesicles and their contributions to the generation of immune tolerance. *J Leukoc Biol.* 2020;108:813–824.

Theofilopoulos AN, Kono DH, Baccala R. The multiple pathways to autoimmunity. *Nat Immunol.* 2017. doi:10.1038/ni.3731.

Turner JA, Stephen-Victor E, Wang S, et al. Regulatory T cell-derived TGF-b1 controls multiple checkpoints governing allergy and autoimmunity. *Immunity.* 2020;53:1202–1214.

Waterfield M, Anderson MS. Clues to immune tolerance: the monogenic autoimmune syndromes. *Ann NY Acad Sci.* 2010;1214:138–155.

Zhang X, Olsen N, Zheng SG. The progress and prospect for regulatory T cells in autoimmune diseases. *J Autoimmunity.* 2020. doi:10.1016/j.jaut.2020.102461.

Loss of Tolerance

Witebsky's Postulates

In 1957, as modern immunology began to stir, German-American scientist Ernest Witebsky proposed four rules (postulates) required to confirm that a disease was truly autoimmune (Box 3.1). Despite the generation of both central and peripheral tolerance, autoimmune diseases are relatively common. They are also highly diverse and can potentially damage or destroy any organ in the body.

Broadly speaking, autoimmune diseases result from a breakdown of tolerance that results in the emergence of clones of rogue lymphocytes. These rogues may either be B cells that make autoantibodies directed against normal body components or T cells with a similar specificity for healthy cells. Tolerance in B and T cells is regulated by multiple mechanisms. These include central tolerance (as a result of negative selection within the thymus), peripheral tolerance (including the need for multiple costimulatory signals and lymphocyte cooperation), and the activities of regulatory cells. These control mechanisms often overlap so that the development of self-reactive rogue clones does not usually occur suddenly. It likely takes multiple accumulated defects acting in diverse regulatory pathways to cause a loss of control of lymphocyte proliferation. As a result of these defects in multiple control systems, autoimmune diseases generally have a multistep pathogenesis.

Given the ubiquity of foreign antigens, especially those resulting from the presence of the normal microbiota on body surfaces, lymphocytes are under constant pressure to respond. Much of the complexity of the immune system results from the need to keep this unwanted and unneeded lymphocyte proliferation in check. The initial trigger that leads to a breakdown of self-tolerance probably involves the recognition of molecular patterns, especially nucleic acids by pattern-recognition receptors. This recognition results in the activation of sentinel cells, the release of proinflammatory cytokines, the development of an inflammatory environment, and the secondary activation of dendritic cells resulting in B- and T-cell activation. While both B and T cells can mediate autoimmune disease, like any other form of immune response, helper T (Th) cells are required for the response to proceed.

The random generation of antigen-binding receptors ensures that many lymphocytes are produced with receptors that can bind self-antigens. It has been estimated that as many as 50% of

29

BOX 3.1 ■ Witebsky's Postulates

Ernest Witebsky (1901-1969) proposed four postulates to confirm that a disease was truly autoimmune. He based these rules on those proposed by Robert Koch for infectious diseases at the dawn of microbiology. Witebsky required that (1) affected individuals must develop antiself-antibodies or cells, (2) the corresponding self-antigen be identified, (3) an analogous autoimmune response be induced in experimental animals, and (4) the experimentally immunized animal must develop a similar disease to the natural one.

These postulates served well for many years but were revised and updated by Noel Rose and Constantin Bona in 1993. These authors, taking into account the great advances in our understanding of immunology in the intervening years, suggested that three kinds of evidence may be used to establish that a disease is truly autoimmune. First, there is direct evidence of the kind that Witebsky required. For example, it is possible to take antibodies from a human with the muscle disease myasthenia gravis, inject them into a mouse, and reproduce the disease in the animal. Second, there is indirect evidence. For example, while it is inappropriate to try and transfer these diseases between humans by means of living cells or purified antibodies, this is readily done in experimental animals. Likewise, some diseases can be induced in experimental animals by immunizing with purified autoantigens. The third form of evidence is circumstantial. This type of evidence applies to many of the diseases of animals described in this book. It can best be summarized as follows: (1) There is an association with other autoimmune diseases in the same animal or related family members, (2) there is a significant lymphocytic infiltration of the affected organ or tissues, (3) a statistical association can be shown with a specific major histocompatibility complex allele or haplotype, and (4) the animal shows a favorable clinical response to immunosuppressive therapy. These four rules have been (largely) followed in considering the diseases to be included in this text.

It is also important to differentiate between autoimmune diseases, autoinflammatory diseases, and immune-mediated diseases. Autoimmune diseases result from adaptive immune responses specifically directed against normal body structures or molecules as a result of a loss of self-tolerance. Autoinflammatory diseases result from dysfunction of the innate immune system, and as a result, cause significant tissue damage, disease, and death. Immune-mediated diseases are primarily directed against foreign antigens such as infectious agents, and any resulting tissue damage is, in a sense, secondary. These classifications overlap because many autoimmune diseases require an innate immune response to trigger their onset, and as pointed out in the accompanying figure, they form a continuum of diseases ranging from pure autoinflammatory to pure autoimmune.

It is also relevant to point out that autoimmune diseases almost always involve inappropriate innate immune responses as well as dysfunctional adaptive immunity. In fact, the diseases discussed here constitute a spectrum of disorders ranging from autoinflammatory disorders at one end to autoimmune diseases at the other. Most diseases discussed in this text involve a pathogenic mixture of inflammatory and autoimmune processes. For example, it is often the case that an inflammatory response can serve as a trigger for adaptive autoimmunity. This may be due to an infection or other environmental stimulus. The importance of these triggering innate responses is highly variable, and there are plenty of these diseases where the trigger is completely unknown. Finally, the eventual damage mediated by autoimmune responses is also often due to hypersensitivity responses triggered by adaptive immunity in addition to secondary inflammation triggered by this tissue damage.

newly produced T and B cells may possess receptors that can bind self-antigens with high affinity. These cells are never completely eliminated. They are, however, usually rigorously suppressed. However, the reasons why some individuals eventually develop autoimmune diseases while others do not remain unclear. Many factors influence susceptibility to autoimmunity. These include sex and age, genetic background, as well as environmental effects such as alterations in the microbiota and virus infections. We also know that the development of autoantibodies is a relatively common event that by itself does not inevitably lead to autoimmune disease. Indeed, some autoantibodies serve a physiologic function.

BOX 3.1 ■ Witebsky Postulates—cont'd

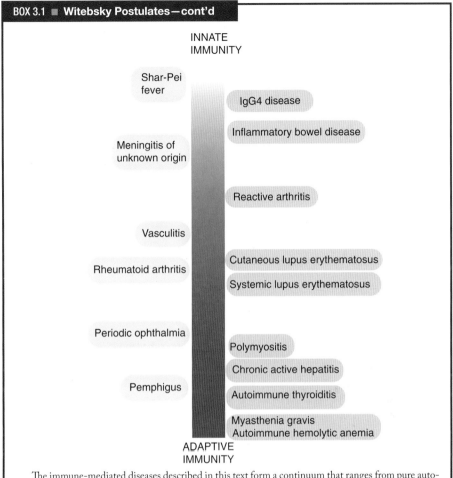

The immune-mediated diseases described in this text form a continuum that ranges from pure auto-inflammatory diseases at one end characterized by a disease such as Shar-Pei fever to pure autoimmune diseases such as myasthenia gravis and autoimmune thyroiditis at the other, mediated exclusively by autoantibodies and T cells. Most immune-mediated diseases, however, fall between these two extremes.

Hayter SM, Cook MC. Updated assessment of the prevalence, spectrum and case definition of autoimmune disease. *Autoimmunity Rev.* 2012;11:754-765.
Rose NR, Bona C. Defining criteria for autoimmune diseases (Witebsky's postulates revisited). *Immunol Today.* 1993;14:426–430.

Because we do not know precisely what triggers autoimmunity, this chapter reviews some of the many different predisposing factors that have been identified or proposed, as well as the mechanisms by which tolerance may be lost (Fig. 3.1). Autoimmune diseases are also complex. Self-reactivity of the immune system ranges from a very low background level that helps maintain lymphocyte homeostasis, to autoimmune responses with detectable autoantibodies with lymphocyte infiltration in tissues but no clinical consequences, to severe organ damage resulting in clinical disease and death. These diseases can involve not only aberrant adaptive responses but often abnormal innate responses as well. These so-called autoinflammatory diseases can result

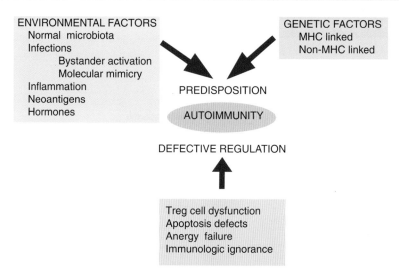

Fig. 3.1   The predisposing factors that influence the development of autoimmunity and the defects in regulatory processes that permit it to develop. In practice, all these factors acting either singly or in combination influence autoimmune disease development. *MHC,* Major histocompatibility complex; *Treg cell,* regulatory T cell.

in the development of uncontrolled inflammation. Thus, in practice, immune-mediated diseases generally result from a combination of inappropriate innate and adaptive responses. The relative contributions of each vary greatly between diseases.

Normal Immune Responses

Although the control of the immune system requires that most self-reactive cells be eliminated or suppressed, it should not be assumed that all autoimmune responses are bad. Some autoimmune responses have physiologic functions. Many low-level autoimmune antibody responses simply reflect a normal B-cell response to an antigen to which the immune system lacks tolerance. Examples include antigens that have been previously hidden from the immune system by hiding within cells or behind tissue barriers. Alternatively, these responses may result from structural identity (cross-reactivity) between an infectious agent and normal body components, a phenomenon called molecular mimicry. Many of these naturally occurring autoantibodies play a role in homeostasis and regulation. They are usually low-titer, low-affinity immunoglobulin M (IgM) or IgG antibodies directed against protein fragments, or proteins damaged by oxidation or enzymes. For example, healthy humans possess low levels of natural autoantibodies against myeloperoxidase, proteinase 3, and glomerular basement membrane type 3 collagen. These have the same specificity as some pathogenic autoantibodies such as the antineutrophil cytoplasmic antibodies and antiglomerular basement membrane antibodies but are not clinically significant. It is abundantly clear that not all self-reactive B-cell clones are purged through central tolerance.

AGED CELLS

Red blood cells must be removed from the blood once they are no longer functional. One way this is accomplished is by the use of autoantibodies. As red cells reach the end of their life span, a senescent cell antigen is generated. This antigen is generated when oxidation activates the proteolytic enzyme caspase 3. The activated caspase 3 acts on an anion transport protein called CD233 (or band 3 protein) located in the cell membrane. As a result, a new structural epitope is generated on the red cell surface. This new senescence antigen is recognized by naturally occurring IgG autoantibodies. When the cells reach the end of their life span, these autoantibodies will bind to the senescent cell antigens on the red cells, activate complement, and so trigger their phagocytosis and destruction by splenic macrophages. CD233 is found on many different cell types, and its exposure on other populations of aged cells and their subsequent removal may also be an important cell elimination pathway.

CRYPTIC ANTIGENS

Some autoimmune responses are triggered when nontolerant T cells encounter previously hidden autoantigens. There are many normal proteins that do not induce tolerance simply because they are hidden within cells or tissues and do not normally encounter T cells. As pointed out in the previous chapter, the autoimmune regulator (AIRE) and other thymic transcription regulators cannot cause the expression of every possible protein made by the body. Thus T cells may remain ignorant of some tissue antigens, especially if they are hidden behind impermeable cellular barriers. These barriers may, however, be disrupted by infections or physical trauma. These antigens are most likely to be found hiding in immunologically privileged sites such as eyes and testes. This phenomenon is called immunologic ignorance (Fig. 3.2).

In the testes, for example, many sperm proteins are only expressed at puberty, long after the T-cell system has developed and become tolerant to other body components. Injury to the testes may permit these proteins to escape and encounter antigen-sensitive cells and so stimulate an autoimmune response. Hidden (or cryptic) antigens are also found inside cells. For example, after a heart attack, autoantibodies may be produced against the mitochondria of cardiac muscle cells. In chronic hepatitis in dogs, animals develop antibodies to liver membrane proteins as a result of cell disruption. In diseases such as trypanosomiasis, Covid-19, or tuberculosis, in which widespread tissue damage occurs, autoantibodies to many different intracellular antigens may be detected in serum. For example, about 40% of tuberculosis patients make antinuclear antibodies and rheumatoid factors (RFs; autoantibodies against IgG) SARS-CoV-2 infection, the cause of Covid-19, triggers the production of antiphospholipid autoantibodies.

NEOANTIGENS

T- and B-cell receptors can bind antigens in two basic ways; thus they can recognize either the specific amino acid sequence of an antigenic peptide or its molecular conformation. As a result, some B cells may be activated by binding to new conformational epitopes generated by alterations in the folding of normal proteins. Two examples of important autoantibodies directed against these neoantigens are the RFs and the immunoconglutinins (IKs, after the German spelling).

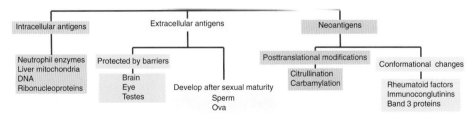

Fig. 3.2 Sources of hidden and neoantigens that may be targets of autoimmune attack. These may be hidden behind barriers, develop later in life, or be generated as a result of posttranslational modifications. Because many of these antigens do not trigger central tolerance, they rely almost exclusively on the maintenance of peripheral tolerance to prevent severe autoimmune disease.

RFs are autoantibodies directed against other immunoglobulins. When an antibody binds to an antigen, the shape of the immunoglobulin molecule changes in such a way that new epitopes are exposed on its Fc region. These new epitopes are recognized by B cells that respond by making RFs. RFs are produced in diseases where large amounts of immune complexes are generated. These include the autoimmune disease of joints called rheumatoid arthritis and systemic lupus erythematosus (SLE), in which B cells respond to many different autoantigens.

IKs are autoantibodies directed against the complement components C2, C4, and especially C3. The conformational epitopes that stimulate IK production are generated when these complement components are activated and so change their shape. The level of IKs in serum reflects the amount of complement activation; this, in turn, is a measure of the antigenic stimulation to which an animal is subjected. IK levels are thus nonspecific indicators of the prevalence of infectious disease within an animal population. Their physiologic role is unclear, but they may enhance complement-mediated opsonization.

It is also important to remember that while the amino acid sequence of any protein is determined by its genes, proteins are often modified after they are formed. This posttranslational modification often involves chemical changes to amino acids. For example, the amino acid serine may be acetylated, methylated, glycosylated, phosphorylated, or sulfated. These changes may, on occasion, result in the generation of neoantigens that can trigger autoimmunity. The best example of this is seen in rheumatoid arthritis, in which the arginine residues in many proteins are deiminated and converted to citrulline. These citrullinated proteins then provoke the production of autoantibodies directed against the new epitopes and so contribute to arthritis development.

RECEPTOR EDITING

Both B- and T-cell antigen receptors are generated by random gene rearrangement. This process inevitably results in the production of both nonfunctional and autoreactive antigen receptors. Once a B cell expresses complete antigen receptors, rearrangement of the cell's receptor genes does not stop. Thus if an immature B cell produces a receptor that binds to a self-antigen, the continuing development of that B cell is normally blocked while its light chain receptor chains continue to undergo recombination. A B cell expressing a specific kappa light chain may restart its V gene rearrangement by switching to the other kappa gene or even switching to either of the lambda light chain genes. This replacement of one light chain by another alters the receptor binding specificity and eventually makes the cells no longer autoreactive. This receptor editing is an important method of preventing the development of cells with receptors that bind to self-antigens.

When the antigen receptors (T-cell receptors [TCRs]) of developing T cells bind to self-antigens, they too undergo receptor editing. Although cell maturation stops once a T cell leaves the thymus, its recombinases remain active, and TCR gene recombination continues to occur. The *TCR* genes continue to diversify so that altered receptors are expressed on newly produced T cells. If a T cell successfully edits its receptors, its maturation can proceed. Failure to generate functional antigen receptors, however, will result in its death. Receptor gene editing is a potentially hazardous process since it can also generate self-reactive T cells that have not passed the negative selection test within the thymus.

EPITOPE SPREADING

When an immune response is initiated, the initial immune response is usually directed against a limited number of epitopes on the inciting antigen. However, as the responding lymphocytes multiply, receptor editing continues, their antigen receptors continue to diversify, and these newly generated receptors may bind other nearby epitopes on the same protein (Fig. 3.3). Eventually these new receptors may be able to bind epitopes on other proteins, including autoantigens. Epitope

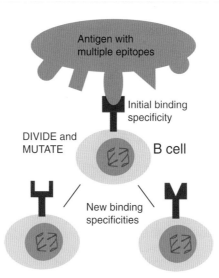

Fig. 3.3 Mechanisms of epitope spreading. Thus B cells responding to antigen undergo cycles of cell division and random mutation of their receptors. These random changes in the B-cell receptors may result in the production of new, self-reactive antibodies that can recognize other nearby epitopes on the same protein.

spreading has been demonstrated in diseases such as thyrotoxicosis, equine recurrent uveitis, and type 1 diabetes mellitus and may account for some of the difficulties encountered in treating these diseases.

BYSTANDER ACTIVATION

Activation of antigen-presenting cells in an inflammatory environment may result in the subsequent activation of autoreactive T and B cells (Fig. 3.4). When viruses destroy cells, previously hidden antigens may be released. These may activate nearby lymphocytes that had not been involved in the initial antiviral response. Additionally, T cells might, in responding to an antigen, produce a mixture of toxic cytokines such as the tumor necrosis factors and nitric oxide, which can kill nearby cells and indirectly trigger an autoimmune response. Viruses may also induce an inflammatory response that results in a flood of cytokines. Pathogens may trigger inappropriate lymphocyte proliferation by acting through pattern-recognition receptors to generate large amounts of costimulatory and proinflammatory cytokines. These cytokines may activate previously naïve T cells. As a result, the newly activated T cells may respond to autoantigens that had previously been ignored. For example, evidence suggests that coxsackievirus–induced diabetes mellitus is mediated in large part through bystander activation. Prolonged infection with some viruses may induce autoimmunity simply as a result of chronic activation of the immune system. Thus prolonged polyclonal B-cell activation may eventually result in the emergence of autoreactive clones. The development of autoantibodies in Covid-19 is probably due to the intense immune stimulation caused by the SARS-2 coronavirus.

ABNORMAL IMMUNE RESPONSES

Central tolerance of B and T cells is not infallible, and it is also clear that some of these cells must escape from peripheral tolerance mechanisms if they are to become pathogenic and trigger autoimmune disease. There are four major regulatory mechanisms that normally maintain peripheral

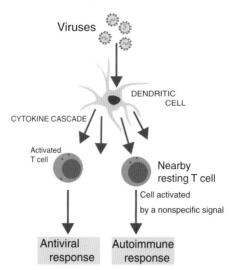

Fig. 3.4 One of the simplest mechanisms by which bystander activation may trigger autoimmunity is through the activation of nearby self-reactive cells by the flood of costimulating cytokines released by dendritic and other cells during a normal immune response.

tolerance and so prevent the activation of autoreactive lymphocytes. These are the production of inhibitory molecules such as cytotoxic T-lymphocyte–associated antigen 4 (CTLA-4), programmed death 1 (PD-1), or Fas; the development of anergy as a result of a lack of appropriate costimulation; T-cell ignorance as a result of antigen sequestration; and active suppression by regulatory T (Treg) cells. However, triggering infections and inflammation, a genetic predisposition, and an animal's age also factor into tolerance loss.

The breakdown of tolerance involves a breakdown in one or more of these regulatory mechanisms. Examples include the severe systemic autoimmune syndrome that results from defects in the CTLA-4 or Fas pathway, the failure of anergy resulting from excessive activation of the CD40–CD40L pathway leading to some forms of systemic lupus, autoimmune orchitis resulting from trauma, and impaired Treg function seen in experimental autoimmune hemolytic anemia.

This last defect can be demonstrated simply by repeatedly injecting mice with rat red blood cells. Following these injections, the mice not only make antibodies to the rat cells but also develop a self-limited and transient autoimmune response to their own red blood cells. In normal mice, this autoimmune response is rapidly controlled by regulatory cells and lasts for only a few days. If, however, Treg cell activity in these mice is impaired, as occurs in the New Zealand Black strain, for example, these autoantibodies can persist and increase to eventually cause red blood cell destruction and anemia (see Chapter 22).

THE EFFECTS OF AGE

Age is a critical feature that influences the development of autoimmunity, especially in very long-lived species such as humans. The gradual accumulation of diverse B cells over time can play a role in triggering many autoimmune diseases. Thus as humans age, the diversity of their B cell repertoire progressively increases. However, some aged individuals generate more diverse B cell populations than others. Those with this "accelerated immune aging" are more likely to develop autoimmune disease. For example, autoantibodies directed against type I interferons are present in about 4% of humans over 70 and their prevalence sharply increases thereafter. These individuals account for about 20% of Covid-19 deaths.

BOX 3.2 ■ MicroRNAs and Autoimmunity

Noncoding RNA molecules occur in the form of microRNAs (miRNAs) of 18 to 23 nucleotides or as long noncoding RNAs (lncRNA) of over 200 nucleotides. MiRNAs bind to messenger RNA, interfere with translation, and silence specific genes. As a result, they can regulate the development and activation of immune cells. LncRNAs are generally transcribed and can then interact with other nucleic acids or proteins. Many different miRNAs have been linked to the development of autoantibodies and inflammation and influence the pathogenesis of these diseases; thus some can cause lymphoproliferation and autoimmunity. Others can reduce expression of antiapoptotic molecules. Some regulate central B-cell tolerance. Some have been identified as potential diagnostic biomarkers. Multiple studies have demonstrated that changes in the levels of some miRNAs and lncRNAs can influence autoimmune disease severity. They have been closely associated with human systemic lupus erythematosus, multiple sclerosis, and rheumatoid arthritis. Their role in naturally occurring autoimmune diseases in animals has rarely been investigated.

Zhang L, Wu H, Zhao M, et al. Clinical significance of miRNAs in autoimmunity. *J Autoimmunity*. 2020. doi.org/10.1016/j.jaut.2020.102438

As an individual's cells age, DNA may accidentally break and need to be repaired. Young, healthy cells possess machinery that senses and repairs these breaks. However, over time, the repair process becomes less and less effective. Inadequate DNA repair may occur in rapidly dividing stem cells, including those generating naïve and memory CD4$^+$ T cells as well as in their mitochondria. This decline in the repair processes results in the accumulation of damaged DNA in the nucleus, at the ends of telomeres, and in mitochondria. MicroRNAs may fail to control gene transcription (Box 3.2). As a result, aged cells may begin to behave abnormally. Changes may develop in the cell cycle, there may be premature loss of telomeres, and there may be cytoplasmic leakage of mitochondrial DNA, resulting in inflammasome activation. As the DNA defects accumulate, they result in T-cell functional changes. They favor cell differentiation into short-lived effector T cells rather than into long-lived memory cells. Unrepaired DNA damage also promotes T-cell apoptosis, exhaustion, and premature aging. It can result in reprogramming of T-cell energy production and biosynthesis. All these changes mean that over time, the tight regulation of adaptive immunity in the young and healthy inevitably becomes less effective and permits the development of T-cell–mediated inflammation and autoimmunity in older individuals.

ROGUE LYMPHOCYTE CLONES

Potentially harmful, self-reactive lymphocytes are normally destroyed in the thymus by apoptosis triggered through the death receptor Fas (CD95). Defects in Fas or its ligand, FasL (CD95L), can result in autoimmunity by permitting abnormal T cells to survive. This is well demonstrated in the *lpr* strain of mice. These animals have a mutation that alters the structure of the intracellular domain of Fas and so blocks its functions. A mutation (called *gld*) in CD95L has a similar effect. Both *lpr* and *gld* mice develop multiple autoimmune lesions accompanied by lymphoproliferation. (This mutation has also been recorded in the cat [see Chapter 22].)

It is also common to find autoimmune diseases associated with lymphoid tumors. For example, myasthenia gravis, an autoimmune disease affecting neuromuscular junctions, is commonly associated with the presence of a thymic carcinoma. In humans, there is a fourfold increase in the incidence of rheumatoid arthritis in patients with malignant lymphoid tumors, and there is evidence for a similar association in other mammals. Since many lymphoid tumors result from a failure in immunologic control mechanisms, a simultaneous failure in self-tolerance may also occur. Alternatively, some lymphoid tumors may consist of cells producing autoantibodies. It is also possible that some lymphoid tumors may develop as a result of chronic overstimulation of the immune system by autoantigens.

INFECTIOUS DISEASES AND MOLECULAR MIMICRY

Autoimmune diseases are triggered by many environmental factors. Among these factors, infections are often identified as initiators or promoters of autoimmunity. The immune system of individuals predisposed to autoimmunity may be pushed over the edge by the additional stimulus provided by infections. There is no doubt that some antiviral immune responses can trigger autoimmunity (Box 3.3); thus some cases of rheumatoid arthritis, autoimmune thyroid disease, and vasculopathies may have an infectious trigger. For example, mice infected with certain reoviruses develop an autoimmune polyendocrine disease characterized by diabetes mellitus and suppressed growth. These reovirus-infected mice make autoantibodies against the anterior pituitary, pancreas, gastric mucosa, thymus, nuclei, glucagon, growth hormone, and insulin. Likewise, persistent infection of NZB mice with a type C retrovirus leads to the production of autoantibodies against nucleic acids and red blood cells. Bacteria such as *Streptococcus pyogenes*, *Borrelia burgdorferi*, and *Leptospira interrogans* may trigger autoimmune heart disease, arthritis, and uveitis, respectively. The protozoan parasite *Trypanosoma cruzi* triggers an autoimmune cardiomyopathy.

Chronic infections not only provoke innate immune responses but also provide a generous supply of antigens to lymphocyte populations and thus long-term stimulation. As a result of chronic inflammation, some susceptible animals may progress through autoimmune or inflammatory diseases to lymphomas and cancers.

Autoimmunity may also result from molecular mimicry, a term used to describe the sharing of structurally similar epitopes (also called mimotopes) between an infectious agent or parasite and a self-antigen. T cells may be activated by several different peptides bound to one or perhaps more major histocompatibility complex (MHC) molecules, provided that they all have a similar shape and charge. As a result, it is possible for otherwise tolerant T cells to respond to microbial antigens that cross-react with some self-antigens.

B and T cells may therefore be triggered by foreign epitopes so that they then respond to normal body components. However, they will only respond to these epitopes if they also receive T-cell help. If nearby Th cells also recognize these microbial epitopes as foreign, they may trigger the production of autoantibodies. Once a B-cell response is triggered in this way, the infectious agent may be removed while the autoimmune response continues—a hit-and-run process.

BOX 3.3 ■ Autoimmunity in Covid-19

Infections often serve as the trigger for autoimmune diseases. One extreme example of this is Covid-19 caused by SARS-2 coronavirus. The clinical course of Covid-19–mediated respiratory disease in humans is highly variable. Most infected individuals never show clinical signs, whereas at the other extreme, individuals develop a rapidly lethal respiratory disease. One reason for these variations in disease severity is the development of autoimmunity. Severe cases of Covid-19 disease are characterized by the production of large amounts of proinflammatory cytokines. This reflects hyperstimulation of both the innate and adaptive immune systems. Consequently, patients may make diverse autoantibodies. Thus about one-third of patients make antinuclear antibodies, about 50% make autoantibodies to phospholipids such as cardiolipin or $\beta2$ glycoprotein 1, and about 10% of patients make autoantibodies against several types of antiviral interferons (IFNs). Most appear to produce neutralizing immunoglobulin G autoantibodies against IFNω and IFNα or both; some make autoantibodies against MDA5 (melanoma differentiation-associated protein 5), an RNA receptor; and some make autoantibodies against neutrophil cytoplasmic antigens. It has been suggested that these autoimmune responses are a reflection of a broader phenomenon (i.e., ASIA syndrome), in which inflammation by infections or proinflammatory stimuli such as vaccine adjuvants may trigger diverse autoimmune and inflammatory diseases.

Bastard P, Rosen LB, Zhang Q, et al. Autoantibodies against type I interferons in patients with life-threatening COVID-19. *Science*. 2020. doi:10.1126/science.abd4585.
Halpert G, Shoenfeld Y. SARS-CoV-2, the autoimmune virus. *Autoimmun Rev*. 2020. doi.org/10.1016/j.autrev.102965.

Many examples of molecular mimicry are now recognized. These include the Epstein-Barr virus DNA polymerase, which cross-reacts with myelin basic protein and may be involved in the induction of multiple sclerosis, and the poliovirus capsid protein VP2, which cross-reacts with the acetylcholine receptor and may induce myasthenia gravis. Antibodies directed against bacterial heat-shock proteins are found in the serum of humans and rats with rheumatoid arthritis, ankylosing spondylitis, and SLE. Injection of killed *Mycobacterium tuberculosis* in Freund's Complete Adjuvant can cause arthritis in rats, and T cells from these animals can transfer arthritis to normal syngeneic recipients. These T cells respond to HSP 60, a mycobacterial heat-shock protein. It has been suggested that molecular mimicry between microbial and mammalian HSP 60 may be an important trigger factor in rheumatoid arthritis.

Group A streptococci are well recognized for possessing cross-reactive antigens that can cause several different human autoimmune diseases as a result of molecular mimicry. Streptococcal immune-mediated sequelae such as acute rheumatic fever are due to antibody and T-cell responses that cross-react with self-antigens. Children infected with certain strains of group A streptococci may develop an autoimmune myocarditis, a glomerulonephritis, or the autoimmune brain disease Sydenham chorea. These cross-reactions appear to result from the presence of similar structures such as alpha helices in the bacterial M protein and in host proteins such as myosin, keratin, tropomyosin, vimentin, and laminin. The streptococcal group A polysaccharides (N-acetyl-glucosamine) are also cross-reactive with cardiac glycoproteins. Antibodies to the bacterial DNA are also cross-reactive. This broad cross-reactivity serves to explain how antistreptococcal antibodies cross-react with the heart, glomerular basement membrane, and brain.

A cell surface protein, integrin CD11a/18 (LFA-1), shares an antigenic determinant with the outer surface protein of the Lyme disease bacterium *B. burgdorferi*. Patients infected with this organism mount an initial immune response that may then develop into autoimmunity. In about 10% of patients with Lyme arthritis, antibiotics fail to resolve the disease, suggesting that once triggered, the autoimmune process proceeds in the absence of the bacterium. Among the autoimmune diseases that have been associated with Lyme disease are dermatomyositis, rheumatoid arthritis, vasculitis, uveitis, immune thrombocytopenia, autoimmune liver disease, and SLE. Many of these associations have been only single case reports and are likely to be coincidental. On the other hand, molecular mimicry and exaggerated immune responses in infected tissues may also contribute to the process.

The situation with spontaneous autoimmune disease is less clear. Many attempts have been made to isolate viruses from patients with autoimmune disease but with mixed results. For example, SLE of dogs and humans has been associated with either a type C retrovirus or a paramyxovirus infection. Small quantities of the Epstein-Barr virus genome can be found in the salivary glands of humans with Sjögren syndrome. Moreover, epidemiologic evidence points to some form of a viral trigger for diseases such as multiple sclerosis, rheumatoid arthritis, and insulin-dependent diabetes mellitus in children. Just how viruses can induce autoimmunity is unclear, but three major mechanisms are recognized: molecular mimicry, epitope spreading, and bystander activation. Other examples include Guillain-Barré syndrome triggered by influenza and other viruses. Coonhound paralysis is an autoimmune polyneuritis of dogs possibly triggered by exposure to an agent from raccoon saliva (see Chapter 7).

In porcine enzootic pneumonia caused by *Mycoplasma hyopneumoniae*, antibodies to the mycoplasma cross-react with pig lungs, and in contagious bovine pleuropneumonia, there is cross-reactivity between *M. mycoides* antigens and normal bovine lung. It is not known to what extent these autoantibodies contribute to the pathogenesis of these diseases. There is a clearer causal relationship between *L. interrogans* infection and the development of periodic ophthalmia, the leading cause of blindness in horses (see Chapter 8).

Some microbial superantigens may trigger autoimmunity through bystander activation. Superantigens bind MHC class II molecules to the V domains of TCRs and so cause T-cell activation irrespective of their antigen-binding specificity. Some of these T cells may be reactive with autoantigens. For example, the superantigen staphylococcal enterotoxin B activates the same T cells that react with myelin and so induces an autoimmune encephalitis. It has been suggested that a bacterial superantigen may trigger rheumatoid arthritis since the T cells in affected joints are enriched in cells bearing specific TCR V domains. The only known agents that can alter V region gene expression in this way are superantigens. Bacterial superantigens have also been implicated in the pathogenesis of inflammatory bowel disease.

Sources of Additional Information

Arvey A, Rowe M, Legutki JB, An G, et al. Age -associated changes in the circulating human antibody repertoire are upregulated in autoimmunity. Immunity Aging 2020; doi.org/10.1186/s12979-020-00193-x.

Cunningham MW. Molecular mimicry, autoimmunity and infection: the cross-reactive antigens of group A streptococci and their sequelae. *Microbiol Spectr.* 2019. doi:10.1128/microbiolspec.

Goodnow CC. Multistep pathogenesis of autoimmune disease. *Cell.* 2007;130:25–35.

Iberg CA, Hawiger D. Natural and induced tolerogenic dendritic cells. *J Immunol.* 2020;204:733–744.

Mackay IR. Clustering and commonalities among autoimmune diseases. *J Autoimm.* 2009;33:170–177.

Moulton VR. Sex hormones in acquired immunity and autoimmune disease. *Front Immunol.* 2018. doi:10.3389/fimmu.2018.02279.

Münz C, Lünemann JD, Teague Getts M, et al. Antiviral immune responses: triggers of or triggered by auto-immunity? *Nat Rev Immunol.* 2009. doi:10.1038/nri2527.

Rodriguez Y, Rojas M, Gershwin ME, et al. Tick-borne diseases and autoimmunity: a comprehensive review. *J Autoimm.* 2018;88:21–42.

Rojas M, Restrepo-Jiminez P, Monsalve DM, et al. Molecular mimicry and autoimmunity. *J Autoimm.* 2018;95:100–123.

Theofilopoulos AN, Kono DH, Baccala R. The multiple pathways to autoimmunity. *Nat Immunol.* 2017;18:716–724.

Xia Y, Kellems RE. Receptor-activating autoantibodies and disease: preeclampsia and beyond. *Expert Rev Clin Immunol.* 2011;7:659–674.

Genetic Factors in Autoimmunity

The development of autoimmune disease in animals is influenced by both environmental and genetic factors. The relative contributions of each differ among diseases. It is unusual for autoimmune diseases to result from single gene mutations that result in a loss of both central and peripheral tolerance. Much more commonly, they result from the interactions between multiple genes and the environment. Thus autoimmunity is one consequence of possessing several common risk gene variants. Each has a relatively small effect, and individually, they cannot trigger disease. However, collectively, they may result in significant susceptibility. Several hundred gene loci have been associated with the development of autoimmunity in humans.

Genome-wide association studies (GWAS) and risk-associated single nucleotide polymorphisms (SNPs) have shown that autoimmune diseases generally depend on the inheritance of multiple gene loci encoding low-risk susceptibility alleles. Linkage studies have shown associations between autoimmune diseases and specific genes. However, by far the strongest association is associated with the genes contained within the major histocompatibility complex (MHC).

MHC Genes

As described in Chapter 1, to trigger adaptive immunity antigens must first be processed. They are captured and broken up inside antigen-presenting cells such as dendritic cells. The resulting peptide fragments are then bound to specialized receptors. These antigen-presenting receptors consist of heterodimeric cell-surface glycoproteins encoded by genes clustered within the MHC. These receptors are therefore called MHC molecules. Antigenic peptides can only trigger helper T (Th) cell responses if they are first bound by these MHC molecules and the peptide-MHC complexes are then presented to T cells (Fig. 4.1). If these complexes also bind to T-cell antigen receptors, then the peptides will trigger an immune response. Thus the MHC heterodimers control antigen presentation and immune responsiveness and so determine resistance or susceptibility to infectious and autoimmune diseases. The genes encoding these MHC molecules therefore determine which antigens can or cannot trigger adaptive immunity.

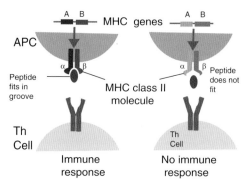

Fig. 4.1   How major histocompatibility complex *(MHC)* genes control immunity. An antigenic peptide can only trigger a helper T-cell *(Th cell)* response if it fits correctly into the binding groove of an MHC class II molecule. *APC,* Antigen-presenting cell.

Each mammalian MHC contains about 200 expressed genes divided into three classes (I, II, and III). The class I genes encode MHC molecules expressed on most nucleated cells. Class I genes can be subdivided into those that are highly polymorphic (class Ia genes) and those that show very little polymorphism (class Ib, Ic, or Id genes). (Polymorphism refers to structural variations between proteins.) As described in Chapter 1, MHC class Ia molecules are antigen-presenting receptors required for cytotoxic T cells to recognize virus-infected cells; therefore, as might be expected, the class Ia genes are often associated with resistance to infectious diseases.

MHC class II genes encode polymorphic antigen-presenting molecules usually restricted to professional antigen-presenting cells (dendritic cells, macrophages, and B cells). MHC class II molecules are required to present processed exogenous antigen fragments to Th cells. They thus determine an animal's ability to respond to any specific epitope. Unsurprisingly, these class II genes are the ones associated with susceptibility or resistance to autoimmune diseases. MHC class III genes encode a mixture of proteins, many of which are important in innate immunity, such as complement components.

Although each MHC contains all three gene classes arranged in distinct regions, their precise gene content and arrangement vary among species. The collective name given to the proteins encoded by MHC genes depends on the species. In humans, they are called human leukocyte antigens (HLA); in dogs, they are called DLA; in cats, FLA; in horses, ELA; and so forth.

MHC CLASS I MOLECULES

The size of the MHC class I region varies among species. Humans and rodents have the largest, and pigs have the smallest. The number of class Ia genes also varies among mammals ranging from more than 60 in rats to 11 in pigs. Not all these genes are functional. The functional polymorphic genes in humans are called *A*, *B*, and *C*. In other mammals, such as dogs, they are usually numbered. Humans, mice, dogs, and cats have relatively few functional MHC class I genes. Thus dogs have only 4 functional class I genes (DLA-88, -12, -64, and -79). Only one of these (DLA-88) is highly polymorphic. Class I genes do not usually play a major role in governing susceptibility or resistance to autoimmune diseases.

MHC CLASS II MOLECULES

Mammals also differ greatly in their expression of MHC class II molecules. In rodents, these molecules are only expressed on the professional antigen-presenting cells such as dendritic cells, macrophages, and B cells. On the other hand, in dogs, cats, and horses, MHC class II molecules are also expressed on nearly all resting adult T cells. The expression of class II molecules is enhanced in rapidly dividing cells and in cells activated by exposure to interferon-gamma (IFNγ).

MHC class II molecules consist of two peptide chains called alpha and beta. The genes for the alpha chains are designated A, and the genes for the beta chains are B. A complete MHC class II region, in theory, contains six genes in three paired loci. For example, in primates, these are called DPA and DPB, DQA and DQB, and DRA and DRB. However, not all mammals possess a complete set of functional genes. For example, dogs lack DPA and DPB.

Canine Class II Genes

Dogs possess four complete and functional class II genes: DRA1, DRB1, DQA1, and DQB1 (Fig. 4.2). They also have two nonfunctional pseudogenes, DRB2 and DQB2. Among the class II genes, DRA1 is unique in that it is monomorphic and thus does not differ between individual dogs. The other three functional class II genes are, however, highly polymorphic, and as a result they collectively encode over 180 different class II alleles and of course many more combinations. For example, DRB1 has at least 100; DQA1 has at least 26, while DQB1 has at least 60 different allelic variants (Box 4.1). Each dog has two sets of these three genes, one set inherited from each parent. The complete set of six alleles found within an individual animal's polymorphic class II MHC is called its MHC haplotype. The antigen-binding site on an MHC molecule is encoded by exon 2, so sequencing of this exon is used to define its MHC haplotype. It has been found that most breeds possess four to five major haplotypes. One is usually at high frequency (50%–70%), with several others ranging from 20% to 1%. Common breeds with large populations are more

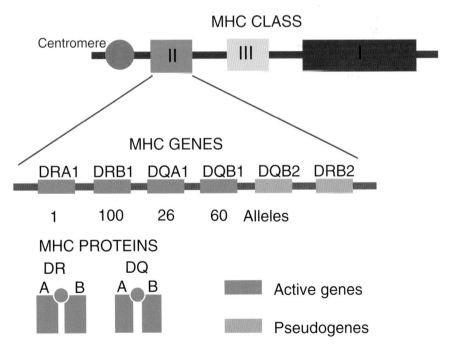

Fig. 4.2 The structure of the canine major histocompatibility complex (MHC) class II region. The number of identified alleles differs greatly between different class II genes. These alleles are classified based on the amino acid sequences lining the antigen-binding grooves in each gene and hence determine which peptides can or cannot bind the groove and trigger an immune response.

BOX 4.1 ■ Rules for Naming Alleles

By international agreement, canine alleles are numbered. They are generally preceded by the name of the specific locus and an asterisk. Five or six digits are used to characterize them. These numbers are based on their amino acid sequences. The first three digits indicate the major type of allele. The fourth and fifth digits indicate the allele subtype; a sixth digit, if necessary, indicates whether the allele is expressed. The designation of the major type of the allele refers to the sequences within the antigen-binding hypervariable regions in exon 2. The subtype designation is based on amino acid differences located within the same exon but located outside the antigen-binding region.

---

diverse and as a result, they tend to have more haplotypes. Conversely, uncommon breeds, especially if they have undergone selective line breeding or gone through recent population bottlenecks, tend to have fewer. There is, however, great interbreed variation. Some haplotypes are ubiquitous and found in many breeds, whereas others are limited to only a few breeds. Some haplotypes may be geographically restricted. Some of these haplotypes are associated with susceptibility or resistance to autoimmune diseases (Table 4.1).

Polymorphism. The variations in amino acid sequence between different MHC alleles are mainly restricted to the deep groove on their surface where antigens bind. For example, MHC class II proteins have an antigen-binding site located between their α_1 and β_1 domains. Its walls are formed by two parallel α-helices, and its floor consists of a β-sheet. Polymorphism results in variations in the amino acids forming the sides of the groove. These variations are generated as a

---

TABLE 4.1 ■ MHC and autoimmunity in dogs: As a species with a remarkably diverse phenotype, dogs have major variations in the amino acids lining the antigen-binding grooves of their major histocompatibility complexes (MHCs). Depending on the population size and breeding history, they have the greatest sequence variation in exon 2 and thus great haplotype variation. Some of these MHC class II haplotypes are associated with susceptibility to immune-mediated disease in dogs, presumably because their amino acid sequence determines whether they can bind to a specific self-antigen. (This data has been derived from multiple sources).

Dog Breed	Disease	Predisposing Haplotypes		
		DRB1	DQA1	DQB1
Collies	Dermatomyositis	00201	00901	00101
Dobermans	Hepatitis	00601	00401	01303
German Shepherds	Superficial keratitis	01501	00601	00301
German Shepherds	Inflammatory bowel disease	01501	00601	00301
Gordon Setters	Systemic lupus erythematosus	01801	00101	00802
Nova Scotia (NS) Tolling Retrievers	Adrenalitis	01502	00601	02301
NS Tolling Retrievers	Rheumatic disease	00601	005011	02001
Pugs	Necrotizing meningoencephalitis	010011	00201	0151
Samoyeds	Diabetes mellitus	015	006	01901
Schnauzers	Thyroiditis	01201	00101	00201
Terrier breeds	Diabetes mellitus	009	001	008
Susceptible breeds	Warm immune-mediated hemolytic anemia (IMHA)	00601	00101	00701
Susceptible breeds	Cold IMHA	01501	00601	00301

(This data has been derived from multiple sources.)

result of mutation and selection. They affect the shape of the antigen-binding site and as a result, determine just which peptides can bind and trigger adaptive immune responses, including auto-immune responses.

MHC CLASS III MOLECULES

The genes within the MHC class III region encode proteins with many diverse functions. Some are important in innate immunity, such as the genes for the complement components C4 and C2. They also include genes that encode tumor necrosis factor-alpha (TNFα), several lympho-toxins, and some natural killer (NK) cell receptors. They do not, in general, appear to be directly associated with susceptibility to autoimmunity.

MHC MOLECULES AND AUTOIMMUNITY

Since the function of MHC molecules is to present antigens to the cells of the immune system, MHC genes regulate immune responses. A peptide that cannot bind to at least one MHC mol-ecule will not trigger an adaptive immune response. Thus possession of specific MHC alleles determines susceptibility to infectious and autoimmune diseases. Because class Ia and class II MHC molecules are structurally diverse, each MHC allele can bind and present a different set of antigenic peptides. The more diversity there is within an animal's MHC, the more antigens it can respond to. Thus an MHC heterozygous animal will express many more alleles and respond to a greater diversity of antigens than a homozygous inbred animal.

The antigen-binding sites of MHC class Ia or II molecules are very nonspecific, and it has been estimated that an average MHC molecule can bind about 2500 different peptides. This is because the MHC groove binds the peptide backbone of the antigenic molecule rather than its amino acid side chains. Nevertheless, structural constraints limit the efficiency of peptide binding to each allele. As a result, it is likely that only one or two peptides from an average antigenic protein can bind to any given MHC molecule. The ability of MHC molecules to bind antigens is therefore a limiting factor in generating adaptive immunity. Increasing the diversity of MHC molecules increases the number of antigens that can be bound and so increases resistance to infectious agents. The number of expressed MHC molecules is, however, constrained because that would also increase the risk that the MHC molecules could bind and present more self-antigens. This would require the elimination of many more self-reactive T cells during the thymic selection process.

When large, outbred populations are examined, no single MHC haplotype predominates. In other words, there is no single MHC haplotype that confers major survival advantages on individual animals. This reflects the futility of the host attempting to recognize all the antigens in a population of invading microorganisms. Microbes can always mutate and evade the immune response faster than mammals can develop resistance. Any changes in an MHC allele may increase resistance to one organism but at the same time might decrease resistance to another. It is more advantageous, therefore, for the members of a population to possess many highly diverse MHC alleles so that any pathogen spreading through a population will have to adapt anew to each individual. Highly adaptable social animals such as dogs, with large populations through which disease can spread rapidly, usually show extensive MHC polymorphism.

Genetic Predisposition to Autoimmunity

Although infectious agents and environmental stimuli may promote autoimmunity, not all affected individuals develop autoimmune disease. This is because genetic factors are key deter-minants of disease susceptibility. GWAS have identified hundreds of loci that encode risk factors for autoimmune diseases. Many of these are shared by multiple diseases and perhaps identify common pathways. It is clear from these studies, however, that the associations so far identified do not account for all genetic effects, and the effect size at any individual locus may be very small. For example, the concordance of autoimmune disease in identical human twins can range from 12% to 67%. This suggests a major role for environmental factors as well as epigenetic events in determining susceptibility.

In mice, at least 25 gene loci that contribute to autoimmunity when deleted or overexpressed have been identified. These include genes that code for cytokines, cytokine receptors, costimulators, molecules that regulate apoptosis, molecules that regulate antigen clearance, and members of cytokine or antigen-signaling cascades. Some diseases result from a defect in a single gene, such as the *lpr* or *gld* mutation. Their gene products play a key role in the destruction of self-reactive T cells. In their absence, excessive T-cell proliferation and autoimmunity result. Other diseases result from inherited complement deficiencies. More commonly, genes influence the severity of disease, and no specific gene is necessary or sufficient for disease expression. Even if an animal has a complete set of susceptibility alleles at multiple loci, the development of overt disease also depends on their genetic and environmental background. This genetic complexity probably also contributes to variations in clinical disease presentation and severity, since these may be determined by different sets of contributing genes. Genetic analysis is also complicated because susceptibility genes may or may not interact with each other. The vulnerability of a target organ or tissue to autoimmune damage may also be genetically determined.

MHC molecules regulate the presentation of processed epitopes. In practice, most MHC alleles have been selected for a strong response to most common infectious pathogens. In contrast, MHC genes' increasing susceptibility to autoimmune diseases in old, postreproductive animals do not offer a selective disadvantage, and MHC-linked predispositions are generally easier to identify. Studies of humans have shown that almost all autoimmune diseases are linked to multiple MHC loci. Presumably, an essential prerequisite for any autoimmune disease is that the autoantigen is appropriately processed and presented on an MHC molecule. Thus the structure of the MHC antigen-binding groove determines whether a specific autoantigen can trigger an immune response. Some MHC alleles appear to protect against autoimmunity, and any predisposition to autoimmunity may be the result of the net effect of both enhancing and protective genes. In addition, most autoimmune diseases are associated with multiple MHC alleles as shown in Table 4.1.

EPIGENETIC MECHANISMS

The development of autoimmunity is also influenced by epigenetic factors (i.e., those factors that regulate gene expression within cells). The most important of these is DNA methylation. The addition of methyl groups to DNA may activate or suppress gene functions and hence either influence autoimmune disease risk or serve as a marker for environmental exposure. Studies on discordant monozygotic twins with type 1 diabetes mellitus (T1DM) or systemic lupus erythematosus (SLE) have found differences in gene methylation patterns between affected and unaffected twins. It is, however, unclear whether these differences are the causes or the results of differences in disease susceptibility.

Epigenetic changes in some genes have been associated with a loss of tolerance. For example, hypermethylation of the insulin gene DNA occurs in T1DM; hypomethylation of peptidylarginine deiminase 2 is recorded in multiple sclerosis, and methylation of the CD40L promoter is seen in primary biliary cirrhosis. Other epigenetic changes include acetylation of histones in SLE and inhibition of histone deacetylases in rheumatoid arthritis, as well as microRNA signaling in many different autoimmune diseases (see Box 3.1). Recent studies suggest that many of these epigenetic changes primarily affect regulatory T (Treg) cells. Autoimmune disease SNPs have been reported to be enriched in CpG-demethylated regions in naïve Treg cells and influence their gene transcription. These epigenetic changes may also explain some of the discordance in autoimmune disease prevalence between identical twins.

BREED PREDISPOSITIONS

While dogs are all descended from wolves, they show quite remarkable variation in size, shape, and colors. Most current dog breeds were created over the past 200 years as a result of aggressive phenotypic selection. In many cases, breeds were developed from a limited number of individuals as a result of aggressive selection for desired characteristics, both structural and behavioral. This selection usually occurred without regard to other genetic characteristics such as disease resistance. This has resulted in inbreeding and a loss of genetic diversity.

Autoimmune diseases are much more common in purebred than in mixed breed dogs. The heritability of some canine autoimmune diseases may be as high as 50%. This lack of genetic diversity has had two effects. First, it has permitted deleterious autosomal recessive genes to be expressed, as is seen in an increased prevalence of immunodeficiency syndromes and other immunologic disorders. Second, it has resulted in a loss of MHC polymorphism. For example, DRB1*04 is found in most Boxers, DRB1*2401 may be restricted to Akitas, DRB1*01 predominates in West Highland White Terriers, and DQA*0203 is restricted to Dobermans. There is a high incidence of DQA*0102 in Irish Wolfhounds and Chows, and DRB1*0101 is common in Irish Setters. This limited haplotype diversity ensures that these breeds will respond to an unusually narrow range of antigens, thus reducing their resistance to infectious agents. It may also increase their susceptibility to immunologic diseases (see Table 4.1).

The three major classes of immune-mediated disease (autoimmunity, immunodeficiency, and atopy) are encountered in some dog breeds more commonly than in others. Old English Sheepdogs are unusually prone to develop autoimmune blood diseases. Certain autoimmune diseases, such as polyarteritis nodosa and hypothyroidism, have familial associations. Many dogs, especially those from rare breeds with small populations, have very restricted MHC polymorphism that increases autoimmune disease susceptibility. These genes may be located in all three MHC regions, but class II genes are by far the most important.

There are several recognized associations between susceptibility to autoimmunity and canine class I MHC alleles. For example, T1DM is associated with possession of DLA-A3, -A7, -A10, and -B4; antinuclear antibody (ANA) production is associated with DLA-A12; SLE is associated with DLA-A7. Possession of an allele of the class I gene DLA-79 (DLA-79*00102) is associated with susceptibility to multiple immune-mediated diseases (hemolytic anemia, thrombocytopenia, polyarthritis, and atopic dermatitis). Canine autoimmune polyarthritis is associated with certain C4 alleles located in the MHC class III region.

Canine diabetes mellitus has features in common with human T1DM. Thus some breeds such as Samoyeds and Cairn Terriers are very susceptible, whereas others such as Boxers, German Shepherd Dogs, and Golden Retrievers are resistant. Several SNPs are also associated with T1DM susceptibility in Miniature Schnauzers, West Highland White Terriers, Border Terriers, and Labradors. Possession of the class II haplotype DQA1*004/DQB1*013 is associated with resistance to canine diabetes. The common alleles found in Samoyeds, Cairn Terriers, and Tibetan Terriers—breeds that are prone to diabetes—are DLA-DRB1*009, DQA1*001, and DQB1*008.

Italian Greyhounds

Italian Greyhounds develop an autoimmune polyendocrine syndrome (see Chapter 6). It is associated with differences in SNPs within the DLA complex. Two specific haplotypes containing DRB1*00203 and DRB1*02901 have been associated with the increased disease risk in some of these dogs.

Nova Scotia Duck Tolling Retrievers

Nova Scotia Duck Tolling Retrievers, a highly inbred breed, have a predisposition to both immune-mediated rheumatic disease (IMRD) and steroid-responsive meningitis-arteritis (SRMA). The rheumatic disease results in a nonerosive polyarthritis, and the dogs also develop ANAs. The inheritance patterns of both the IMRD and the SRMA in this species are complex and involve multiple genes. Their MHC class II locus is also closely associated with the development of SLE-related disease. Thus one MHC haplotype (DLA-DRB1*00601/DQA1*005011/DQB1*02001) is found in increased frequency in ANA-positive IMRD dogs. Only 13 MHC genotypes have been found in the entire tested population, and the genotype homozygous for the abovementioned haplotype was found in 48.5% of IMRD dogs compared to 11.5% of control dogs.

Portuguese Water Spaniels

Primary hypoadrenocorticism (Addison disease) in Portuguese Water Spaniels is significantly affected by these genetic realities. This breed originated with only 31 founders, and 10 animals are responsible for 90% of the current gene pool. The breed-specific disease incidence is 1.5%. They have two disease-associated loci on chromosomes 12 and 27. One locus is within the MHC, whereas the other is associated with cytotoxic T-lymphocyte–associated antigen 4 (CTLA-4) production.

Bearded Collies

Two autoimmune diseases, primary adrenocorticism and symmetric lupoid onychodystrophy, occur in multiple dog breeds, but Bearded Collies have an especially high prevalence of these diseases. Predisposing MHC risk haplotypes that have been identified in this breed include DQA1*00101 in association with DQB1*00201 or in association with DQB1*00802. These risk haplotypes are also associated with the development of diabetes mellitus and hypothyroidism in other breeds.

German Shepherd Dogs

Canine chronic superficial keratitis is an autoimmune disease affecting the eyes of dogs. While it may affect many breeds, it is most prevalent in female German Shepherd Dogs. Investigations have shown that affected dogs frequently possess the MHC class II haplotype DLA-DRB1*01501/DQA1*00601/DQB1*00301. Both overall homozygosity and homozygosity of this haplotype increase the risk of a dog developing keratitis. Homozygosity of this haplotype increases the risk over more than eightfold.

Monogenic Diseases

On occasion, mutations in a specific gene encoding a critical regulatory protein may trigger autoimmune diseases. For example, *AIRE* mutations result in the development of autoimmune polysystemic syndrome-1 in humans. Another example is the autoimmune lymphoproliferative syndrome that develops due to a defect in the gene encoding one form of the TNF receptor. In mice, both *lpr* (lymphoproliferation) and *gld* (generalized lymphoproliferative disease) are loss-of-function mutations in the genes encoding Fas and FasL, respectively. Both mutations block apoptosis, and as a result activated T cells accumulate and accelerate autoimmune diseases (see Chapter 22).

Other important single gene mutations include those affecting the CTLA-4 pathway and so impairing Treg functions. Among the genes that appear to influence canine susceptibility to T1DM are SNPs associated with the promoter of the gene encoding CTLA-4 (see Box 2.2). Another example occurs when mutations in the *NOD2* gene that normally controls the initiation of innate immunity play an important role in the development of inflammatory bowel disease. Other such genes include those encoding the interleukin-23 receptor (*IL23R*), the Treg transcription factor FoxP3 (*FOXP3*), and some complement components (*C1Q* and *C4A*).

Vitamin D deficiency is recognized as a risk factor for many autoimmune diseases in humans, and there is a link between low serum vitamin D levels and autoimmunity. Thus blacks African-Americans have low vitamin D levels and are two to three times more likely to develop SLE than Caucasians. Likewise, multiple sclerosis and inflammatory bowel disease increase in prevalence as one moves away from the equator. Mutations in the genes involved in vitamin D transport and metabolism have been associated with an increased incidence or severity of autoimmune disease. For example, the gene that encodes the vitamin D3 receptor *(VDR)* is expressed on most immune system cells, including neutrophils, macrophages, and T cells. Binding of vitamin D to this receptor on T cells downregulates IFNγ and IL2 expression and promotes Th2 responses. It also promotes Treg cell differentiation in the skin. Binding to the vitamin D receptor on macrophages, in contrast, promotes their activation and the production of cathelicidin and β-defensin-2. The *VDR* gene is overexpressed in joints affected by rheumatoid arthritis. *VDR* gene polymorphisms also appear to influence both T-cell responses and T-cell–dependent inflammatory diseases.

SEX GENES

Sex hormones have significant effects on immune function, and it is unsurprising therefore that they influence the development of autoimmune diseases. This is especially obvious in humans, where SLE and rheumatoid arthritis are especially prevalent in women. Estrogen and prolactin play a role in SLE by promoting B-cell proliferation. Testosterone and other prolactin inhibitors have an opposite effect. Sex hormones can also alter the expression pattern of programmed death 1 (PD-1). Genes on the X chromosomes also play an important role in SLE and autoimmune thyroid disease as exemplified by the Yaa mouse (see Chapter 22).

Studies in mice have also demonstrated that females produce more immunoglobulins, respond more vigorously to vaccines, and generate more autoantibodies, making them more susceptible to autoimmune diseases. Sex hormones also have an effect on expression of the *AIRE* gene. Androgens enhance *AIRE* transcription, whereas estrogens have an opposite effect. As a result, tolerance develops more readily in men, while women are more likely to develop autoimmune diseases. One possible reason for the increased predisposition of females to develop autoimmune diseases may be attributed to the gene encoding the pattern-recognition receptor TLR7. This gene is located on the X chromosome so that females have two copies, while males have only one. SNPs in the *TLR7* gene are closely linked to the development of SLE.

In the field of veterinary medicine, there are four distinct genders: intact and neutered males and intact and spayed females. The relationship between spaying/neutering and the development of autoimmune disease has been investigated in a population of over 90,000 dogs. Compared to intact dogs, spayed/neutered dogs had a significantly greater risk of developing hypoadrenocorticism, hypothyroidism, immune-mediated hemolytic anemia, and thrombocytopenia. Spayed females were at greater risk than neutered males for hypothyroidism and thrombocytopenia. Spayed females also had a greater risk of developing SLE when compared to intact females. There was no significant difference in risk between neutered and intact dogs for immune-mediated polyarthritis, myasthenia gravis, or the pemphigus complex.

Neutering increases the risk of hypoadrenocorticism, autoimmune hemolytic anemia, hypothyroidism, inflammatory bowel disease, and thrombocytopenic purpura in both males and females. In diseases where both males and females were at higher risk, neutered females had up to twice the risk of neutered males. Addison disease was a greater risk for neutered males than for neutered females. Unlike humans, intact female dogs had only a slightly greater risk of developing autoimmune disease than intact dogs. Neutering is associated with increased life expectancy, but neutered/spayed dogs have an increased risk of developing some autoimmune diseases.

Sources of Additional Information

Gershony LC, Belanger JM, Short AD, et al. DLA class II risk haplotypes for autoimmune diseases in the bearded collie offer insight to autoimmunity signatures across dog breeds. *Canine Genet Epidemiol.* 2019. doi:10.1186/s40575-019-0070-7.

Gough A, Thomas A, O'Neill D. *Breed Predispositions to Disease in Dogs and Cats.* 3rd ed. Hoboken, NJ: Wiley Blackwell; 2018.

Gutierrez-Arcelus M, Rich SS, Raychaudhuri S. Autoimmune diseases—connecting risk alleles with molecular traits of the immune system. *Nat Rev Genet.* 2016. doi:10.1038/nrg.2015.33.

Al Holder, Kennedy LJ, Ollier WER, et al. Breed differences in development of anti-insulin antibodies in diabetic dogs and investigation of the role of dog leukocyte antigen (DLA) genes. *Vet Immunol Immunopathol.* 2015;167:130–138.

Inshaw JRJ, Cutler AJ, Burren OS, et al. Approaches and advances in the genetic causes of autoimmune disease and their implications. *Nat Immunol.* 2018;19:674–684.

Jokinen P, Rusanen EM, Kennedy LJ, et al. MHC class II risk haplotype with canine chronic superficial keratitis in German Shepherd dogs. *Vet Immunol Immunopathol.* 2011;140:37–41.

Kennedy LJ, Barnes A, Short A, et al. *Canine DLA diversity: 3. Disease studies. Tissue Antigen.* 2007;69:292–296.

Kennedy LJ, Davison LJ, Barnes A, et al. Identification of susceptibility and protective major histocompatibility complex haplotypes in canine diabetes mellitus. *Tissue Antigen.* 2006;68:467–476.

Marson A, Housley WJ, Hafler DA. Genetic basis of autoimmunity. *J Clin Invest.* 2015;125:2234–2241.

Montgomery TL, Künstner A, Kennedy JJ, et al. Interactions between host genetics and gut microbiota determine susceptibility to CNS autoimmunity. *Proc Natl Acad Sci USA.* 2020. doi:10.1073/pnas.2002817117.

Sundburg CR, et al. Gonadectomy effects on the risk of immune disorders in the dog: a retrospective study. *BMC Vet Res.* 2016;12:278. doi:10.1186/s12917-06-0911-5.

Wilbe M, Jokinen P, Hermanrud C, et al. *Immunogenetics.* 2009;61:557–564.

Wiles BM, Llewellyn AM, Evans KM, et al. Large-scale survey to estimate the prevalence of disorders for 192 Kennel Club registered breeds. *Canine Genet Epidemiol.* 2017. doi:10.1186/s40575-017-0047-3.

Xiang Z, Yang Y, Chang C, et al. The epigenetic mechanism for discordance of autoimmunity in monozygotic twins. *J Autoimm.* 2017;83:43–50.

The Microbiota and Autoimmunity

It is abundantly clear that the prevalence of autoimmune diseases is increasing in the developed world. In searching for reasons for this increase, attention has focused on changes in the composition and behavior of the intestinal microbiota. It is now well accepted that the intestinal, respiratory, and skin microbiota have profound effects on adaptive immunity and the development of autoimmune diseases. This is especially true of those autoimmune diseases that require an innate immune response to trigger their onset.

The microbiota and the animal body have different goals. The microbiota needs to protect itself against destruction caused by the host's innate and adaptive responses. Conversely the host needs to monitor the microbiota and prevent any potential invaders from penetrating the epithelial barriers and causing disease.

Microbial components and metabolites are continually released into the body where they regulate immune cell function. Depletion of the gut microbiome, especially as a result of antibiotic treatment, can significantly affect both innate and adaptive immunity. When the microbiota is disturbed, the immune system is disturbed. If the populations of commensal microorganisms on body surfaces are significantly altered, a process called dysbiosis, this can promote the development of autoimmune and inflammatory diseases. Microbial dysbiosis has been linked to the development of multiple autoimmune diseases such as rheumatoid arthritis (RA), type 1 diabetes mellitus, multiple sclerosis (MS), Crohn disease, and autoimmune liver disease.

The situation is complex, however. Autoimmune responses can be both stimulated and inhibited by the commensal microbiota. In fact, the influence of the microbiota can range from being required for the onset of autoimmunity to having no apparent effect. Some commensals may even protect against autoimmune disease.

The Hygiene Hypothesis

The surfaces of the body are stable, nutrient-rich ecosystems where microbes thrive. Each surface is populated by enormous numbers of commensal bacteria, archea, fungi, and viruses; these are collectively termed the microbiota. Bacteria inhabit the skin, the respiratory tract, parts of the genitourinary tract, and even live within some organs, but the vast majority are found within the gastrointestinal tract. It has been estimated that in an animal body, at least half of all the cells are microbial. As a result of their lifelong, intimate association with body surfaces, the microbiota can be considered an integral part of the body. As such, they influence both innate and adaptive immunity, and conversely they are influenced by signals generated by the immune system. These bacteria not only influence immunity on body surfaces, but they are also integrated into the overall regulation of systemic immune responses. This has given rise to the concept that animals and their microbiota together form superorganisms that share nutrition and exchange energy and metabolites, whose complex interactions are regulated in large part by immune mechanisms (Fig. 5.1). Microbial signals in the form of certain key metabolites are conveyed from the intestine to the thymus and other organs, and as a result they influence the development of the immune system. They do this by influencing the balance between the major helper T cell subsets: Th1, Th2, Th17, and Treg cells.

The hygiene hypothesis at its simplest suggests therefore that the recent increases in the prevalence of allergic and autoimmune diseases are a result of changes in Western lifestyles and diets as well as increased antibiotic usage over the last half-century. Diets rich in meats and processed foods and low in fiber cause changes in the intestinal microbiota. These microbial changes in turn have resulted in an increased prevalence of immune-mediated diseases, including allergies and autoimmunity. It is perhaps relevant to point out here that there is a connection in humans between the occurrence of allergic disease such as atopic dermatitis and the development of autoimmune diseases. This linkage is related not only to diseases of the skin such as dermatitis herpetiformis, alopecia areata, or chronic urticaria, but also to gastrointestinal diseases such as celiac disease, Crohn disease, and ulcerative colitis and to systemic inflammatory diseases such as systemic lupus erythematosus (SLE) and rheumatoid arthritis.

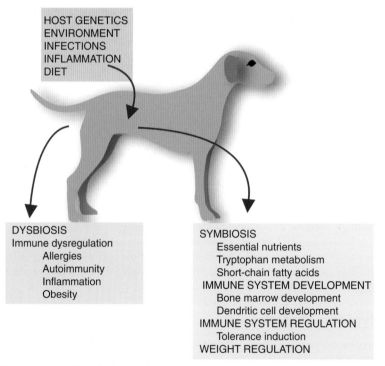

Fig. 5.1   The factors that affect the intestinal microbiota in addition to the many different roles played by the microbiota in maintaining the health of an animal and the consequences of dysbiosis.

The Normal Microbiota

INTESTINAL TRACT

The intestinal microbiota consists of huge numbers of diverse microorganisms. The most obvious of these are trillions of bacteria belonging to hundreds of different species. It has been estimated that the canine small intestine harbors more than 200 different bacterial species, and the canine colon may be home to as many as 1000 species. In dogs and cats these populations are dominated by three phyla, the Firmicutes (~50%), the Actinobacteria (~25%), and the Bacteroidetes (~14%). There are also lesser numbers of Actinobacteria, Spirochaetes, Fusobacteria, Tenericutes, and Verrucomicrobia. The Firmicutes mainly consist of gram-positive bacteria, many of which are spore forming. Important members include the *Clostridia* that may be beneficial or pathogenic (called pathobionts). They also include other pathobionts such as *Streptococci* and *Staphylococci*. The Actinobacteria are gram-positive bacteria with a different nucleotide content than the Firmicutes. The Bacteroidetes are gram-negative bacteria that ferment indigestible plant carbohydrates to produce short-chain fatty acids (SCFAs). The Proteobacteria include gram-negative pathobionts such as *Escherichia coli* and *Klebsiella* (Box 5.1).

Each individual's microbiota is unique. Its composition is determined by diet, antibiotic exposure, genetic factors, and environmental factors. The composition of the microbiota also differs along the gastrointestinal tract under the influence of nutrient availability and local environmental factors such as pH and oxygen tension.

The horse with its enormous cecum and colon requires its microbiota to utilize its cellulose-rich diet. As a result, the horse gut may contain up to 10^{15} bacterial cells. The anterior digestive tract contains many environmental bacteria such as the Proteobacteria consumed with the forage. In the hindgut, the predominant resident bacteria include Firmicutes, Bacteroidetes, and Verrucomicrobia. Firmicutes constitute 40% to 90% of this microbiota and include *Clostridia* and *Bacilli*. The horse cecum also contains a dense population of methanogenic archaea. These organisms are potent sources of SCFAs such as butyrate. As in other species, diets influence the composition of the microbiota, thus a high-starch diet in horses may result in proliferation of lactobacilli resulting in lactic acidosis and the development of laminitis.

Immunosuppression

Given the size, diversity, and importance of the commensal populations on body surfaces, it is in everyone's interests to try to live together in peace. An animal would gain nothing if its immune system were to aggressively attack its microbiota. To ensure that this does

---

BOX 5.1 ■ The Firmicutes/Bacteroidetes (F/B) Ratio

While the role of the intestinal microbiota in controlling immunity appears to be incredibly complex and confusing, one way of obtaining an overview is to determine the relative ratio of the two major phyla that make up 90% of the gut microbiota in humans, the Firmicutes (F) and the Bacteroidetes (B). This F/B ratio appears to be affected by aging and obesity as well as several different inflammatory diseases. For example, obesity has been associated with an increase in Firmicutes and/or a drop in Bacteroidetes. Obesity is also associated with a generalized inflammatory state. The F/B ratio in humans increases steadily from 0.4 in infancy to 10.9 in adulthood. The ratio then decreases from 10.9 in middle age to 0.6 in elderly humans, a feature consistent with the development of chronic inflammation in the elderly (inflammaging). An increased F/B ratio is also associated with the development of systemic lupus erythematosus in humans and the development of inflammatory bowel disease in dogs.

De Luca F, Shoenfeld Y. The microbiome in autoimmune diseases. *Clin Exp Immunol.* 2018;195:74-85.

not happen the microbiota is actively but selectively immunosuppressive. On normal body surfaces it prevents immune attack by promoting immunoregulatory pathways, especially by inducing large numbers of Treg cells. If, however, the composition of the microbiota changes and dysbiosis follows, then Treg numbers may be reduced. The immune system will respond by upregulating its defensive responses. In practical terms, the balance shifts, the immune systems become activated, and as a result allergic, inflammatory, and autoimmune responses may begin to develop.

Evolutionary pressures ensure that the body strikes a balance between protecting itself from invasion and maintaining an environment where beneficial commensal microorganisms can survive and thrive. This mutually advantageous situation needs to be managed by constant cross-talk and negotiations. If the negotiations break down, then confusion and misunderstanding are sure to follow. In effect, the immune system depends on signals from the microbiota to determine its appropriate level of activity. Conversely, immunologic attack on the microbiota increases their expression of stress proteins and suppresses their carbohydrate metabolism while increasing amino acid metabolism. In addition, the immune system produces immunoglobulin A (IgA) that influences the composition of the microbiota.

IMMUNOREGULATION

Bacteria, whether on the skin, respiratory tract, genital tract, or intestine, communicate directly and effectively with their host's immune system. For example, an appropriately balanced microbiota generates antiinflammatory molecules such as SCFAs (Fig. 5.2).

Dietary plant fibers contain complex carbohydrates, especially cellulose. When digested by *Clostridia, Ruminococci,* and *Bacteroides fragilis* in the cecum and colon, these complex carbohydrates are broken down into SCFAs such as formic, butyric, propionic, succinic, and acetic acids. Butyric acid is the most important of these since it has significant antiinflammatory effects. It acts on mast cells to inhibit FceR1 signaling and hence their degranulation. Butyric acid boosts Treg cell numbers and interleukin-10 (IL10) production throughout the body. Likewise, the production of propionate by intestinal bacteria suppresses lung dendritic cell (DC) function, inhibits Th2 responses, and protects from allergic airway disease. As a result, high-fiber diets play a key role in regulating inflammation in the intestine and lung. In carnivores such as dogs and cats,

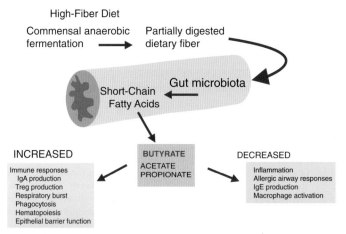

Fig. 5.2 The key roles played by microbial short-chain fatty acids in suppressing both innate and adaptive immune responses. These fatty acids are derived either from a fiber-rich diet, as in herbivores, or from proteins in carnivores. Butyrate appears to be the most important. *Ig,* Immunoglobulin; *Treg,* regulatory T cell.

butyrate is also generated from proteins through the butyrate kinase pathway by organisms such as *Clostridium perfringens* and *Fusobacterium varium*.

Humans that consume large amounts of fiber have a lower prevalence of colitis and inflammatory bowel disease (IBD). Conversely Western diets low in fiber increase pathogen susceptibility in mice and increase the prevalence of allergic disease and autoimmunity in humans. SCFAs are also a source of energy for the epithelial cells in the large intestine. Butyric acid therefore promotes intestinal barrier function by stimulating enterocyte growth and increasing both goblet cell differentiation and mucous production. SCFAs are also important nutrients for other commensal bacteria.

Other groups of intestinal bacteria play important roles in regulating immune responses. One such group are classified as *Clostridia* clusters, which generate SCFAs and so induce Treg cell activity and IL10 production in the gut. The *Clostridia* can also form biofilms over the epithelium and enhance the release of immunosuppressive cytokines such as transforming growth factor-β (TGFβ) from enterocytes. In addition to the *Clostridia*, some subtypes of *B. fragilis* produce large amounts of capsular polysaccharide A, which can convert $CD4^+$ T cells into IL10-producing Tregs. It therefore reduces the production of proinflammatory Th17 cells in diseases such as experimental colitis and experimental autoimmune encephalomyelitis (EAE).

Some commensal bacteria actively suppress intestinal inflammation. For example, Lactobacilli and Bacteroides inhibit the innate signaling pathways triggered by toll-like receptors (TLRs) and other pattern-recognition receptors. A common commensal, *Bacteroides thetaiotaomicron* inhibits NF-κB signaling, while intestinal lactobacilli prevent degradation of the NF-κB inhibitor IκB (see Fig. 2.4).

Intestinal T-Cell Functions

The intestinal tract is home to the largest population of immune cells in the body. These cells play a critical defensive role and guard against microbial invasion from the gut. The intestinal immune system must, however, be relatively unresponsive to the commensal microbiota and ingested food antigens while still being able to respond to invasion by pathogens. It is therefore tightly regulated and selective in the magnitude and nature of its responses. The key to successful accommodation with the intestinal microbiota depends on the body's ability to control immune responses in the gut while at the same time maintaining an effective barrier against invasion. This is achieved by adjusting T-cell populations so that a balance is maintained between each of the proinflammatory helper T-cell types (Th1, Th2, and Th17) and antiinflammatory Treg cells (Table 5.1).

TABLE 5.1 ■ Experimental Animal Models of Autoimmune Disease Shown to Be Directly Affected by the Presence or Absence of the Intestinal Microbiota

Disease Model	Germ-Free Animals	Conventional Animals
NOD diabetic mice	Develop severe disease	Resistant
EAE in mice	Resistant	Susceptible
Dextran sulfate colitis in C3H mice	Develop severe disease	Resistant
TSA-induced mouse colitis	Resistant	Susceptible
IL10-deficiency colitis	Resistant	Susceptible
Experimental autoimmune uveitis	Resistant	Susceptible
Adjuvant-induced experimental autoimmune arthritis	Develop severe disease	Resistant
Arthritic GFK/BxN mice	Resistant	Susceptible

EAE, Experimental autoimmune encephalomyelitis; *IL*, interleukin; *TSA*, trinitrobenzene sulfonic acid.

Intestinal helper T-cell phenotypes are "plastic," and Th0 precursor cells can differentiate into many other types of T cells. This differentiation is regulated by signals from the microbiota. In effect the microbiota manage these T-cell populations to optimize and balance their function (Fig. 5.3). SCFAs produced by the gut microbiota promote the differentiation of naïve T cells into Tregs by suppressing histone deacetylases. As a result, FoxP3 transcription factors are acetylated resulting in Treg activation.

It is possible to derive mice by cesarean section and raise them in a sterile environment. On analysis, these germ-free animals have low levels of Treg and Th17 cells and elevated levels of Th2 cells. This situation can be reversed if the mice are colonized with a normal mouse microbiota within the first 3 weeks of life. Some selected microbial species can also reduce this imbalance although they are generally less effective than a complete, complex, mixed microbiota.

In addition to microbial regulation, helper T-cell differentiation is also regulated by exposure to cytokines and nutrients. For example, the development of both Tregs and Th17 cells is promoted

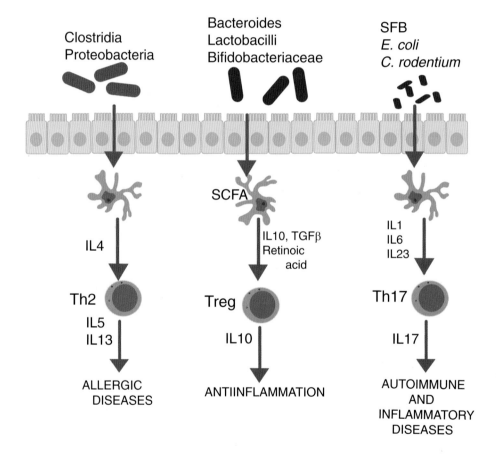

Fig. 5.3 While in general a healthy microbiota is immunosuppressive, not all organisms act in the same way. Different microbial species can influence different forms of T-cell responses. Clearly, when all are growing together within the intestinal tract, the sum of their effects on the immune responses can be complex. Likewise, the loss of some species in dysbiosis will result in significant changes in the levels of immune activity. *IL,* Interleukin; *SCFA,* short-chain fatty acid; *SFB,* segmented filamentous bacteria; *TGFβ,* transforming growth factor-beta; *Th,* helper T cell; *Treg,* regulatory T cell.

by TGFβ. Treg cells require TGFβ plus retinoic acid and IL2, whereas Th17 cells require TGFβ plus IL6 and IL23.

Treg Cells. A healthy microbiota is a powerful promoter of Treg cell function and immune tolerance. Treg populations are maintained by signals from both the microbiota and enterocytes (Fig. 5.4). However, the Treg phenotype is not stable, and cytokines may convert them from one cell type to another simply by turning selected genes on and off. For example, intestinal viral infections may trigger a local interferon (IFN) response. This IFN can turn Treg cells off thus enabling the virus to be attacked and destroyed by a local type 1 immune response. In other infections the Treg cells may be converted to Th2 cells and promote a B-cell switch to IgA production. Indeed about 75% of the IgA directed against the microbiota is produced through a pathway controlled by these Treg cells.

One feature of the Tregs produced under the influence of microbial antigens is their use of a novel transcription factor called RORγt. It appears that one way microbial products regulate the

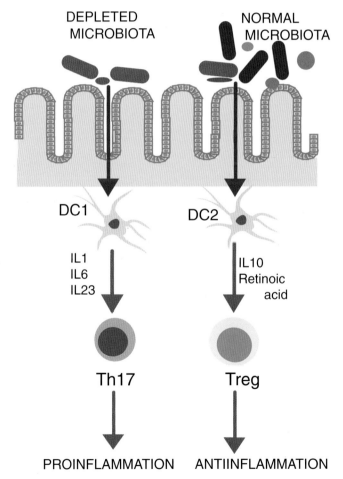

Fig. 5.4 The microbiota and Treg cells. In an animal with a normal, healthy microbiota, Treg production predominates and unwanted inflammation is effectively suppressed. On the other hand, in an animal with a depleted microbiota, Th17 cells may come to predominate and so provoke autoimmunity, allergies, and inflammatory diseases. *DC,* Dendritic cell; *IL,* interleukin; *Th,* helper T cell; *Treg,* regulatory T cell.

Treg/Th17/Th2 balance is by altering RORγt levels. RORγt$^+$ Tregs and Th17 cells are profoundly reduced in germ-free or antibiotic-treated mice so that the mice are significantly skewed toward Th2 responses

Mucosal inflammation is actively suppressed by large numbers of IL10-producing Treg cells. Under stable conditions, the production of Treg cells is favored, while that of effector T cells is suppressed. In the absence of Treg cells, however, uncontrolled effector responses are directed against the antigens of the microbiota and as a result will trigger IBD. IL10-deficient mice develop chronic unremitting colitis driven by IL23 and the Th17 pathway.

Treg cells generated by exposure to bacterial products in the intestine do not only act locally but also emigrate to distant tissues and so determine the body's overall T-cell balance. For example, the presence of *Clostridia* clusters in the colon results in an increase in the numbers of IL10-producing Treg cells in the spleen and lung where they presumably suppress unwanted immune responses. It is clear that excessive immune function and a consequent increase in inflammatory and autoimmune diseases involving the skin and respiratory tract results from a decline in the activities of these systemic Treg cells. This is in large part a result of intestinal dysbiosis.

Th17 Cells. While a healthy microbiota is generally immunosuppressive, its effects may be more complex than simply generating Treg cells. For example, Th17 cells are a subset of CD4$^+$ T cells that promote inflammation, maintain the intestinal epithelial barrier, and mount type 17 responses to defend mucosal surfaces against pathogens. They are abundant in the lamina propria of the intestine. Under the influence of IL23 they produce the proinflammatory cytokines IL17A, IL17F, and IL22. Like Treg cells the development of Th17 cells is regulated by signals from both the microbiota and tissue cytokines. This is especially the case if microbial invasion of the gut wall occurs and triggers inflammation. Thus Treg cells, when acted on by proinflammatory cytokines, can convert to IL17 effectors and so break tolerance. Under these circumstances, the Th17 cells may develop into IFNγ producers that functionally resemble Th1 cells, and it is likely that many intestinal Th1 cells develop through this pathway.

IL17 production is specifically stimulated by the attachment of segmented filamentous bacteria (SFB) to enterocytes. SFB cause enterocytes to produce serum amyloid A (SAA). The SAA acts as a cytokine and stimulates IL23 production by macrophages leading to secretion of IL22 and IL17. These in turn promote the development of Th17 cells. Lamina propria macrophages and DCs can also detect SFB-derived molecules through their TLRs and produce IL23 and TGFβ so promoting further Th17 cell differentiation. Th17 cells in turn regulate the abundance of SFBs by stimulating the production of antibacterial peptides such as β-defensins, lipocalins, and calprotectin by enterocytes.

Excessive Th17 responses have been implicated in many human and animal autoimmune diseases such as RA, encephalomyelitis, and IBD. It is also believed that under some circumstances Th17 cells activated by intestinal infections can enter joints and cause reactive arthritis (see Chapter 17).

THE SKIN MICROBIOTA

The skin harbors a dense and diverse commensal population. Its composition varies across different skin ecosystems as a result of differences in moisture, temperature, and sebum secretion. As in the intestine, it is not in the body's best interests to mount an aggressive attack on the commensals that inhabit healthy skin. Commensal skin bacteria, like their intestinal counterparts, produce SCFAs that act as antiinflammatory agents, thus reducing the skin pH and making the microenvironment less attractive to potential pathogens. Some skin bacteria also induce keratinocytes to secrete antibacterial peptides that influence the composition of the microbiota and enhance resistance to pathogens.

Studies comparing the transcriptome of the skin of germ-free mice with normal mice have found major differences in the genes encoding both innate immunity and antimicrobial proteins. Commensal colonization of hair follicles is needed to recruit Treg cells to the skin, and skin microbial dysbiosis is associated with a loss of Tregs. This may be of relevance to the pathogenesis of the autoimmune skin diseases. For example, lupus patients show consistent reductions in the diversity of their skin microbiota compared to healthy patients.

The microbiota also control the balance between effector and regulatory T cells within the skin. They influence keratinocyte production of IL1 and its effects on epidermal DCs and thus influence local T-cell responses. Some skin bacteria can activate antigen-specific T-cell subsets across intact epithelium. *Staphylococcus epidermidis* is known to stimulate DCs to secrete the immunosuppressive cytokine IL10.

Skin contains the highest concentrations of Treg cells in the body. Most of these cells are localized around hair follicles where the bacterial population tends to be most dense. The presence of Treg cells in neonatal skin mediates tolerance to commensal bacteria at a time when the skin is establishing its microbiota. In human infants but not adults, colonization with *S. epidermidis* results in an influx of activated Treg cells. If this Treg influx is blocked, then tolerance to commensals (and perhaps self-antigens) will not occur. Thus Treg cells play a key role in regulating the skin's response to microorganisms.

DYSBIOSIS

It is important to note that dysbiosis does not necessarily involve the absolute loss of individual bacterial species, although the composition of the microbiota may change, and its diversity may be greatly reduced. Major differences in the intestinal microbiota depend not only on diet but also on the environment in which an animal is raised. These differences influence the expression of their immune system genes. For example, pigs raised in a very clean indoor environment have reduced microbial diversity and express more genes related to inflammation such as those encoding type 1 interferons, major histocompatibility complex (MHC) class I, antibacterial peptides, and chemokines. Conversely, pigs housed in outdoor pens develop a much more diverse microbiota and express more genes linked to T-cell function such as TCR and CD8 as well as the polymeric immunoglobulin receptor pIgR.

Antibiotic treatment is an important cause of dysbiosis. It can radically alter the composition of the intestinal microbiota, increase the risk of developing infections with resistant organisms such as *Clostridioides difficile*, and permit the overgrowth of other pathogens. Antibiotics may alter the composition of the microbiota resulting in an increased risk of obesity. (Obese individuals have more Firmicutes and fewer *Bacteroides* than lean ones.) Antibiotic use in infants may result in a dysbiosis that predisposes to allergic diseases. In many animal models of autoimmunity, antibiotic use predisposes to the development of experimental autoimmune disease. Likewise, with the notable exception of IBD, there is minimal evidence that antibiotic treatment is of benefit in treating autoimmune diseases; however, much remains to be learned about this very complex subject.

The Microbiota and Autoimmunity

As discussed, intestinal dysbiosis influences the development of many different autoimmune diseases such as RA, ankylosing spondylitis, type 1 diabetes mellitus, and experimental autoimmune encephalitis. In some experimental mouse arthritis models, changes in the gut microbiota induced by antibiotic treatment exacerbate the disease. Antinuclear antibody production in mice is also influenced by the microbiota, especially by increased colonization with SFB.

Many intestinal bacteria continuously shed peptidoglycans from their cell walls. These molecules can penetrate the intestinal epithelial barrier and enter the circulation. Peptidoglycans are barely detectable in the serums of germ-free mice indicating that they originate in the microbiota. These bacterial peptidoglycans promote the development of autoimmunity since their neutralization halts the progression of several autoimmune disease models in mice. When peptidoglycan concentrations in the blood were measured in human patients with SLE or RA they were found to be very much higher than those in healthy control patients. Studies were then conducted in mice with experimental collagen-induced arthritis (see Chapter 22). Increasing the serum concentration of the peptidoglycan muramyl-L-alanine-D-isoglutamine (MDP) exacerbated the experimental disease, while treatment with a specific MDP-neutralizing monoclonal antibody reduced its severity. It is known that MDP is recognized by the pattern-recognition receptor NOD2, so it is believed that it influences these autoimmune diseases by promoting NOD2 signaling. The bacterial peptidoglycan appears to act as a natural immune potentiator. In animals in which pattern recognition receptors such as TLRs and NODs are deficient, the defense of the intestine against invading organisms is impaired.

Molecular mimicry also plays an important role in the influence of the microbiota on autoimmune immune responses. This mimicry has long been recognized as critical in some autoimmune syndromes such as Guillain-Barré syndrome, periodic ophthalmia, and rheumatic fever. In addition, computer-based searches have identified epitope mimicry between some conserved bacterial proteins and the Ro autoantigen. Ro is a highly conserved RNA-binding protein found in both commensals and mammals. Lupus patients make high levels of antibodies to Ro. Ro-containing commensals are found in the human skin, oral, and gut microbiota. When these bacteria colonized germ-free lupus-prone mice, the mice developed anti-Ro antibodies. However, while these Ro-positive commensals are common, lupus is rare. It is speculated that some lupus patients may lack central tolerance and rely to a great extent on peripheral tolerance mechanisms. Molecular mimicry may also be the reason why certain gut bacteria can induce antiphospholipid antibodies and trigger a systemic vasculitis (see Chapter 18). Given the enormous diversity of the commensal microbiota, it is highly likely that molecular mimicry is a common factor in the development of many autoimmune diseases.

Unresolved low-grade inflammation underlies the development of many forms of autoimmune disease. This also appears to be associated with changes in the gut microbiota and its metabolites since dysbiosis affects immune function both within the gut and systemically.

Given all this evidence it is clear that recent increases in the prevalence of autoimmune diseases are a consequence of changes in the intestinal microbiota. These in turn are a collective result of dietary changes, a Western lifestyle, and increased use of antibiotics.

RHEUMATOID ARTHRITIS

RA is an inflammatory disease that affects humans and dogs. Its precise etiology remains unclear, but like other such diseases it is probably multifactorial. One feature of the joint inflammation in RA is an excessive Th17 response associated with suppressed Treg activity. The development of RA is influenced by the gut microbiota. The microbiota of RA patients differs significantly from normal healthy individuals. RA patients show decreased gut microbial diversity when compared to controls. For example, the Actinobacteria are decreased, and the Lactobacilli and Prevotella are increased. Periodontal disease caused by *Porphyromonas gingivalis* is also associated with the development of RA. It is still unclear, however, whether these changes in the microbiota are causes or consequences of RA.

Partial depletion of the gut microbiota with Baytril (enrofloxacin) in experimental mice suffering from collagen-induced arthritis results in increased disease severity. Depending on the experimental model and strain of mice used, germ-free mice with experimental adjuvant-induced arthritis may be more (or less) resistant to disease development! Studies following the introduction of different bacterial species into germ-free animals have shown that some species are proarthritogenic, and others are antiarthritogenic. For example, introduction of *Lactobacillus bifidus* into arthritic mice decreased the severity of disease. Likewise, introduction of a single species of SFB into their gut increased Th17 numbers, and arthritis developed rapidly. These discrepancies need to be pursued because it remains unclear whether dysbiosis is a cause or a consequence of RA.

SYSTEMIC LUPUS ERYTHEMATOSUS

SLE is a multisystemic autoimmune and inflammatory disease that affects humans, dogs, cats, and horses. It is clinically diverse, depending on the organ systems involved. It is associated with a loss of control of both T and B cells. Gut microbial dysbiosis with reduced bacterial diversity and changes in community structure have been reported in human patients. This is reflected by a marked change in the ratio of Firmicutes to Bacteroidetes. Lupus patients also have a decrease in Proteobacteria and an increase in Ruminococcaceae. Among the disordered microbiota, *Streptococci*, *Campylobacter*, and *Veillonella* were positively correlated with lupus activity, and *Bifidobacterium* was negatively associated with disease activity. Like other dysbioses, these changes correlate with a reduction in butyrate production and its suppressive effects on Treg cells. Lupus patients also have a lower microbial diversity, both in their intestine and on their skin. Studies on lupus mouse models have suggested that dysbiosis may in fact cause the disease.

SPONDYLOARTHRITIS

The microbiota influences the development of several different immune-mediated arthritic diseases, especially those related to IBD. Ankylosing spondylitis is an autoimmune arthritis of humans that affects the sacroiliac joints, spine, and peripheral joints. Patients also develop acute anterior uveitis (inflammation of the iris and neighboring structures in the eye). More than 95% of humans with ankylosing spondylitis possess the MHC class I allele HLA-B27; in the normal population, the prevalence of this allele is less than 8%. It is suggested that the disease results from molecular mimicry between the hypervariable region of the HLA-B27 molecule and antigens found in *Klebsiella pneumoniae* and related bacteria. *K. pneumoniae* is found more frequently than normal in the intestinal microbiota of patients with active ankylosing spondylitis and uveitis, and patients with active disease have elevated levels of IgA against *Klebsiella* in their sera. Cloning of HLA-B27 into mice and subsequent infection of these animals with *K. pneumoniae* causes an acute spondylitis. HLA-B27–associated ankylosing spondylitis has been described in gorillas. Up to 20% of wild gorillas may have spondylitis, and the disease has also been described in a gibbon, in baboons, and in rhesus macaques.

NEUROLOGIC DISEASE

Gut microorganisms play a role in the human autoimmune disease MS and its mouse experimental counterpart, EAE. It has been calculated that about 30% of the risk of MS is genetic. The remaining 70% is likely due to environmental factors. The gut microbiota is one of the most important of these environmental factors. As with other autoimmune diseases, the microbiota of MS patients differs significantly from that of their normal counterparts. One obvious difference is the loss of SCFA-producing bacteria. It appears that a loss of the suppressive signals from gut microorganisms may permit activation of autoreactive T cells in the small intestine. These can then mount an immune response against myelin oligodendrocyte glycoprotein. Thus mice colonized with intestinal lactobacilli expressing peptides that mimic the myelin glycoprotein develop more severe EAE. It has even proved possible to transfer the intestinal microbiota from MS patients into transgenic mice expressing a myelin-autoantigen–specific T-cell receptor and so induce central nervous system–specific autoimmunity. These affected recipient mice produced significantly less IL10 than control animals.

Studies on EAE in mice elicited by immunization with myelin peptides have revealed the complexity of the links between the microbiota and this disease. Analysis has shown that specific gut bacteria and their SCFA metabolism influence disease severity across multiple mouse genotypes. *Lactobacillus reuteri* has been shown to exacerbate EAE. Conversely, germ-free or antibiotic-treated mice are resistant to the disease, while those with a wild-type microbiota are susceptible. It is also of interest to note that the gut microbiota progressively changes in mice with the experimental disease; thus they lose *Lactobacilli* but gain *Clostridia*.

Meningoencephalomyelitis in dogs has an unknown etiology but is believed to be autoimmune in nature (see Chapter 7). When the fecal microbiota of dogs with this disease is compared to that of normal dogs, it has been found that Prevotellaceae were considerably less abundant in dogs with meningoencephalitis. (A similar finding has been reported for MS in humans.) There was no evidence of any other significant differences in the microbiota between groups. It should be noted, however, that the Prevotellaceae are organisms that produce abundant butyrate under appropriate circumstances and are thus normally immunosuppressive.

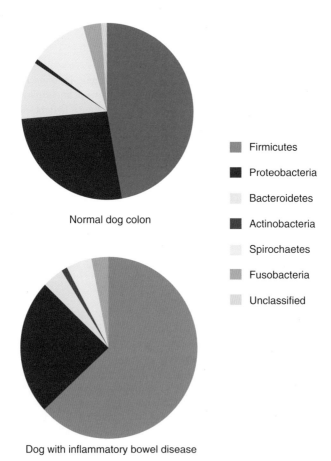

Fig. 5.5   Changes in the composition of the colonic microbiota of dogs with inflammatory bowel disease as compared to the colon of normal dogs. (Courtesy Dr. P. Xenoulis.)

INFLAMMATORY BOWEL DISEASE

Investigations of human IBD have identified many potential pathobionts such as *E. coli, B. fragilis, Campylobacter,* and *Yersinia enterocolitica* in the affected intestine. However, surveys of the complete intestinal microbiota have also revealed a significant dysbiosis. For example, there is a consistent reduction in the diversity of the microbial community. Persons with IBD carry about 25% fewer microbial genes than those with a healthy intestine. There are also major shifts in the abundance of Firmicutes and especially some *Clostridia*. Some species were up 5 to 10 times more abundant in healthy intestines. Other studies have compared the microbiota in different clinical forms of IBD and found not only differences between Crohn disease and ulcerative colitis, but also changes occurring between different locations within the intestine. The most obvious effects of dysbiosis are on IBDs such as Crohn disease and ulcerative colitis in humans. Studies have revealed major changes in the microbiota of these cases, including a loss of beneficial microbes such as *Clostridia* and *B. fragilis*. The loss of these organisms may have a significant effect because they generate SCFAs by the fermentation of dietary fibers. Similar drastic changes have been recorded in dogs with IBD (Fig. 5.5). It is difficult to escape the conclusion that the microbiota plays a major role in suppressing excessive immune functions. In cases of dysbiosis, this immunosuppressive activity is reduced. As a result, autoimmunity and inflammation are prone to develop.

Sources of Additional Information

Bach J-F. The hygiene hypothesis in autoimmunity: the role of pathogens and commensals. *Nat Rev Immunol.* 2017. doi:10.1038/nri.2017.111.

Berer K, Gerdes LA, Cekanaviciute E, et al. Gut microbiota from multiple sclerosis patients enables spontaneous autoimmune encephalomyelitis in mice. *Proc Natl Acad Sci USA.* 2017;114:10719–10724.

Chen B, Sun L, Zhang X. Integration of microbiome and epigenome to decipher the pathogenesis of autoimmune diseases. *J Autoimm.* 2017;83:31–42.

Chervonsky AV. Microbiota and autoimmunity. *Cold Spring Harb Perspect Biol.* 2013;5:a007294.

Forbes JD, Van Domselaar G, Bernstein CN. The gut microbiota in immune-mediated inflammatory diseases. *Front Microbiol.* 2016. doi:10.3389/fmicb.2016.01081.

Huang C, Yi X, Long H, et al. Disordered cutaneous microbiota in systemic lupus erythematosus. *J Autoimm.* 2019. doi:10.1016/j.jaut.2019.102391.

Huang Z, Wang J, Xu X, et al. Antibody neutralization of microbiota-derived circulating peptidoglycan dampens inflammation and ameliorates autoimmunity. *Nat Microbiol.* 2019. doi:10.1038/s41564-019-0381-1.

Jeffrey N, Barker AK, Alcott CJ, et al. The association of specific constituents of the fecal microbiota with immune-mediated brain disease in dogs. *PlosOne.* 2017. doi:10.1371/journal.pone.0170589.

Pilla R, Suchodolski JS. The gut microbiome of dogs and cats and the influence of diet. *Vet Clin Small Anim.* 2021. doi:10.1016/j.cvsm.2021.01.002.

Rogers GB. Germs and joints: the contribution of the human microbiome to rheumatoid arthritis. *Nat Medicine.* 2015;21:839–841.

Ruff WE, Dehner C, Kim WJ, et al. Pathogenic autoreactive T and B cells cross-react with mimotopes expressed by a common human gut commensal to trigger autoimmunity. *Cell Host Microbe.* 2019;26:100–113.

Vieira SM, Hiltensperger M, Kumar V, et al. Translocation of a gut pathobiont drives autoimmunity in mice and humans. *Science.* 2018;359:1156–1161.

Wu H-J, Ivanov II, Darce J, et al. Gut-residing segmented filamentous bacteria drive autoimmune arthritis via helper T17 cells. *Immunity.* 2010. doi:10.1016/j.immuni.2010.06.001.

Xenoulis PG, Palculict B, Allenspach K, et al. Molecular phylogenetic characterization of microbial communities imbalances in the small intestine of dogs with inflammatory bowel disease. *FEMS Microb Ecol.* 2008;66:579–589.

Xu H, Liu M, Cao J, et al. The dynamic interplay between the gut microbiota and autoimmune diseases. *J Immunol Res.* 2019. doi:10.1155/2019/7546047.

Autoimmune Endocrine Diseases

Autoimmune diseases that affect a single organ or tissue presumably result from the development of a rogue clone of B or T cells resulting in an immune response directed against a small number of self-antigens. They do not necessarily reflect complete loss of tolerance in the adaptive immune system. All tissues of the body are potentially susceptible to this form of immunologic attack. Nevertheless, autoimmune diseases directed against endocrine organs, skin, blood, and the nervous system tend to be most common in animals. Their prevalence depends to a great extent on the species and breed of an animal as well as its age.

Among the commonest targets of organ-specific autoimmunity in animals are the endocrine organs. Although companion animals develop autoimmune endocrine diseases, they tend to differ from humans insofar as these are primarily targeted at single organs rather than involving multiple endocrine glands. On occasion, dogs may experience two or more autoimmune endocrine disorders simultaneously (autoimmune polyglandular syndrome), usually affecting both the thyroid and adrenals, but this is uncommon.

Lymphocytic Thyroiditis

Autoimmune thyroid diseases result from the interplay of genetic, environmental, and endogenous factors. The thyroid appears to be especially vulnerable to these diseases. In humans, it is clear that their prevalence has increased significantly over the past 30 years. As a result, a form of lymphocytic thyroiditis called Hashimoto thyroiditis is now one of the most common human autoimmune diseases.

Dogs also suffer from an autoimmune lymphocytic thyroiditis. This is also the most common cause of primary hypothyroidism in dogs. Up to 80% of canine hypothyroid cases are a result of autoimmune attack. The disease has both clinical and histologic similarities to Hashimoto thyroiditis in humans and results from the production of autoantibodies directed against the thyroid hormone thyroglobulin.

In humans, Hashimoto disease is caused by the production of autoantibodies against two autoantigens, thyroglobulin and thyroid peroxidase. Thyroglobulin is a 660-kDa glycoprotein stored within the thyroid follicles that serves as the source of the secreted thyroid hormones. Thyroid peroxidase is a glycoprotein that iodinates tyrosine residues in the thyroglobulin. These are then cleaved by follicular proteases and released as the thyroid hormones triiodothyronine (T3) and thyroxine (T4). Antibodies against thyroglobulin cross-react with T3 and T4. The major autoantigen found in Hashimoto disease in humans is thyroid peroxidase, but antiperoxidase antibodies are only found in about 17% of affected dogs. Antibodies directed against the thyroid-stimulating hormone (TSH) receptor cause hyperthyroidism in humans but have not been reported in dogs. Uncharacterized thyroid microsomal antibodies have been detected in some animals. The antithyroglobulin autoantibodies can bind to thyroid follicular cells and cause their destruction by both complement-mediated lysis and antibody-dependent cellular cytotoxicity.

Some dogs may develop a lymphocytic thyroiditis in the absence of detectable autoantibodies, and it is believed that in these cases, T-cell–mediated cytotoxic responses are responsible for the thyroid destruction. Immunoglobulin G4 (IgG4)–mediated thyroiditis is a variant of autoimmune thyroiditis in humans and may occur in dogs (see Chapter 14).

In humans, there is an association between the development of autoimmune thyroiditis and infection with the bacterium *Helicobacter pylori*. This is believed to result from molecular mimicry since some *H. pylori* epitopes are structurally similar to an ATPase found in the thyroid. In the absence of peripheral tolerance, this antigen may stimulate a helper T type 1 (Th1) response that results in thyroid follicular cell damage. It has also been shown that infection rates with *H. pylori* are higher in patients with autoimmune thyroiditis than in control patients. There is also evidence that hepatitis C virus may contribute to the development of lymphocytic thyroiditis in humans, but the mechanism of this is unclear. It has been suggested that the virus may act by triggering an inflammatory response that suppresses regulatory T (Treg) cell activity.

Thyroid follicular cells that produce thyroglobulin are especially susceptible to autoimmune attack. They secrete cytokines such as interleukin-1 (IL1), IL6, and IL12; growth factors; adhesion molecules; and inflammatory mediators such as nitric oxide and prostaglandins. They can express major histocompatibility complex (MHC) class II molecules and thus act as antigen-presenting cells.

LESIONS

Affected thyroid glands are infiltrated with macrophages, plasma cells, and lymphocytes, and germinal centers may also form (Fig. 6.1). This results in progressive cellular destruction, resulting in reduced size and numbers of thyroid follicles as well as atrophied epithelium. The surviving follicular epithelium may be hypertrophic with granular, brown cytoplasmic pigmentation. Focal accumulations of macrophages, lymphocytes, and plasma cells associate with the remaining follicles. The infiltrating lymphocytes are predominantly CD4$^+$ and CD8$^+$ T cells. Eventually the collapsed follicles are replaced with fibrous connective tissue and scattered clusters of inflammatory cells. Affected thyroids become diffusely atrophic and in severe cases, they may be difficult to find.

GENETICS

Predisposed breeds include Dobermans, Golden Retrievers, Borzois, Giant Schnauzers, Akitas, and Irish Setters. Other affected breeds include English Setters, English Pointers, Skye Terriers, German Wirehaired Pointers, Old English Sheepdogs, Boxers, Maltese Terriers, and Kuvasz.

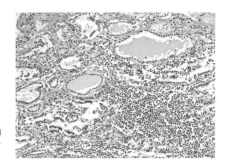

Fig. 6.1 A lymphocytic nodule in the thyroid of a dog suffering from a lymphocytic thyroiditis. Original magnification × 100. (Courtesy of Dr. G. Stoica.)

Females are more likely to develop antithyroid antibodies than males. The disease is less common on outbred mongrels. Relatives of affected animals may have antithyroglobulin antibodies while remaining clinically normal. Dogs from high-risk breeds such as Dobermans tend to develop the disease when young, whereas dogs from low-risk breeds tend to develop it when older.

English Setters and Rhodesian Ridgebacks share a specific dog leukocyte antigen (DLA) class II haplotype containing DLA-DQA1*00101. This doubles the risk of these dogs developing hypothyroidism. Giant Schnauzers with the haplotype DLA-DRB1*01201/DQA1*00101/DQB1*00201 also have an increased risk. The same haplotype has been found in other susceptible breeds, including Dobermans and Labradors; however, it is not found in all susceptible breeds.

The DLA alleles most closely associated with hypothyroidism in English and Gordon Setters are DLA-DQB1*00201 and DQA1*00101. In Gordon Setters, one DLA haplotype (DLA-DRB1*01801/DQA1*00101/DQB1*00802) is associated with protection against hypothyroidism. In a series of 173 hypothyroid dogs, there was also a significant association with possession of the DLA-DQA1*00101 allele. Thus many different genes may play a role in determining canine susceptibility to lymphocytic thyroiditis.

CLINICAL DISEASE

The onset and destructive process of canine lymphocytic thyroiditis is generally slow and insidious. Thyroglobulin autoantibodies usually develop well before the onset of clinical hypothyroidism. As a result, the preclinical period can be very long (i.e., months to years).

Lymphocytic thyroiditis develops in stages. In the first stage, the lymphocytic infiltration within the gland tends to be focal as autoantibodies first appear. When the follicle cell destruction reaches about 60%, the falling T4 level triggers an increased TSH response, but the disease remains subclinical. Only when about 75% of the functional thyroid tissue has been destroyed and T4 production cannot be maintained will clinical signs appear. Finally, when the thyroid atrophies and is replaced by adipose and fibrous tissue, the inflammation subsides as the lymphocytes and antibodies run out of targets.

Affected animals develop the classical clinical signs of hypothyroidism. They gain weight and become lethargic and exercise intolerant. They become obese (even with reduced appetite) and develop a patchy, symmetric bilateral alopecia involving the flanks and tailhead. The alopecia is associated with excessive scaling, slow hair regrowth, and hyperpigmentation. The remaining hair is dry, dull, coarse, and brittle. Other common skin problems include myxedema and pyoderma. Other signs include myopathy, hyperlipidemia, hypothermia, galactorrhea, diarrhea or constipation, and polyneuropathy. Affected dogs may also develop hypercholesterolemia as well as a low-grade normochromic normocytic anemia. Estrus cycles become irregular, and there may be prolonged periods of anestrus. Affected animals become cold intolerant. Hypothyroid dogs have an increased risk of developing thyroid follicular adenocarcinomas.

DIAGNOSIS AND TREATMENT

There is an understandable reluctance to biopsy otherwise healthy dogs to confirm the occurrence of autoimmune thyroiditis. A biopsy will, however, show the characteristic follicular atrophy, lymphocytic infiltration, and secondary fibrosis. As a result, it is more usual to measure the appropriate hormone levels in a serum sample. Seven different assays are normally conducted in a thyroiditis screen. These include assays for autoantibodies against thyroglobulin (TgAA), triiodothyronine (T3AA), thyroxine (T4AA), free and total triiodothyronine (FT3 and TT3), and free and total thyroxine (FT4 and TT4). Most cases of lymphocytic thyroiditis have TgAA in their serum. As many as 35% may also have T3AA, and about 14% have T4AA. These T3 and T4 autoantibodies are directed against epitopes on thyroglobulin and are, in effect, subsets of TgAA. Both T3AA and T4AA can interfere with the measurement of total TT3 and TT4 and must also be assayed to get an accurate result. Some consider serum total T4 as the most reliable single indicator of hypothyroidism. Others believe that free T4 is more reliable. T3 levels may remain within the reference range in up to 15% of hypothyroid animals. These assays for T4 or T3 can only confirm that levels are significantly reduced, thus supporting a diagnosis of hypothyroidism.

Thyroid scintigraphy is a useful diagnostic procedure, but it is expensive and not widely available. A TSH response test is potentially more useful and reliable because it can confirm the inability of the affected thyroid to respond to stimulation. This involves intravenous administration of TSH. Plasma T4 levels are measured immediately before and 6 hours after injection of TSH.

It is important to perform a TgAA assay when screening breeding stock since up to 80% of dogs with low thyroid hormone levels may have TgAA. As pointed out earlier, there is poor correlation between antithyroid antibody titers and disease severity, reflecting the importance of cell-mediated processes in this disease. These antithyroid antibodies are usually detected in serum using an enzyme-linked or chemiluminescent immunosorbent assay (ELISA), immunoblot, or an indirect fluorescent antibody test (see Chapter 20).

Management of affected dogs involves replacement therapy with sodium levothyroxine (synthetic T4). Improvement should be seen within 4 to 6 weeks. There is no cure for this disease, and success depends on effective replacement therapy.

AUTOIMMUNE THYROIDITIS IN CHICKENS

The obese strain (OS) of chickens is characterized by the development of a lymphocytic thyroiditis. Developing chicks become hypothyroid within a few weeks of hatching as a result of mounting a strong autoimmune response against thyroglobulin. These antibodies are synthesized by B cells within the thyroid gland itself. T cells also play a significant role in the pathogenesis of this thyroiditis (see Chapter 22).

HYPERTHYROIDISM

Hyperthyroidism is a disease of old cats. Autoantibodies to thyroid peroxidase have been demonstrated in almost one-third of cases of feline hyperthyroidism, and about 10% of these animals also have circulating antinuclear antibodies. Lymphocytic infiltration of the thyroid is also observed in about one-third of cases. It is believed that these changes are secondary to the disease process and not its primary cause.

Lymphocytic Parathyroiditis

Primary hypoparathyroidism is an uncommon endocrine disorder in dogs and cats. Affected animals usually have a history of abrupt onset neurologic or neuromuscular disease, especially seizures. On investigation, these animals are profoundly hypocalcemic, have mild to

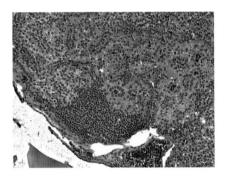

Fig. 6.2 A lymphocytic parathyroiditis in a 14-year-old dog with a parathyroid adenoma. Original magnification × 20. (Courtesy of Dr. G. Dominique Wiener.)

moderate hypophosphatemia, and their serum parathormone levels are severely reduced. One possible cause of this disease is immune-mediated destruction of the glands. In a large study conducted at the University of California–Davis, 18 canine cases were examined. The disease affected mainly middle-aged female animals. Of 12 dogs whose tissues were submitted for histopathology, all 12 had their normal parathyroid tissue replaced by a massive infiltration of lymphocytes and a few plasma cells (Fig. 6.2). There were also a few neutrophils present. Thus it is plausible that these cases are immune mediated. Parathyroid fibrosis is the end result of this autoimmune process. Once hypocalcemic tetany is controlled, these animals may be treated with oral vitamin D and calcium. There has been at least one report on the apparent resolution of a case of primary hypoparathyroidism following immunosuppressive treatment with prednisolone and cyclosporine. Unfortunately, hypocalcemia is a potential complication of steroid therapy in these patients. Antiparathyroid antibodies have been detected in humans with this condition.

Type 1 Diabetes Mellitus

CANINE DIABETES

Canine diabetes mellitus is a relatively common disease. Its prevalence has increased significantly over the past 15 years in the United States. Thus the 2016 State of Pet Health Report noted that in dogs it had climbed from 13.1 cases per 100,000 in 2006 to 23.6 cases per 100,000 in 2015. Certain breeds, especially Samoyeds, Cairn Terriers, and Tibetan Terriers, appear to be very susceptible; other breeds, such as Boxers, are resistant. These breed differences imply a genetic basis for disease development.

In humans, diabetes mellitus is classified according to its pathogenesis. A major distinction is made between type 1 diabetes mellitus (T1DM) and type 2 diabetes mellitus (T2DM). T1DM is an autoimmune disease caused by a permanent insulin deficiency resulting from T-cell–mediated destruction of the beta cells in the pancreatic islets. T2DM, in contrast, usually develops in older adults and is caused by a progressive reduction in islet cell insulin secretion accompanied by reduced insulin sensitivity of target tissues. T2DM is commonly associated with obesity and inactivity and is not considered to be immune mediated. There is a third form of diabetes recognized in adult humans. It resembles T2DM but occurs in individuals who are not overweight and some of whom possess autoantibodies. This form of the disease is called latent autoimmune diabetes of adults. It is of gradual onset as compared to the sudden overwhelming autoimmune response in T1DM patients.

Diabetes mellitus is a spontaneous syndrome in dogs, and most cases have an unknown etiology. It has been classified into insulin-dependent and noninsulin-dependent disease, but its pathogenesis remains unclear. It is probably best classified into insulin-deficiency diabetes where animals produce insufficient insulin and insulin-resistant diabetes where dogs produce sufficient insulin, but this is antagonized by other hormones. Insulin-deficient diabetes is most common. It typically affects dogs between 5 and 12 years of age. The cause of the insulin deficiency is unclear in most cases.

Because diabetic dogs suffer from an insulin deficiency, they require exogenous insulin. In its absence, dogs develop ketoacidosis. In some ways, diabetes in dogs resembles the latent autoimmune disease in adult humans, since it primarily occurs in middle-aged dogs and is of relatively slow onset. Some cases of canine diabetes are secondary to inflammatory disease in the exocrine pancreas or result from immune-mediated destruction.

Immunology

Autoimmune diabetes mellitus appears to be uncommon in dogs. The usual form of canine disease is associated with a decrease in islet numbers, pancreatic islet atrophy, and a loss of beta cells, accompanied by vacuolation and degeneration. In only a small proportion of cases are the islets infiltrated by lymphocytes. Likewise, only a small proportion of canine diabetic cases develop autoantibodies to islet cells, although published numbers have varied greatly.

In those dogs that have both spontaneous diabetes mellitus and autoantibodies, the autoantibodies are directed against the same major islet autoantigens that are found in humans. These are insulin, glutamic acid decarboxylase (GAD), and insulinoma-antigen-2 (IA-2). Some dogs also make autoantibodies to proinsulin. Thus in one survey, 4 of 30 diabetic dogs had anti-GAD reactivity, while 3 had antibodies to IA-2. Two dogs reacted to both antigens. Insulin-specific T cells have been detected in both diabetic and normal dogs. Experimentally, it has been shown that mononuclear cells from some diabetic dogs can suppress insulin production by cultured mouse islet cells in vitro. Additionally, the serum from some diabetic dogs can lyse islet cells in the presence of complement. When diabetic dog serum was tested for antibodies against cultured beta cells by immunofluorescence, 9 of 23 dogs showed strongly positive reactions, and an additional 3 showed weak reactions. Only 1 of 15 normal dog sera gave a positive response in this assay.

Genetics

Human T1DM has a genetic predisposition associated with the MHC, thus 30% of human disease susceptibility is attributed to MHC genes compared to only 9% for loci located elsewhere in the genome. A similar situation occurs in the dog where sequencing of exon 2 has found that certain DLA class II haplotypes are more prevalent in susceptible breeds such as the Samoyed, Tibetan Terrier, and Cairn Terrier; however, these haplotypes are not uncommon in other less susceptible breeds. They include DLA-DRB1*009/DQA1*001/DQB1*008, DLA-DRB1*015/DQA1*006/DQB1*023, and DLA-DRB1*002/DQA1*009/ DQB1*001. One haplotype, DLA-DQA1*004, is underrepresented in diabetic dogs. A DLA class Ia predisposition to neonatal diabetes mellitus has also been observed in Keeshonds, where it appears to be controlled by a single autosomal recessive gene. Boxers, German Shepherd Dogs, and Golden Retrievers rarely get the disease. The DLA-DRB1*009/DQA1*001/DQB1*008 haplotype shows the strongest association with susceptibility but is rare in these resistant breeds. Other single nucleotide polymorphisms that appear to influence susceptibility to canine diabetes include those in the genes encoding the cytotoxic T-lymphocyte–associated antigen 4 (CTLA-4) promoter and in those encoding interferon-gamma, IL12, IL4, tumor necrosis factor-alpha, and IL10. IL4 polymorphisms appear to play a role in the development of diabetes in Collies, Cairn Terriers, and Schnauzers, whereas IL10 appears to play role in Cavalier King Charles Spaniels. Breed-specific associations have also been identified in the canine insulin gene. Polymorphisms in the canine immunoglobulin heavy chain gene cluster have also been determined to influence the development of insulin-deficiency diabetes, possibly by preventing the production of certain variable domains.

Clinical Disease

As with autoimmune thyroiditis, the emergence of autoimmunity and the production of autoantibodies against islet cell antigens long precedes the development of hyperglycemia and clinical disease. Dogs between 5 and 12 years of age classically present with polydipsia, polyphagia, and polyuria as a result of hyperglycemia and glycosuria. Virtually all dogs require lifelong exogenous insulin to manage their hyperglycemia. The loss of beta cells is irreversible. About one-third of diabetic dogs with diabetes may suffer from a concurrent pancreatitis. In such cases, islet destruction is likely secondary to the pancreatitis.

FELINE DIABETES

As in dogs, the prevalence of diabetes mellitus in cats has climbed significantly over the past 15 years. The predominant form of diabetes mellitus in cats is believed to be T2DM. Its occurrence is often associated with inactivity and obesity. T1DM is very rare in cats, and lymphocytic infiltration of the islets has been described in only a few cases. There is a tendency for more lymphocytes to be present in the islets of diabetic cats than in normal cats, but when present, the infiltration is usually mild.

BOVINE DIABETES

Diabetes mellitus has been reported to occur in cattle, pigs, sheep, horses, and bison. It is uncommon in cattle. Animals typically show weight loss, polydipsia, polyuria, poor hair coat, ketonuria, and hyperglycemia. While glycosuria is present, the disease is most commonly diagnosed on necropsy. Affected calves have a lymphocytic pancreatitis and reduced numbers of islets, together with a partial or complete loss of beta cells. Lymphocytes and plasma cells commonly infiltrate the remaining islets; thus their histopathology resembles T1DM and suggests that the disease may be immune mediated. The occurrence of diabetes in calves has been associated with simultaneous infection with bovine viral diarrhea virus (BVDV); however, the correlation is not absolute, although BVDV may serve as a disease trigger in some cases.

EQUINE DIABETES

While horses do develop diabetes mellitus, it most closely resembles T2DM. Thus it is associated with equine metabolic syndrome, and as in humans, it is associated with obesity, a high carbohydrate diet, and lack of exercise. There is no evidence that diabetes mellitus is immune mediated in this species.

Autoimmune Adrenalitis

Naturally occurring primary hypoadrenocorticism (Addison disease) is an uncommon disease in dogs. It results from a lymphocyte-mediated destruction of all the cell layers within the adrenal cortex (Fig. 6.3). As a result, affected dogs suffer from both a mineralocorticoid and a glucocorticoid deficiency. The severity of the disease varies, ranging from very mild and subclinical to a severely affected animal that develops shock. While uncommon in the general dog population, with a prevalence ranging from 0.36% to 0.5%, some breeds are genetically predisposed to autoimmune adrenalitis with frequencies ranging from 1.5% to 9%. Predisposed breeds include Standard Poodles, Bearded Collies, Nova Scotia Duck Tolling Retrievers, Leonbergers, Portuguese Water dogs, Labradoodles, and West Highland White Terriers. Standard Poodles and Bearded Collies may have a disease prevalence of up to 9%. The Standard Poodle disease appears to be caused by a single autosomal recessive trait. The disease in Nova Scotia Duck Tolling Retrievers is associated

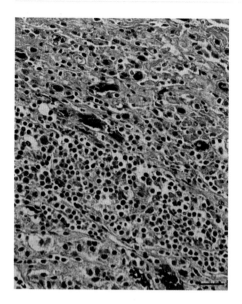

Fig. 6.3 An adrenal gland from a dog with confirmed Addison disease. The adrenal capsule is at the upper right and the medulla at the lower left. The adrenal cortex is devoid of cortical cells and consists of macrophages and numerous lymphocytes in collapsed stroma. H&E stain. Bar = 25 mm. (Frank CB et al. Correlation of inflammation with adrenocortical atrophy in canine adrenalitis. J Comp Pathol. 2013; 149:268-279.)

with possession of one haplotype, DLA-DRB1*01502/DQA*00601/DQB1*02301. In this breed, homozygous dogs develop the disease at a younger age than heterozygous dogs.

The antiadrenal autoantibodies that develop in humans are directed against two autoantigens found in the adrenal cortex: 21-hydroxylase and 17-alpha hydroxylase. 21-hydroxylase is a member of the cytochrome p450 enzyme superfamily. It converts 17-alpha-progesterone and progesterone into 11-deoxycortisol and deoxycorticosterone. 17-alpha hydroxylase is also a key enzyme in the pathway that produces diverse glucocorticoids. Other adrenal enzymes that act as autoantigens have been reported in humans. It is assumed that similar autoantibodies are produced in dogs. These antibodies can be detected and measured by direct immunofluorescent assays in dogs, but their antigenic specificity has yet to be characterized.

Affected dogs develop a lymphoplasmacytic infiltration of the adrenal cortex. This results in severe atrophy of the adrenal cortical layers as a result of progressive immune-mediated destruction. All three layers (zona glomerulosa, zona fasciculata, and zona reticularis) are attacked, so the cortical thickness is reduced to about one-tenth or less of its original size. The animals are functionally deficient in aldosterone and cortisol.

CLINICAL DISEASE

The clinical syndrome only becomes apparent when at least 85% of the adrenocortical tissue is destroyed so that corticosteroid levels drop below functional levels. Initially symptoms may only be apparent in times of stress.

The median age at diagnosis of hypoadrenocorticism is 4 to 5 years with a range from 4 weeks to 16 years of age. It appears to be most prevalent in young female dogs. There are no pathognomonic clinical signs. Affected animals present with many nonspecific signs. Anorexia, lethargy/depression, and vomiting are common. Other signs include weak pulse, bradycardia, abdominal pain, diarrhea, dehydration, weight loss, and hypothermia. As a result of excessive sodium and chloride loss, animals develop hypovolemia and acidosis, leading to circulatory shock, hyponatremia, hyperkalemia, and cardiac arrhythmias. Blood corticosteroid levels are low in these animals. Abdominal sonograms may show atrophic adrenals. In some cases, the disease may be episodic.

DIAGNOSIS AND TREATMENT

Low serum cortisol levels following adrenocorticotropic hormone (ACTH) stimulation can be used as a measure of adrenal cortical function. Affected dogs have low baseline serum cortisol, and they generally respond poorly to ACTH stimulation.

Treatment is lifelong since animals must be supplemented with mineralocorticoids and glucocorticoids as needed. Long-term maintenance therapy involves use of the mineralocorticoid desoxycorticosterone pivalate administered every 25 to 28 days. Electrolytes should be measured to calibrate the optimal dose and duration of action. Some dogs may also require oral glucocorticoid therapy for maintenance.

Autoimmune Hypophysitis

Autoimmune hypophysitis is a rare disease in humans and a very rare disease in dogs. Its defining property is an infiltration of the pituitary gland with lymphocytes. This is usually a diffuse infiltration, but lymphoid follicles have been reported to develop within the gland. The clinical manifestations in humans reflect the functions of the pituitary. Thus patients also suffer from autoimmune thyroiditis, while smaller numbers of cases develop autoimmune polyendocrine syndrome type 2 (APS2), systemic lupus erythematosus, Sjögren syndrome, or T1DM. The only autoantigen identified so far appears to be a 49-kDa cytosolic pituitary protein called alpha-enolase.

Similar cases have been recorded in dogs. Thus one case in a Scottish Terrier presented with a localized pituitary mass. On necropsy, the dog had a lymphoplasmacytic hypophysitis. This animal may have suffered from secondary hypoadrenocorticism. In another canine case, a Great Pyrenees with hypothyroidism and hypoadrenocorticism (APS2) had an enlarged pituitary. It was found to have a lymphocytic hypophysitis that consisted mainly of B cells.

Multifocal lymphocytic hypophysitis has also been reported in horses. One such case occurred in an Appaloosa gelding with clinically diagnosed pituitary pars intermedia dysfunction. The presence of small numbers of scattered lymphocytes appears to be a normal feature of the equine pituitary gland.

Autoimmune Polyendocrine Syndromes

In humans, autoimmune polyendocrine diseases are a diverse and complex mixture of autoimmune endocrinopathies. For example, autoimmune polyendocrine syndrome type 1 (APS1) is an autosomal recessive disease resulting from mutations in the autoimmune regulator gene (*AIRE*) and is discussed in Chapter 2. It has not yet been recorded in domestic animals.

APS2, on the other hand, was first described by Schmidt in 1926 and is sometimes called Schmidt syndrome. It is a combination of any two of three endocrinopathies: hypothyroidism, adrenal insufficiency, and T1DM. It is marked by a lymphocytic infiltration in both the thyroids and adrenals. While rare, it has been reported to occur in dogs. Its pathogenesis generally involves dysfunction of the genes involving key regulatory proteins, especially within the MHC or the major regulatory pathways such as CTLA-4.

Autoimmune polyendocrine syndrome type 3 is a combination of an autoimmune thyroiditis and another organ-specific autoimmune disease such as T1DM, pernicious anemia, vitiligo, and myasthenia gravis. The adrenal is not involved. It typically affects middle-aged women and has yet to be reported in domestic animals.

Studies on animal polyendocrine syndromes suggest that they occur as comorbidities with other endocrine disorders, but these are not necessarily immunologic in origin. Dogs with polyendocrine disease accounted for 0.3% of total canine cases and 2.3% of cases with endocrine disease. Most of these cases occurred in Miniature Schnauzers, but it has also been reported in Dobermans and Boxers. The most common combinations are hypothyroidism plus diabetes mellitus or hypothyroidism plus Addison disease. A concurrent thyroiditis and orchitis has been reported in a Beagle colony.

In one study of 187 dogs with hypoadrenocorticism, 15% had at least one other endocrinopathy. These were, in order, hypothyroidism, T1DM, hypoparathyroidism, and azoospermia. Several dogs had more than two such disorders. In another retrospective study of 38 dogs with polyendocrinopathy, 80% had two conditions and 20% had three. The following combinations occurred (Fig. 6.4): diabetes + Addison disease, 20/35 (57%); Addison disease + hypothyroidism, 8/35 (23%); diabetes + hypothyroidism, 10/35 (29%). These diseases were not usually diagnosed simultaneously, and several months often elapsed between the first and second diagnosis.

Italian Greyhounds appear to suffer from more than their fair share of autoimmune diseases. A syndrome has been described in this breed that resembles APS2 in humans. This is not a random collection of unlinked diseases but a syndrome with a common etiology and diverse clinical manifestations. It involves mainly endocrine tissues such as the adrenals, thyroid, and gonads, as well as the pancreas and skin. It tends to occur in female dogs at midlife (2–15 years). Affected dogs suffer attacks of lupuslike disease, autoimmune hemolytic anemia, thrombocytopenia, hypoadrenocorticism, thyroiditis, masticatory myositis, and pemphigus. Commonly, a sire, dam, or sibling may develop a similar or different autoimmune disease. Two specific MHC haplotypes (DLA-DRB1*00203, DRB1*02901) have been associated with increased risk in about one-third of affected dogs. Some affected dog lines may be very homozygous.

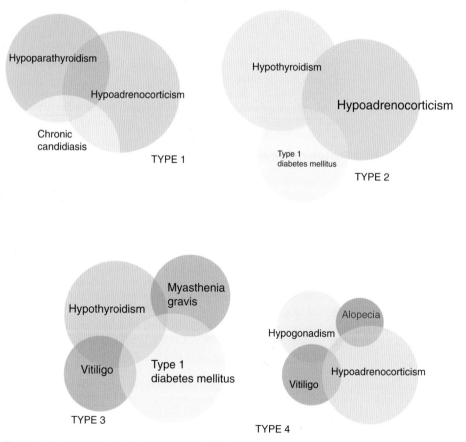

Fig. 6.4 Autoimmune polyendocrine syndromes (APS). APS type 2 has been encountered in dogs. There is no reason why the others might not occur in domestic mammals.

Sources of Additional Information

Diabetes Mellitus

Catchpole B, Adams JP, Holder AL, et al. Genetics of canine diabetes mellitus: are the diabetes suscepti-bility genes identified in humans involved in breed susceptibility to diabetes mellitus in dogs?. *Vet J*. 2013;195:139–147.

Davison LJ, Weenink SM, Christie MR, et al. Autoantibodies to GAD65 and IA-2 in canine diabetes mellitus. *Vet Immunol Immunopathol*. 2008;126:83–90.

McAllister M, Breuninger K, Spofford N, et al. *State of Pet Health Report*. Albany, NY: Connections; 2016:1–21.

Short AD, Catchpole B, Kennedy LJ, et al. T cell cytokine gene polymorphisms in canine diabetes mellitus. *Vet Immunol Immunopathol*. 2009;128:137–146.

Taniyama H, Shirakawa T, Furuoka H, et al. Spontaneous diabetes mellitus in young cattle: histologic, immu-nohistochemical, and electron microscopic studies of the islets of Langerhans. *Vet Pathol*. 1993;30:46–54.

Hypoadrenocorticism

Chase K, Sargan D, Miller K, et al. Understanding the genetics of autoimmune disease: two loci that regulate late onset Addison's disease in Portuguese water dogs. *Int J Immunogenet*. 2006;33:179–184.

Frank CB, Valentin SY, Scott-Moncrieff JCR, et al. Correlation of inflammation with adrenocortical atrophy in canine adrenalitis. *J Comp Path*. 2013;149:268–279.

Klein SC, Peterson ME. Canine adrenocorticism. Pt 1. *Can Vet J*. 2010;51:63–69.

Hypoparathyroidism

Bruyette DS, Feldman EC. Primary hypoparathyroidism in the dog: report of 15 cases and review of 13 previ-ously reported cases. *J Vet Intern Med*. 1988;2:7–14.

Warland J, Skelly B, Knudsen C, et al. Apparent resolution of canine primary hypoparathyroidism with immu-nosuppressive treatment. *J Vet Intern Med*. 2015;29:400–404.

Hypophysitis

Adissu HA, Hamel-Jolette A, Foster RA. Lymphocytic adenohyophysitis and adrenalitis in a dog with adrenal and thyroid atrophy. *Vet Pathol*. 2010;47:1082–1085.

Polledo L, Oliviera M, Adamany J, et al. Hypophysitis, panhypopituitarism and hypothalamitis in a Scottish Terrier dog. *J Vet Intern Med*. 2017;31:1527–1532.

Pancreatitis

Brenner K, Harkin KR, Andrews GA, et al. Juvenile pancreatic atrophy in greyhounds: 12 cases (1995-2000). *J Vet Intern Med*. 2009;23:67–71.

Wiberg ME, Saari SAM, Westermarck E. Exocrine pancreatic atrophy in German Shepherd dogs and rough-coated collies: an end result of lymphocytic pancreatitis. *Vet Pathol*. 1999;36:530–541.

Polyglandular Disease

Blois SL, Dickie E, Kruth SA, et al. Multiple endocrine diseases in dogs: 35 cases (1996-2009). *J Amer Vet Med Assoc*. 2011;12:1616–1621.

Cartwright JA, Stone J, Rick M, et al. Polyglandular endocrinopathy type II (Schmidt's syndrome) in a Doberman pinscher. *J Small Anim Pract*. 2016;57:491–494.

Pedersen NC, Liu H, Greenfield DL, et al. Multiple autoimmune disease syndrome in Italian greyhounds. *Vet Immunol Immunopathol*. 2012;145:264–276.

Thyroiditis

Graham PA, Nachreiner RF, Refsal KR, et al. Lymphocytic thyroiditis. *Vet Clin NA Small Anim*. 2001;31:915–933.

Happ GM. Thyroiditis—a model canine autoimmune disease. *Adv Vet Sci Comp Med*. 1995;39:97–139.

Kennedy LJ, Huson HJ, Leonard J, et al. Association of hypothyroid disease in Doberman pinscher dogs with a rare major histocompatibility complex DLA class II haplotype. *Tissue Antigens*. 2006;67:53–56.

Autoimmune Neurologic Diseases

For many years, it was believed that the brain was uniquely immunologically privileged and that immune and inflammatory responses within the brain were actively suppressed. It was thought that the blood-brain barrier limited the entry of leukocytes into the brain parenchyma. That is no longer considered the case. Apart from astrocytes, leukocytes are largely absent from healthy brain tissue. Nevertheless, antigens in the brain can be captured and processed just as in any other organ. Likewise, potential autoantigens are expressed not only within the brain and central nervous system but also in peripheral nerves. Interactions between the brain and the immune system occur at several sites on the borders of the brain, including the perivascular spaces, the choroid plexus, and in the sinuses of the dura mater. As a result, cell- or antibody-mediated autoimmune attacks do occur and can give rise to many distinct clinical syndromes, depending on the target of the attack.

The two most important neurologic autoimmune diseases in humans are Guillain-Barré syndrome (GBS) and multiple sclerosis (MS). GBS is triggered by infections and tends to be a self-limiting disease. MS is a much more severe and progressive disease. MS is an immune-mediated neurologic disease that has no precise counterpart in domestic animals; however, it has provided the stimulus for extensive animal studies on the nature of autoimmune diseases within the central nervous system.

Peripheral Nervous System

In 1880, the French microbiologist Louis Pasteur began to develop a rabies vaccine. Pasteur sought to attenuate the rabies agent. (He did not know it was a virus!) To make this vaccine, he infected rabbits with rabies and showed that the agent was present in their spinal cords. Once the rabbits developed disease, he removed their spinal cords and air-dried them to attenuate the virus, then injected infected emulsified rabbit spinal cord into recipients. He began by using the driest cords but gave repeated injections of cords dried for progressively shorter periods until the recipient eventually received fresh infected cord material. The method worked, and in July 1885 he used the vaccine to save the life of Joseph Meister, a boy who had been savaged by a rabid dog. However, within 3 years, as Pasteur's vaccination procedure became more widely employed, it was found that some recipients developed a severe and sometimes lethal neuroparalytic disease. It was initially assumed that the attenuated virus was responsible. In 1919, a killed, brain-derived rabies vaccine was introduced, but the complications persisted. It was eventually determined by studies on monkeys that repeated injection of the rabbit spinal cord myelin induced autoantibodies and triggered an immune attack on the patient's own nerves. Further investigations showed that antibodies directed against a protein called myelin basic protein correlated with both central and peripheral neurologic complications. Autoantibodies to myelin cerebrosides and gangliosides also contributed to the pathologic process. As a result, newer myelin-free vaccines were developed.

GUILLAIN-BARRÉ SYNDROME

GBS is a polyneuritis of humans. The most frequent form of the syndrome in Western countries is an acute inflammatory polyneuropathy. Clinically, it presents as a rapid-onset, acute or subacute motor and sensory dysfunction in the limbs, resulting in an ascending muscle weakness and paralysis. It is associated with a mononuclear cell infiltration, demyelination, and an axonopathy of peripheral nerves. The disease may be relapsing-remitting or progressive. The disease is most severe about 8 weeks after onset. As it increases in severity, it may eventually be life threatening as affected individuals develop weakness in their respiratory muscles and require mechanical ventilation. Damage to autonomic nerves may also result in lethal changes in blood pressure and heart rate. Weakness affecting the legs can result in paraplegia and paralysis. GBS also affects sensory nerves and can, as a result, be very painful. The disease is usually treated with immunosuppressive drugs but is often self-limiting. About 5% of GBS patients die as a result of the disease or its complications.

Although the triggering mechanisms of GBS are incompletely understood, the underlying lesion results from a T-cell attack on neuronal myelin sheaths. The attack is specifically directed against gangliosides located on the neuronal surface. It is believed that these antiganglioside antibodies are produced as a result of molecular mimicry. In about two-thirds of individuals, GBS is usually triggered by an infection, a common feature of nervous system autoimmunity. These are often gastrointestinal or respiratory in origin. In about one-third of cases, the disease is triggered by the surface lipooligosaccharide of the enteric pathogen *Campylobacter jejuni*. This molecule structurally mimics the gangliosides of the peripheral nervous system. The prevalence of GBS dropped in New Zealand after major efforts were made to reduce *Campylobacter* transmission from chickens. About 10% of cases are triggered by cytomegalovirus infection. Other cases may be triggered by influenza or SARS (severe acute respiratory syndrome) coronavirus.

Polyneuritis

POLYNEURITIS EQUI

Equine polyneuritis (neuritis of the cauda equina) is an uncommon disease syndrome affecting the cranial, sacral, and coccygeal nerves. Affected horses show hyperesthesia, followed by progressive paralysis of the tail, rectum, and bladder. Loss of sensation in sacral dermatomes may be accompanied by hyperesthesia in the surrounding skin. In about 80% of cases, the disease also affects the cranial nerves. It mainly attacks the vagus nerve and so causes dysphonia. This is also associated with facial and trigeminal paralysis. Although sacral and lumbar involvement is usually bilateral, the cranial nerve involvement is often unilateral. The cranial nerve problems often precede development of the sacral lesions.

Affected nerves are thickened and discolored. Early lesions are characterized by infiltration with lymphocytes, multinucleated giant cells, and plasma cells. The predominant lymphocytes in the infiltrate are CD8+ cytotoxic T cells with some B cells and plasma cells. These are gradually replaced by abundant neutrophils and macrophages. Affected nerves develop demyelination of the sacrococcygeal and lumbosacral nerve roots. Chronic granulomatous inflammation eventually develops in the region of the extradural nerve roots. Perineural fibrosis and perivascular lymphocyte cuffs with hemorrhage are found in the affected nerves (Fig. 7.1). Areas of demyelination and remyelination are present. There is a loss of myelinated axons; in severe cases, the nerve trunks may be almost totally destroyed. Affected horses develop autoantibodies to a peripheral myelin protein called P2.

The etiology of polyneuritis equi is unknown, but like GBS and experimental allergic neuritis (EAN), it is probably triggered by an infection through molecular mimicry. Candidate triggers include *Campylobacter,* equine adenovirus 1, and equine herpesvirus 1. As mentioned earlier, *Campylobacter* infection is regarded as a major contributor to GBS in humans. Another possible contributor is *Sarcocystis neurona.* It is interesting to note that horses diagnosed with equine protozoal myeloencephalitis also make autoantibodies against P2. They appear to share a common antigenic determinant; thus polyneuritis may reflect molecular mimicry between *S. neurona* and myelin.

Clinical Disease

Polyneuritis has been reported in adult horses of many breeds. It presents as a slowly progressive paralysis of the tail, rectum, anus, and bladder. Hindlimb weakness and ataxia develop progressively. This may result in urine scalding, as well as hyperesthesia and hind muscle fasciculations. Muscle atrophy may result, but this is variable. When cranial nerves are involved, the lesions are often asymmetric. It generally affects nerves V, VII, and VIII. This may be reflected in facial muscle paralysis, head tilt, nystagmus, tongue paralysis, and dysphagia.

Diagnosis and Treatment

Diagnosis of polyneuritis is based on clinical signs, history, and exclusion of other possibilities. While affected horses have autoantibodies against P2-myelin protein, this test is not available commercially. Serum chemistry may show evidence of chronic inflammation such as elevated C-reactive protein (CRP) levels. While not specific, these CRP levels may be useful in following

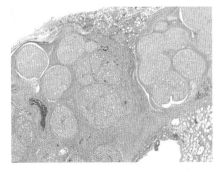

Fig. 7.1 Histologic nerve lesions from a case of polyneuritis equi. Note the massive peri- and intraneuronal mononuclear cell infiltrate. Original magnification × 4. H&E stain. (Courtesy of Dr. Brian Porter.)

the disease course. Cerebrospinal fluid (CSF) analysis may show xanthochromia and elevated protein and cell counts (neutrophil pleocytosis). Definitive diagnosis is based on necropsy findings.

Palliative treatment includes managing the cystitis, urinary and fecal incontinence, and urinary scalding. If the dysphagia is severe, horses may require tube feeding. Because of the severe nerve damage, immunosuppressive or antiinflammatory therapy is rarely successful. The disease is progressive, and the prognosis is poor.

CANINE POLYNEURITIS

Polyneuropathies affecting motor, sensory, or autonomic nerves occur in dogs. There are multiple possible causes of these conditions. They may be secondary, occurring in response to toxins or infectious agents. Possible infectious agents include *Toxoplasma gondii* and *Neospora caninum*. The polyneuritis may also associated with other autoimmune diseases such as systemic lupus erythematosus (SLE) or myasthenia gravis. Many cases appear to be breed related. Many also have an unknown etiology and appear to be immune-mediated primary diseases.

In a study of dogs with polyneuritis conducted in Australia, dogs with polyradiculoneuritis were almost 10 times more likely to carry *Campylobacter* spp. in their feces (48%) compared to 23% in the control group. In addition, there was a significant association between the occurrence of this disease and the consumption of raw chicken (96% of owners with neuritis-affected dogs reported feeding raw chicken compared to 26% of owners of normal dogs). *Campylobacter*, it should be noted, are normal members of the intestinal microbiota in chickens and the leading cause of poultry-associated food poisoning in humans. They are also considered a major trigger of GBS.

A characteristic acute polyradiculoneuritis may develop in dogs 7 to 10 days after fighting with a raccoon. Acute canine polyradiculoneuritis (ACP) or coonhound paralysis affects dogs following a bite or scratch from a raccoon, and it is assumed due to some factor/agent in raccoon saliva. Coonhound paralysis primarily affects ventral nerve roots. There is minimal dorsal root pathology, and the changes in the dorsal roots are invariably milder than in the corresponding ventral roots. Affected ventral root nerves show segmental demyelination and axonal degeneration with macrophage infiltration. Demyelination appears to occur in nerves from which macrophages are absent, suggesting that macrophages do not initiate the demyelination. An acute polyneuritis similar to coonhound paralysis has also been described as developing 1 to 2 weeks following vaccination of dogs with rabies or other vaccines.

The sera of 25 ACP dogs and 15 epileptic control dogs were screened for the presence of autoantibodies to 10 different glycolipids. Immunoglobulin G (IgG) antibodies directed against GM2 gangliosides were detected in 14/25 ACP dogs, and antibodies to GA1 glycoside were detected in a single dog. GM2 is a ganglioside normally located on the abaxial side of Schwann cell membranes, thus ACP appears to share antiganglioside-mediated autoimmunity with GBS. The precise role of raccoons remains unclear. It proved possible to experimentally reproduce the disease by injecting raccoon saliva into a hound that had previously suffered two spontaneous attacks of the disease but had been held in isolation for a year. Polyneuritis also occurs in countries where raccoons are absent, so raccoons are not essential. Interestingly, the form of the disease that occurs in Europe is much milder than that in North America and lasts for only a few weeks.

Clinical Disease

The signs of coonhound paralysis in dogs usually appear suddenly. Animals first show weakness in their hindlimbs. As a result they develop an abnormal gait and tire easily. This progresses to incoordination and ataxia. Motor impairment is much more severe than sensory impairment. It presents as an ascending, symmetric flaccid paralysis. The bitten limb is usually affected first, but the disease is progressive and will worsen for 10 to 12 days following the raccoon bite. Animals cannot stand or lift their heads. In severe cases, the dog may develop flaccid quadriplegia and lose the ability to swallow, bark, or breathe. If autonomic nerves are also affected, then laryngeal or pharyngeal paralysis may result in lethal aspiration pneumonia.

Dogs remain alert and afebrile. Decreased muscle tone is obvious. Electromyographic studies show signs of denervation and decreased conduction velocity in some nerves. Reflexes are decreased or absent. Motor function in the perineal area may be retained and the dog may be able to wag its tail. It is rare for the head muscles to be involved, but some animals show decreased blinking. If the diaphragm is affected, dogs may require mechanical ventilation. If sensory nerves are also affected, animals may exhibit hyperesthesia. Over time, muscle atrophy occurs. The prognosis is good, and most dogs recover in 2 to 3 months, but disabilities may persist for up to 6 months. The disease is, however, self-limiting, and if respiration is not impaired, dogs usually recover completely.

Diagnosis and Treatment

History and clinical signs provide a tentative diagnosis; however, it must be distinguished from botulism. A biopsy of the affected nerve roots may show lymphocytic infiltration (Fig. 7.2). CSF analysis will show evidence of inflammation with increased cellularity and protein levels.

Supportive care is required as the inflammation subsides and nerves begin to heal. Soft bedding and good nutrition are needed. Assistance may be required for defecation and urination. Veterinarians treating canine polyneuritis have traditionally administered corticosteroids, but their effectiveness is unclear and possibly misadvised until its pathogenesis is clarified.

FELINE POLYNEURITIS

Several different polyneuropathies have been described in cats. These are mainly secondary to metabolic diseases and toxins. Cats have also been reported to suffer from a primary neuropathy of presumed immunologic origin. Necropsy in these cases shows a generalized peripheral motor neuropathy. There is a mononuclear cell infiltration of affected nerves. The lesions are restricted to the ventral roots at the spinal cord. The dorsal roots and dorsal ganglia are normal. There is moderate to severe axonal degeneration. Clinically, these diseases resemble GBS.

Clinical Disease

There is no apparent gender predisposition. Affected cats are generally between 3 months and 4 years of age. Some cases may be breed associated, and the disease may present as an acute or chronic disease. The cats present with paresis of the hindlimbs that rapidly develops within 24 to 48 hours into acute tetraparesis and loss of spinal reflexes. Affected cats retain pain perception. The first signs of improvement appear between 7 and 21 days. Cats usually recover completely within 4 to 6 weeks in the absence of treatment and show no residual disabilities. Some, however, may develop severe dyspnea and respiratory complications that require euthanasia.

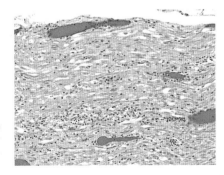

Fig. 7.2 Histologic nerve lesions from a case of canine polyradiculoneuritis. A mild mononuclear cell infiltration is present. Original magnification × 20. H&E stain. (Courtesy of Dr Brian Porter.)

Diagnosis and Treatment

Biopsy and teased nerve fiber preparations show invasive mononuclear cell infiltrates. CSF is unremarkable. Tests for *Toxoplasma,* feline leukemia virus, and feline immunodeficiency virus are negative. Treatment involves appropriate nursing care.

CENTRAL NERVOUS SYSTEM

Meningoencephalitis

Three somewhat similar immune-mediated forms of meningoencephalitis are recognized in dogs. These are necrotizing meningoencephalitis (NME), necrotizing leukoencephalitis (NLE), and granulomatous meningoencephalomyelitis (GME) (Table 7.1). These three diseases are collectively classified as meningoencephalitis of unknown origin (MUO). Collectively, they constitute up to about 25% of canine central nervous system diseases. Antemortem diagnosis of specific MUOs is often difficult and requires several different types of tests, including CSF analysis, imaging, and exclusion of other causes such as infectious diseases. The precise form of the disease may only be established by histopathology. MUO can affect the meninges, the brain, and/or the spinal cord. Each of its subsets has its own distinct lesions, clinical manifestations, and breed predispositions. The clinical signs associated with these diseases are similar and generally reflect the location of the lesions within the central nervous system. In general, as in so many autoimmune diseases, females are overrepresented. Dogs with granulomatous disease tend to be older than dogs with necrotizing lesions.

As in most immune-mediated diseases, the development of MUO is likely a result of many factors, both environmental, and genetic. They all appear to result from T cell dysfunction and the release of a proinflammatory cytokine mixture into brain tissues. They differ primarily in the nature and location of the lesions within the brain. These differences appear to be determined by the different cytokine mixtures produced by T cell subpopulations. In addition, some animals produce autoantibodies whose contribution to the disease process remains quite unclear. As discussed earlier, the presence of autoantibodies in a sick animal does not automatically mean that the disease is of autoimmune origin. Studies on dogs with MUO have demonstrated the presence of autoantibodies in some but not all cases. For example, high-titered autoantibodies in the CSF against astrocytes and the astrocyte protein glial fibrillary acidic protein (GFAP) appear to be a consistent feature of NME and GME, as well as in some cases of dogs with intracranial tumors.

NECROTIZING MENINGOENCEPHALITIS

There are two distinct forms of necrotizing encephalitis recognized in dogs, one in which the lesions are predominantly cortical and meningeal (NME) and the other in which the lesions are located predominantly in the white matter (NLE). While the affected sites are distinctly different, their clinical presentations overlap, and they may be better classified simply as necrotizing encephalitis.

Canine NME has been described in several toy breeds, most notably young female Pugs. Other breeds such as Papillons, Shih Tzu, Cotons de Tuléar, Maltese and Yorkshire Terriers, Pekingese, and Chihuahuas have also been affected. Pugs are highly inbred, with 87% of them being traced to a single ancestor. A study of Pugs indicated that NME had a heritability of between 0.52 and 0.82. Genetic analysis indicates that the disease associates with genes located in the dog leukocyte antigen (DLA) major histocompatibility complex (MHC) class II region on chromosome 12. The most significant linked haplotype is DRB1*010011/DQA1*00201/DQB1*0151. This haplotype is present in 70% of affected dogs versus 25% of clinically normal dogs. Two disease-associated gene regions have also been identified by single nucleotide polymorphism (SNP) analysis on

TABLE 7.1 ■ **Meningoencephalitis of Unknown Origin in Dogs**

Syndrome	Predisposed Breeds	Location of Lesions	Histopathology	Immune Abnormalities
Necrotizing meningoencephalitis	Pugs, Chihuahuas, small terrier breeds	Cortex and meninges of the cerebrum and brainstem	Necrosis, cavitation, liquefaction, demyelination, and perivascular cuffing; infiltration with macrophages, T cells, dendritic cells, neutrophils	Excessive Th1 cell activity; antibodies against glial fibrillary acidic protein
Necrotizing leukoencephalitis	Yorkshire Terriers, French Bulldogs	Periventricular cortical white matter and brainstem	Large areas of necrosis resulting in cavitation	As above
Granulomatous meningoencephalitis	Poodles, Terriers	White matter of the cerebrum, cerebellum, caudal brainstem, and cervical spine; coalescing perivascular lesions are found throughout the central nervous system	Multifocal perivascular granulomas; accumulations of T cells, macrophages, plasma cells, and few neutrophils	Excessive Th17 cell activity
Greyhound encephalitis	Greyhounds	Caudate nucleus, cortical gray matter of the cerebrum the anterior brainstem; milder lesions in caudal brainstem, anterior spinal cord, and cerebellum	Diffuse and focal gliosis and mononuclear cell perivascular cuffing; lymphocytoplasmic meningitis; no demyelination	Unknown
Eosinophilic encephalomyelitis	Young male large-breed dogs	Diffuse meningitis with atrophy of the cortical gray matter; bilateral symmetric lesions in the cortical gray matter	Eosinophils in the lesions and the cerebrospinal fluid; some dogs have a peripheral eosinophilia	Excessive Th2 cell activity

Th, Helper T cell.

chromosomes 4 and 15 in Pugs, Chihuahuas, and Maltese Terriers. One of these genes has been identified as that encoding the interleukin-7 (IL7) receptor.

The characteristic necrotic lesions are multifocal and asymmetric, restricted to the gray and white matter in the cerebrum and brainstem, and are accompanied by a severe meningitis. The foci are characterized by cavitation, necrosis, liquefaction, demyelination, and perivascular cuffing (Fig. 7.3). Macrophages predominate in the lesions, but scattered T cells, dendritic cells, and a few neutrophils are also present. B cells are restricted to the meninges.

Dogs with NME may have autoantibodies to GFAP in their CSF, but their significance is unclear. GFAP is a 52-kDa protein normally found within the cytoplasm and processes of astrocytes. The diagnostic sensitivity of an anti-GFAP assay is 91% and its specificity is 73%, making their detection a useful test. These antibodies are nonspecific, however, since they can also be found in the CSF of dogs with GME, some with brain tumors, and even in some clinically normal dogs. Interestingly, many healthy Pugs and some dogs with NME have high levels of free GFAP in their CSF, suggesting that Pug astrocytes may be fragile and prone to leakage. NME has been reported in a West Highland White Terrier that also suffered from an antiglomerular basement membrane glomerulonephritis, a combination that supports the hypothesis that NME is immune mediated.

As with many putative autoimmune diseases, the gut microbiota (feces) in dogs with MUO has been reported to contain significantly lower numbers of the bacteria Prevotellaceae than that in normal dogs. Attempts to prove a viral etiology have been unsuccessful.

Clinical Disease

NME usually develops in Pugs under 7 years of age, but younger animals are more commonly affected. The average age at death is 16 months. The disease may be acute or chronic. It characteristically presents as lethargy and depression followed by seizures with ataxia, head pressing, circling, blindness, and neck pain. Seizures occur in almost all cases, while cerebellar lesions and brainstem involvement are each present in about half. The acute form is rapidly progressive, and status epilepticus or coma may develop within days or weeks. Dogs affected by the chronic disease develop recurrent seizures and eventually persistent neurologic defects.

Diagnosis and Treatment

Hematology is usually normal in these cases. CSF analysis consistently shows increased protein (>25 mg/dL cisternal) and cell counts (>5 cells/mm^3). These are primarily lymphocytes, and neutrophils are uncommon. Radiography is not diagnostic but may be used to rule out fractures, tumors, or spondylitis. Magnetic resonance imaging (MRI) is often used, and there are many reports in the veterinary literature regarding its findings and interpretation. Likewise, tests should be performed to exclude any potential infectious causes. Definitive diagnosis requires biopsy or necropsy.

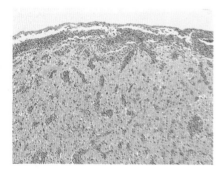

Fig. 7.3 Histopathology of the cerebral cortex in a dog with necrotizing meningoencephalitis. There is a diffuse mononuclear cell infiltration of the leptomeninges with extension into the cortical parenchyma. Original magnification 10 × . H&E stain. (Courtesy of Dr Brian Porter.)

The prognosis is poor for affected animals. Steroid therapy may provide temporary relief, but there is no record of long-term recovery. Most dogs die or are euthanized within 6 months, although some may survive for much longer.

NECROTIZING LEUKOENCEPHALITIS

Some investigators consider NLE to be a variant of NME with a similar pathogenesis. The histologic differences between the two possibly reflect the different genetic background of the affected dogs rather than a different pathogenesis. In contrast to NME, the lesions of NLE spare the cerebrum and meninges and primarily affect the periventricular cortical white matter. Lesions are also found in the brainstem. Areas of necrosis may coalesce to form large areas of cavitation. Neurons in the gray matter appear largely unaffected.

Clinical Disease

NLE has been reported in Yorkshire Terriers and French Bulldogs. It generally develops between 6 months to 10 years of age with a mean age of onset of 4 to 5 years. Clinical signs are similar to NME. These include depression, seizures, circling, ataxia, and blindness, leading to death. The characteristic distribution of the lesions may be observed on imaging. Treatment is the same as NME.

GRANULOMATOUS MENINGOENCEPHALOMYELITIS

The third form of canine MUO is GME. While occurring in many breeds, it appears to be most common in young adult Poodles and Terriers. GME is characterized by the formation of multifocal inflammatory cell granulomas surrounding blood vessels in the cerebellum and brainstem (Fig. 7.4). T cells and macrophages predominate in the lesions, but plasma cells and a few neutrophils may also be present. GME may be disseminated, focal, or ocular.

The disseminated form of GME is most common. In this form, coalescing perivascular lesions are mainly located in the white matter of the cerebrum, cerebellum, caudal brainstem, and cervical spine. The focal form of GME generally consists of a single discrete granuloma usually located in the cerebral white matter, cerebellum, or brainstem. These dogs may, however, also have small, inapparent disseminated lesions. The ocular form presents as sudden blindness resulting from a bilateral optic neuritis.

The etiology of GME is unknown. It is speculated that it may be a virus-mediated disease, but investigations have failed to reveal a specific cause. Its female predisposition suggests an immunologic origin. The lymphocytes found within the granulomas are predominantly T cells. One suggestion is that it is a T-cell–mediated autoimmune disease or at least a consequence of immune

Fig. 7.4 A section of brain from a dog with granulomatous meningoencephalitis. Note the presence of multifocal inflammatory cell accumulations surrounding blood vessels in the brainstem. T cells and macrophages predominate in the lesions, but plasma cells are also present. Original magnification 4 × . H&E stain. (Courtesy of Dr Brian Porter.)

dysregulation. Antiastrocyte antibodies have been detected in the CSF of affected dogs, but as in so many brain diseases, it is unclear whether these are causes or consequences.

Based on immunofluorescence studies, the IL17 in GME appears to be produced by microglia rather than T cells. Its production and that of the chemokine receptor CCR2 are greatly increased in the tissues of GME dogs. In contrast, interferon-gamma (IFNγ) and the chemokine receptor CXCR3 appear to be increased in the brains of dogs with NME. Thus, the differences between these diseases may have their origins in the specific populations of T cells activated: helper T (Th) type 17 cells and macrophages in GME, and Th1 cells in NME.

Clinical Disease

GME is a progressive disease of acute onset. It is most common in dogs between 4 and 8 years of age. It affects both sexes and all breeds, but females and toy and terrier breeds are overrepresented. Dogs with the disseminated disease sometimes deteriorate rapidly and die within a few weeks. Dogs with the focal form decline slowly over a period of many months. Signs include ataxia, nystagmus, seizures, depression, and apparent cervical pain. Some may develop a fever accompanied by systemic signs such as vomiting or diarrhea. Dogs may eventually become paretic. Dogs with optic nerve involvement have dilated and unresponsive pupils, retinal detachment, and secondary glaucoma, optic disk edema, and chorioretinitis.

Diagnosis and Treatment

The CSF may show increased protein, albumin, and a significant mononuclear pleocytosis (Fig. 7.5). The focal and diffuse forms of GME may be recognized on computed tomography (CT) or MRI. Definitive diagnosis requires a biopsy or necropsy with appropriate histopathology. This shows perivascular mononuclear cell infiltrates (macrophages mixed with lymphocytes and plasma cells), accumulating in masses together with local edema and necrosis.

The prognosis of GME is variable, although aggressive treatment with corticosteroids and other immunosuppressive medication may be beneficial. Thus prednisolone and/or cytarabine, mycophenolate, or cyclosporine may stabilize the condition. However, while most patients respond well to therapy, relapses are common, and many affected animals develop disabilities that eventually require euthanasia.

EOSINOPHILIC MENINGOENCEPHALITIS

Another sporadic idiopathic inflammatory disease of the central nervous system that tends to be most common in young male large-breed dogs is an eosinophilic meningitis/encephalitis. Animals develop a diffuse meningitis with atrophy of the cortical gray matter. Bilateral symmetric lesions develop in the cortical gray matter, and affected dogs develop ataxia together with seizures. Eosinophils are found in the lesions and, in the CSF, and some dogs have a peripheral eosinophilia. Eosinophils

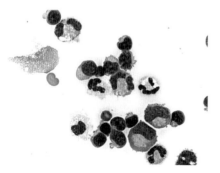

Fig. 7.5 Cerebrospinal fluid from a dog with granulomatous meningoencephalomyelitis. Note the mixed cell pleocytosis, consisting mostly of lymphocytes but with frequent neutrophils and large mononuclear cells that are probably macrophages. (Courtesy of Dr Mark Johnson.)

are normally very rare in the CSF, and their presence may be a response to the presence of migratory parasites such as *Dirofilaria, Toxocara,* or even *Toxoplasma.* Affected animals respond well to immunosuppression.

GREYHOUND MENINGOENCEPHALITIS

An MUO has been reported as occurring in 4- to 18-month-old Greyhounds. Head tilting, recumbency, circling, and blindness are commonly observed. Dehydration and weight loss result. On necropsy, the dogs show both diffuse and focal gliosis and mononuclear cell perivascular cuffing in the caudate nucleus, the cortical gray matter of the cerebrum, and the anterior brainstem. Milder lesions may be found in the caudal brainstem, anterior spinal cord, and cerebellum. They also may have a lymphocytoplasmic meningitis but no demyelination. The cause of this disease is unknown, but its occurrence in a single breed implies a genetic predisposition. Many viruses have been tested for, but none have been detected.

EXPERIMENTAL MODELS

A rat model of experimental autoimmune encephalitis (EAE) resembling MUO (and MS) has been established. In this case, rats were injected with rat cerebral or cerebellar extracts in Freund's complete adjuvant. The animals that received cerebral extracts developed vacuolar and malacic changes in their cortex. The lesions were infiltrated with T cells, and autoantibodies against GFAP were found in their sera. The pathology was consistent with GME. In contrast, rats immunized with the cerebellar extract developed lesions in the cerebellum, brainstem, and spinal cord that resembled typical experimental autoimmune encephalomyelitis in laboratory animals and not the dog diseases.

An experimental model of canine necrotizing encephalitis has been established in the same way. Dogs were immunized with a canine forebrain homogenate emulsified in Freund's complete adjuvant. Seven of 12 injected dogs developed clinical neurologic disease. This included decreased activity, hypothermia, anorexia, paresis, nystagmus, facial palsy, and seizures. On necropsy, inflammatory lesions were found in the white matter, but two dogs also showed cerebral involvement. Most brains had a dense neutrophil infiltration, while one had a lymphocytic infiltration. Their CSF showed elevated proteins and a leukocytosis primarily involving neutrophils and macrophages. The authors suggested that the lesions were comparable to NME and NLE.

STEROID-RESPONSIVE MENINGITIS-ARTERITIS

Steroid-responsive meningitis-arteritis (SRMA) is also known by other names such as necrotizing vasculitis, Beagle pain syndrome, and juvenile polyarteritis syndrome. It is not an encephalitis but has a distinct pathology characterized by inflammation of the cervical leptomeninges and the meningeal arteries (Fig. 7.6). The cause is unknown, and no infectious agents have yet been associated with it.

SRMA is characterized by cervical hyperesthesia, depression, and fever. While the inflammatory lesions primarily affect leptomeningeal arteries, they may also affect vessels in the heart and mediastinum as well as the thyroid. Two clinical forms of SRMA are recognized. In the acute form, affected dogs develop anorexia, fever, stiff gait, lameness, and listlessness, followed by progressive cervical rigidity; hyperesthesia along the vertebral column; generalized cervical or spinal pain; and ataxia. The typical disease course consists of severe episodes with periodic symptom-free remissions. Dogs may assume a hunched posture in an effort to "guard" the head and neck, since they may be in extreme pain. The CSF contains elevated protein as well as many neutrophils and erythrocytes as a result of vascular leakage. Radiographs are normal, but MRI or CT scans

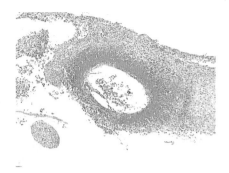

Fig. 7.6 A meningeal artery from a case of steroid-responsive meningitis-arteritis in a dog. Note the fibrinoid degeneration, medial necrosis, and hyalinization of this meningeal artery. Original magnification 10 × . H&E stain. (Courtesy of Dr Brian Porter.)

may show enhancement of the meningeal images. A less-common, chronic form of SRMA may develop following relapses of the acute disease or after inadequate treatment.

On necropsy, the spinal meningeal arteries show fibrinoid degeneration, intimal or medial necrosis, and hyalinization, and are infiltrated with lymphocytes, plasma cells, macrophages, and a few neutrophils. Complete obliteration of the blood vessel lumina may occur. Rupture and thrombosis of inflamed vessels may lead to hemorrhage, compression, and infarction. On histology, there is a severe arteritis and necrosis of meningeal arteries with necrosis of the leptomeninges. There is wallerian degeneration of the white matter in the spinal cord underlying the meningeal lesions. In chronic cases, the CSF contains predominantly mononuclear cells. Meningeal fibrosis may occur secondary to the inflammation and affect blood or CSF flow.

Analysis of the blood mononuclear cells in affected dogs shows reduced expression of the Th1 cytokines, IFNγ, and IL2, and increased expression of the Th2 cytokine IL4. IL6, transforming growth factor-beta (TGFβ), and vascular endothelial growth factor (VEGF) levels are significantly increased in CSF. These changes in IL6 levels promote Th17 cell differentiation. As a result, high levels of IL17 are also found in the CSF. They are especially elevated in dogs with acute disease or in relapse. It is believed therefore that activated Th17 cells are involved both in the production of this IL17 and disruption of the blood-brain barrier. IL17 levels correlate well with the degree of cellular pleocytosis. It should also be noted that Th17 cells mediate neutrophil immigration via IL6; thus these Th17 cells may also be responsible for the cellular infiltrate so characteristic of this disease. The CSF in acute cases of SRMA also contains high IgA and IL8 levels as well as mature neutrophils. Serum IgA, CRP, and alpha-2 macroglobulin are also elevated. About one-third of these dogs have a positive SLE cell test but no detectable antinuclear antibodies. Some autoantibodies have been detected in affected dogs, but these are generally considered a consequence rather than a cause of the inflammatory process (Box 7.1).

In addition to the increased IL17, affected dogs possess high levels of CD40L in their CSF. CD40L is a key stimulant of adaptive immune pathways. It is normally expressed on the surface of activated CD4+ T cells. It is also produced in a soluble form that binds to CD40 on B cells (see Chapter 2).

The cause of SRMA is unknown. Affected animals possess activated T cells suggesting some sort of antigenic trigger. The response is primarily of the Th17 and Th2 types, and this explains the elevated IgA especially in the central nervous system.

Recent studies have found that the normal meninges in mice and humans contain IgA-secreting plasma cells. These cells are located adjacent to venous sinuses. These plasma cells originate within the intestine since prolonged antibiotic treatment of experimental animals results in their depletion in both the intestine and the brain. They play an essential role in blocking microbial invasion from the venous sinuses. (It may be relevant to note here that gut microbiota-specific IgA+ B cells are also present within the brain and CSF in active cases of MS in humans. It appears that they, too, traffic from the intestine to the brain.)

> **BOX 7.1 ■ Th17 Cells, the Microbiome, and Autoimmunity in the Central Nervous System**
>
> Th17 cells producing the cytokines interleukin-17A (IL17A) and IL17F are clearly implicated in the pathogenesis of experimental autoimmune encephalitis (EAE) and multiple sclerosis. They are present in the brain lesions and almost certainly mediate much of the brain damage. Mice that are deficient in IL17A and IL17F are resistant to developing EAE. However, their Th cells still retained the ability to cause encephalitis when passively transferred between animals! These IL17-deficient animals also developed significant changes in their intestinal microbiota. Surprisingly, the IL17-deficient animals could regain their susceptibility to EAE by housing them together with a wild-type mouse population (and hence altering their microbiota) or by introducing IL17 directly into their gut epithelium. Thus it appears that the IL17 is not a direct mediator of encephalitis. It does so indirectly by modulating the gut microbiota. It appears to be the intestinal microbiota that actually determines resistance or susceptibility to autoimmune encephalitis.
>
> ---
>
> *Th,* Helper T cell.
>
> Regen T, Isaac S, Amorim A, et al. IL-17 controls central nervous system autoimmunity through the intestinal microbiome. *Sci Immunol.* 2021;6:eaaz6563.

Clinical Disease

Large dogs such as Boxers, Weimaraners, Nova Scotia Duck Tolling Retrievers, and Bernese Mountain Dogs are commonly affected, although the disease has also been reported in Beagles, Border Collies, Jack Russell Terriers, and Whippets. The disease occurs most commonly in dogs under 18 months of age. Unlike MUO cases, affected animals generally show more systemic signs such as fever and leukocytosis, The acute disease is characterized by fever, stiffness, lethargy, and acute neck pain.

Diagnosis and Treatment

Diagnosis is primarily based on clinical examination, complete hematology, analysis of CSF, and imaging The presence of fever is characteristic. Cervical radiographs must be used to rule out neck injury, fractures, and discospondylitis. SRMA patients characteristically have increased IgA levels in both CSF and blood serum, as well as an acute-phase response as reflected by an elevated CRP. Other immunoglobulins may also be elevated in the CSF. The neutrophils in the CSF may also show pleocytosis.

Treatment of SRMA is based on reducing inflammation through the use of immunosuppressive doses of glucocorticosteroids. The prognosis in young dogs is good, since aggressive antiinflammatory and immunosuppressive therapy leads to rapid clinical improvement. Once the disease is in remission, the steroid dose should be gradually reduced to the minimum necessary to prevent relapses. Treatment may be stopped 6 months after clinical status, CSF, and blood cell counts return to normal, although elevated IgA levels may persist. Given the significant adverse events associated with prolonged high-dose glucocorticoid treatment, a combination of a steroid such as prednisolone given together with azathioprine works well, with a shorter duration of treatment and a corresponding reduction in adverse events. Relapses occur in about one-third of treated dogs, especially in animals that have persistently high CRP levels.

Some dogs with SRMA may also suffer from concurrent immune-mediated polyarthritis. Thus it is not uncommon for dogs with polyarthritis to exhibit signs of spinal pain. This has generally been attributed to spinal arthritis. A survey of 62 cases of dogs with polyarthritis indicated that 18 also exhibited evidence of spinal pain. CSF analysis demonstrated that five of these dogs were suffering from concurrent SRMA.

FELINE MENINGOENCEPHALOMYELITIS

Meningoencephalomyelitis of unknown origin also occurs in cats. In a study of 16 cases, onset ranged from 10 months to 12 years. The median age at onset was 9.4 years. There was no evidence of breed or gender susceptibility. The onset of disease was acute. Clinical signs included ataxia, proprioceptive defects, seizures, and spinal hyperesthesia. Affected cats also showed fever, weight loss, anorexia, and leukocytosis. The CSF cell count was increased (median 70.7 cells/µL) with mixed pleocytosis. The CSF protein concentration was also increased in almost all affected cats. MRI showed infiltrative, ill-defined lesions throughout the brain. Histopathology showed a multifocal lymphohistiocytic meningoencephalitis or in one case, a myelitis. There was focal neural necrosis as well as mononuclear perivascular cuffing. The most obvious infectious agents were excluded, so it is assumed to be of immune origin. Treatment with glucocorticoids such as dexamethasone or prednisolone resulted in a good recovery rate.

FELINE LIMBIC ENCEPHALITIS

Limbic encephalitis associated with the production of autoantibodies against voltage-gated potassium channel complexes (VGKC) has been recognized in both humans and cats. These autoantibodies are directed against two components of the complexes, leucine-rich glioma inactivated-1 (LGI-1) and contactin-associated protein-like 2 (CASPR2). Histopathology shows degeneration and inflammation located primarily in the hippocampus. The feline lesions closely resemble those observed in humans. Serum from cats suffering from acute disease was investigated for the presence of autoantibodies to VGKC. Of the affected cats, 5/14 but none of 19 control animals had detectable antibodies to VGKC. Four also had antibodies directed against LGI-1. It is believed that both the human and feline diseases are autoimmune in nature.

Clinical Disease

Limbic encephalitis is of acute onset and presents with both confusion and cluster seizures involving the facial muscles. MRI often shows high signal intensity in the region of the hippocampus. Clinically, the cats present with distinctive complex partial cluster seizures that consist of facial twitching, salivation, motionless staring, lip smacking, chewing, swallowing, mydriasis, and vocalization. These episodes are short lived, lasting for only a few seconds to 1 minute. They may be followed by behavioral changes, including fear and aggression. Affected cats often respond poorly to antiepileptic drugs but may respond well to immunosuppression.

Other Neurologic Diseases
CEREBELLAR DEGENERATION

Cerebellar degeneration has been observed in Coton de Tuléar puppies between 12 and 14 weeks of age. On necropsy, their cerebellum is shrunken, and histopathology reveals a loss of cerebellar granular cells. Marked gliosis and occasional inflammatory foci are present. The affected tissue is, however, diffusely infiltrated with T cells. Microglial cells are also present in the lesions, but B cells are absent. There is T-cell–mediated destruction of the granular cell layer and microglial cell activation. Cotons de Tulear are highly inbred, so it is assumed that the disease is primarily genetic in origin. The condition closely resembled human T-cell–mediated paraneoplastic cerebellar degeneration. Immune-mediated cerebellar ataxias in humans are often associated with the presence of extraneural tumors.

NARCOLEPSY

Narcolepsy is a disabling sleep disorder that affects both humans and dogs. It is characterized by sudden-onset daytime sleepiness, often accompanied by sleep paralysis and a loss of muscle tone in response to emotional stimulation (cataplexy). Victims, both human and canine, suddenly fall into rapid eye movement sleep. Recent studies in humans have confirmed that sporadic narcolepsy is an autoimmune disease. In these cases, cytotoxic CD8+ T cells target and kill hypocretin-secreting neurons. Hypocretins are sleep-modulating neurotransmitters that regulate sleep-wake cycles. The T cells specifically target antigens presented by the disease-associated MHC allele HLA-DQB1*0602.

In dogs, two distinct forms of narcolepsy are seen. One form is inherited as a result of a mutation in the gene encoding hypocretin receptor 2. The second form results from an induced hypocretin deficiency. Thus in Dobermans with the inherited form of the disease, the hypocretin neurons and their contents appeared normal. On the other hand, in dogs with the sporadic form of the disease, hypocretin was undetectable in their CSF. Narcolepsy has also been reported in a dog with a brainstem MUO. While autoimmunity has not yet been demonstrated in narcoleptic dogs, it may be that affected dogs would benefit from immunosuppressive therapy.

EXPERIMENTAL AUTOIMMUNE ENCEPHALITIS AND MULTIPLE SCLEROSIS

No discussion on autoimmune neurologic disease would be complete without briefly mentioning EAE and MS. MS is an autoimmune disease of humans. The autoimmune response targets neurons, myelin sheaths, and astrocytes within the brain. This results in demyelination, a loss of neurons, and significant impairment to the sensory, motor, visual, and autonomic nervous systems. MS is a progressive disease. It generally starts as a relapsing-remitting disease but may eventually shift to a secondary progressive form. Some cases may be progressive from the onset. As it progresses, disabilities accumulate. This progression may be accompanied by dysbiosis of the intestinal microbiota.

The etiology of MS is complex and not yet fully understood. As a result, there has been extensive reliance on the use of animal models. The most common of these models is EAE, which like its peripheral counterpart EAN can be induced by immunizing animals with brain tissue or neural peptides (see Chapter 22). Encephalitogenic peptides such as proteolipid protein, spinal cord homogenate, myelin basic protein, or oligodendrocyte proteins are emulsified in Freund's complete adjuvant and used to immunize the animals. In response, the animal generates cytotoxic T cells that can cross the blood-brain barrier. Within the central nervous system, these cells recruit dendritic cells and macrophages that generate proinflammatory cytokines and reactive oxygen species, and activate complement. These in turn damage and destroy the myelin sheaths, resulting in progressive clinical disease. In some patients, B cells also participate in this process.

Studies using EAE have identified many important factors that contribute to the complex MS syndrome, including the gut microbiota, age, genetic background, and gender. They have also provided the starting points for some successful drug treatments of MS. As pointed out earlier, human MS patients may share similar genetic alterations with Pugs with meningoencephalitis.

It has been suggested that postdistemper demyelinating leukoencephalopathy in dogs may also be of autoimmune origin. Up to 97% of spontaneous canine cases develop autoantibodies against central nervous system myelin. However, the presence of these autoantibodies or T-cell responses does not correlate with the course of the disease. Likewise, the lesions that develop in dogs with EAE are distinctly different from those with distemper-mediated demyelination. Thus the myelin loss in dogs with distemper is focal and periventricular, whereas the lesions of canine EAE are disseminated and perivascular. It is unlikely that autoimmunity contributes significantly to the pathogenesis of distemper demyelinating encephalomyelitis. The production of antimyelin antibodies appears to be common response to central nervous tissue damage, regardless of its cause.

BOX 7.2 ■ Sydenham Chorea and Pediatric Acute-Onset Neuropsychiatric Syndrome

Following a group A streptococcal infection, some children develop rheumatic fever. This is an autoimmune inflammatory disease that affects the heart, joints, skin, and brain in susceptible individuals. The disease generally develops as a result of the development of cross-reactive antibodies (molecular mimicry) between the streptococcal group A carbohydrate antigen and host antigens. About 25% of rheumatic fever victims may develop neurologic disease. In the brain, these antibodies can bind to neuronal cell surface glycolytic enzymes, lysogangliosides, and type 2 dopamine receptors as well as intracellular antigens such as tubulin. They alter signal transduction in the brain, so causing Sydenham chorea (historically called St. Vitus dance). This disease presents as rapid involuntary movements affecting the feet, hands, and face. Most children recover within 2 to 6 months.

A subgroup of children exposed to group A streptococci may develop pediatric acute-onset neuropsychiatric syndrome (PANS). These children develop acute-onset neuropsychiatric disturbances such as obsessive-compulsive disorder, eating disorders, polyuria, sleep issues, and motor abnormalities. This may become a relapsing-remitting disorder or a chronic condition. A subset of PANS patients develop pediatric autoimmune neuropsychiatric disorders (PANDAS) within 2 to 3 days of group A streptococcal infections such as strep throat or scarlet fever. The autoantibodies in PANDAS cases react against tubulin, lysoganglioside Gm1, and dopamine receptors D1 and D2 in the basal ganglia. It should be pointed out, however, that the existence of PANS/PANDAS is controversial.

Ben-Pazi H, Stoner JA, Cunningham MW. Dopamine receptor autoantibodies correlate with symptoms in Sydenham's chorea. *PlosOne.* 2013. doi:10.1371/journal.pone.0073516; Chang K, Frankovich J, Cooperstock M, et al. Clinical evaluation of youth with pediatric acute-onset neuropsychiatric syndrome recommendations from the 2013 PANS consensus conference. *J Child Adolesc Psychopharm.* 2015;25:3-13.

Recent studies have begun to clarify the precise pathogenesis of MS. For example, over 99% of MS patients have antibodies against the human herpesvirus – Epstein-Barr virus (EBV). It also appears that there is molecular mimicry between EBV and certain key antigens in the brain. An EBV transcription factor closely resembles human glial cell adhesion protein, GlialCAM. MS patients therefore make autoantibodies against GlialCAM on microglia and so trigger demyelination.

Sources of Additional Information

Polyneuritis Equi

Aleman M, Katzman SA, Vaughan B, et al. Antemortem diagnosis of polyneuritis equi. *J Vet Intern Med.* 2009;23:665–668.

Canine Polyneuritis

Cummings JF, de Lahunta A, Holmes DF, et al. Coonhound paralysis: further clinical studies and electron microscopic observations. *Acta Neuropathol.* 1982;56:167–178.

Martinez-Anton L, Marenda M, Firestone SM, et al. Investigation of the role of Campylobacter infection in suspected acute polyradiculoneuritis in dogs. *J Vet Intern Med.* 2018;32:352–360.

Vitale S, Foss K. Immune-mediated central nervous system disease—current knowledge and recommendations. *Topics Comp Anim Med.* 2019;34:22–29.

Feline Polyneuritis

Chrisman CL. Polyneuropathies of cats. *J Small Anim Pract.* 2000;41:384–389.

Steroid-Responsive Meningitis-Arteritis

Freundt-Revilla J, Maiolini A, Carlson R, et al. Th17-skewed immune response and cluster of differentiation 40 ligand expression in canine steroid-responsive meningitis-arteritis, a large animal model of neutrophilic meningitis. *J Neuroinflamm.* 2017. doi:10.1186/s12974-016-0784-3.

Moore SA, Kim MY, Maiolini A, et al. Extracellular hsp70 release in canine steroid responsive meningitis arteritis. *Vet Immunol Immunopathol*. 2012;145:129–133.

Stafford EG, Kortum A, Castel A, et al. Presence of cerebrospinal fluid antibodies associated with autoimmune encephalitis of humans in dogs with neurologic disease. *J Vet Intern Med*. 2019;33:2175–2182.

Necrotizing Meningoencephalitis

Greer KA, Schatzberg SJ, Porter BF, et al. Heritability and transmission analysis of necrotizing meningoencephalitis in the pug. *Res Vet Sci*. 2009;86:438–442.

Multiple Sclerosis

Lanz TV, Brewer RC, Ho PP, Moon J-S, et al. Clonally expanded B cells in multiple sclerosis bind EBV EBNA1 and GlialCAM. *Nature*. 2022. doi:10.1038/s41586-022-04432-7.

Moon J-H, Jung H-W, Lee H-C, et al. A study of experimental autoimmune encephalomyelitis in dogs as a disease model for canine necrotizing encephalitis. *J Vet Sci*. 2015;16:203–211.

Park E-S, Uchida K, Nakayama H. Th1-, Th2-, and Th17-related cytokine and chemokine receptor mRNA and protein expression in the brain tissues, T cells, and macrophages of dogs with necrotizing and granulomatous meningoencephalitis. *Vet Pathol*. 2013;50:1127–1134.

Shibuya M, Matsuki N, Fujiwara K, et al. Autoantibodies against glial fibrillary acidic protein (GFAP) in cerebrospinal fluids from pug dogs with necrotizing meningoencephalitis. *J Vet Med Sci*. 2007;69:241–245.

Talarico LR, Schatzberg SJ. Idiopathic granulomatous and necrotizing inflammatory disorders of the canine central nervous system: a review and future perspectives. *J Small Anim Pract*. 2010;51:138–149.

Uchida K, Park E, Tsuboi M, et al. Pathological and immunological features of canine necrotizing meningoencephalitis and granulomatous meningoencephalitis. *Vet Jour*. 2016;213:72–77.

Eosinophilic Meningoencephalitis

Windsor RC, Sturges BK, Vernau KM, et al. Cerebrospinal fluid eosinophilia in dogs. *J Vet Intern Med*. 2009;23:275–281.

Greyhound Meningoencephalitis

Callanan JJ, Mooney CT, Mulcahy G, et al. A novel nonsuppurative meningoencephalitis in young Greyhounds in Ireland. *Vet Pathol*. 2002;39:56–65.

Feline Meningoencephalitis

Negrin A, Spencer S, Cherubini GB. Feline meningoencephalomyelitis of unknown origin: a retrospective analysis of 16 cases. *Can Vet J*. 2017;58:1073–1080.

Nessler J, Wohlisein P, Junginger J, et al. Meningoencephalomyelitis of unknown origin in cats. A case series describing clinical and pathological findings. *Front Vet Sci*. 2020. doi:10.3389/fvets.2020.00291.

Narcolepsy

Tonokura M, Fujita K, Nishino S. Review of pathophysiology and clinical management of narcolepsy in dogs. *Vet Rec*. 2007;161:375–380.

Autoimmune Eye Diseases

The function of the eye is to provide visual signals to the brain. Local inflammation, especially if it damages or kills cells, may therefore have devastating consequences. Even minor damage can profoundly affect vision. The eyes must therefore protect the visual pathways from damage induced by excessive inflammation. This is done through careful, rigorous but local regulation of both innate and adaptive immune responses.

Immune Privilege

Eye tissues resist the development of inflammation through a process called immune privilege (Fig. 8.1). Immune privilege is both a passive and active process that strengthens local immune tolerance mechanisms while minimizing any damage resulting from innate or adaptive immune responses.

The tissues within the eye use three major mechanisms to regulate innate immune responses and limit inflammation. The first is the establishment of a blood-ocular barrier in the uveal tissues. These intraocular blood vessels are nonfenestrated. This means that there are continuous tight junctions between the vascular endothelial cells that line these vessels. These tight junctions inhibit the emigration of leukocytes and selectively control the movement of macromolecules in and out of the vessels. These intraocular vessels do not express adherence molecules such as the integrins on their endothelial cells. As a result, circulating leukocytes and macromolecules are largely prevented from leaving these blood vessels and entering eye tissues. This is not an absolute barrier but is selective, admitting some cells and excluding others. The net result, however, is to reduce local inflammatory responses to minor insults.

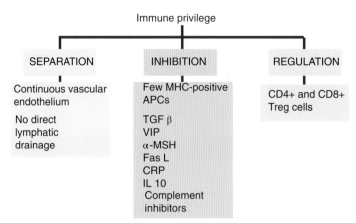

Fig. 8.1 The mechanisms of immune privilege within the eye. These can be classified as separation as a result of physical barriers, inhibition as a result of the presence of diverse suppressive molecules, and regulation as a result of the activities of regulatory T cells. *APCs*, Antigen Presenting Cells; *TGF*, Transforming growth factor; *VIP*, Vasoactive intestinal peptide; *MSH*, Melanocyte stimulating hormone; *CRP*, C-reactive protein; IL, Interleukin.

The second mechanism of immune privilege involves inhibition of both innate and adaptive immunity. Thus the aqueous humor contains many soluble regulatory and antiinflammatory molecules. Collectively, these regulatory molecules suppress inflammation, induce antiinflammatory cytokines, and promote the suppressive functions of both macrophages and T cells. Examples of these negative regulators include cytokines such as transforming growth factor-beta (TGFβ, present in microgram quantities) and interleukin-10 (IL10) that suppress T-cell, natural killer (NK) cell, and macrophage activation; neuropeptides such as vasoactive intestinal peptide, alpha melanocyte-stimulating hormone, calcitonin gene-related peptide, and somatostatin that also inhibit T-cell activation; enzymes such as indoleamine 2,3-dioxygenase (IDO) and L-arginase; and regulatory proteins that inhibit complement activation. In addition, many eye cells express surface molecules such as Fas-ligand, programmed death ligand 1 (PD-L1), and tumor necrosis factor (TNF)–related apoptosis-inducing ligand (TRAIL) that can cause apoptosis in any T cells that venture to attack them.

The third mechanism of privilege relies on the presence of CD4$^+$ and CD8$^+$ regulatory T (Treg) cells plus regulatory B cells. Together they ensure that the eye is uniquely capable of suppressing T-cell–mediated responses. This phenomenon is called anterior chamber-associated immune deviation (ACAID).

Immune privilege is not, however, a panacea. It may be sufficient to control naïve T cells, but if antigen-primed helper T type 1 (Th1) and Th17 cells develop and gain access to the eye, they can cause significant damage. Privilege may also be overcome after microtrauma or when infectious agents invade and pattern-recognition receptors are strongly stimulated. Likewise, hidden intraocular antigens often fail to induce peripheral tolerance. In addition, the existence of multiple overlapping immunosuppressive mechanisms runs the risk of developing an immunologic blind spot and thus a site of vulnerability to microbial invasion. For example, relatively few class II major histocompatibility complex (MHC)–positive, antigen-presenting cells are found within the normal eye.

Autoimmune Diseases of the Cornea and Conjunctiva

CHRONIC SUPERFICIAL KERATITIS

Chronic superficial keratitis (CSK) is a common disease of dogs and horses in which granulation tissue containing a mixture of blood vessels, fibroblasts, lymphocytes, plasma cells, and melanocytes invades the superficial corneal stroma (Fig. 8.2). Immunoglobulin deposits may be present in

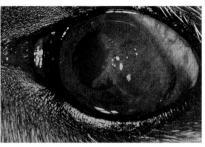

Fig. 8.2 The left eye of a 6-year-old German Shepherd Breed name is German Shepherd Dog with chronic superficial keratitis advancing from the dorsolateral aspect of the cornea. (Andrew SE. Immune-mediated canine and feline keratitis. *Vet Clin Small Anim.* 2008;38:269–290.)

the granulation tissue. The stroma is infiltrated with CD4⁺ T cells, many of which produce IFNγ, and much smaller numbers of CD8⁺ cells. They are followed by macrophages, plasma cells, and neutrophils. There is also aberrant MHC class II expression in the central cornea. Eventually the growing granulation tissue mass blocks vision.

Like other immune-mediated diseases, some dogs have a genetic predisposition to develop CSK. For example, the MHC class II haplotype DLA-DRB1*01501/DQA1*00601/DQB1*00301 is significantly associated with disease development.

The prevalence of CSK is correlated with altitude. It is more prevalent in dogs living at high altitudes, suggesting that exposure to ultraviolet light is an environmental predisposing factor. Dogs living at over 7000 ft altitude are more than 7.75 times more likely to develop the disease than dogs living between 3000 and 5000 ft.

Clinical Disease

CSK is most prevalent in German Shepherd Dogs, but it has been reported in many other breeds, and Greyhounds are reported to develop it at a younger age. Females are also overrepresented. This bilateral disease generally develops between 3 and 6 years of age. It first presents as conjunctival hyperemia near the temporal limbus, followed by superficial vascularization and pigmentation of the temporal peripheral cornea. With chronicity, the lesion progresses with extensive vascularization, edema, and pigment deposition toward the central cornea.

This type of lesion is known as pannus, a layer of fibrovascular granulation tissue. Dogs also develop hyperplasia of the corneal epithelium with basement membrane thickening. As the disease progresses, the pannus flattens and spreads. The advancing border of the lesion may contain a line of white crystalline corneal deposits or cellular infiltrate within the clear corneal stroma. In some dogs, this is self-limiting. In others, the pannus may spread to cover the entire cornea. The disease is not ulcerative, so the lesions are not painful. CSK is often accompanied by depigmentation and thickening of the leading edge of the third eyelid, often referred to as atypical pannus (see Nictitans Plasmacytic Conjunctivitis, later). Immunohistochemical staining of affected corneas showed that MHC class II–positive cells are abundant in the limbus but not on the cells of the central cornea. These positive cells appeared to be Langerhans cells. Within the pannus, there are also many MHC-positive cells. Some are lymphocytes, while others appear to be dendritic cells (DCs).

Diagnosis and Treatment

Diagnosis of CSK is based on clinical observations and breed predisposition. Corneal cytology shows increased numbers of lymphocytes, plasma cells, and mast cells. It is important to ensure that the cornea is not ulcerated or dry.

CSK is controllable but not curable. The more extensive the lesion, the slower the recovery and the poorer the prognosis. The condition often recurs and requires lifelong therapy. CSK is responsive to topical steroids (prednisolone or dexamethasone) and/or topical immunomodulatory therapy (cyclosporine or tacrolimus).

EQUINE IMMUNE-MEDIATED KERATITIS

Horses can also develop an immune-mediated nonulcerative keratitis (IMMK). It results in chronic corneal opacity without ulceration, uveitis, or overt ocular discomfort. The lesions are usually unilateral, and their severity depends on the depth of the corneal lesion. The lesions may be classified by anatomic level. They may be epithelial, superficial stromal, midstromal, or endothelial. Almost half of the cases are superficial stromal; about one-fourth are midstromal and another fourth are endothelial, while epithelial keratitis is rare.

Epithelial IMMK is characterized by the development of punctate opacities in the ventral corneal epithelium. Superficial IMMK is a relapsing-remitting corneal opacity consisting of a subepithelial yellow-white infiltrate surrounded by superficial corneal vascularization. Midstromal disease differs from the superficial disease in its location. It tends to have a more dense cellular infiltrate and less vascular branching. Endothelial IMMK shows a slowly progressive diffuse ventral area of corneal edema. An endothelial cellular infiltrate may be apparent at the edge of the edematous lesion. In general, the endothelial form does not respond well to immunosuppressive medications and has a poor prognosis. On the other hand, horses with the more superficial forms of IMMK may respond well to topical antiinflammatory therapy.

In superficial stromal IMMK, the cellular infiltrate consists of predominantly T cells with some plasma cells, macrophages, and few neutrophils. Both CD4+ and CD8+ T cells are present as are immunoglobulin G (IgG), IgM, and IgA deposits. The most damaging form of IMMK is endotheliitis, in which the cornea becomes markedly edematous. Autoantibodies are present and have been shown to be directed against the protein maspin. Maspin is expressed on corneal stromal keratocytes and is responsible for inhibiting corneal vascularization, cell migration, and adhesion to the intracellular matrix during wound healing. No breed or gender predisposition has been noted. Diagnosis is based on exclusion of other causes such as infections and the presence of concomitant uveitis. Treatment consists of topical steroids and/or cyclosporine. Surgical removal of the lesion (keratectomy) may be effective for persistent superficial or midstromal lesions.

NICTITANS PLASMACYTIC CONJUNCTIVITIS

Swelling of the nictitating membrane as a result of plasma cell infiltration may be referred to as a plasmoma or atypical pannus in dogs. It is not neoplastic but is believed to be immune mediated. It commonly occurs in association with CSK and may be part of the same disease syndrome. It can also occur in the absence of any corneal disease. As with CSK, German Shepherd Dogs appear to be most commonly affected.

The disease initially presents with follicle formation at the margin of the anterior surface of the nictitating membrane. However, owners may not present animals to a veterinarian, as the condition is not painful. Follicles progressively increase in size and coalesce, eventually resulting in diffuse thickening and depigmentation across the entire surface of the membrane. Histologically, the lesions are characterized by a dense plasmacytic infiltration with some lymphocytes and pigment dispersion. Diagnosis involves both the classical clinical signs and possibly a biopsy.

Treatment consists of topical or subconjunctival corticosteroids in combination with topical cyclosporine or tacrolimus. Once resolution is obtained, medication is slowly tapered to the lowest effective dose.

SUPERFICIAL PUNCTATE KERATITIS

This rare canine disease presents as bilateral multiple punctate superficial corneal opacities with or without epithelial defects. It is seen almost exclusively in Dachshunds and Shetland

Sheepdogs. The lesions may develop into erosions or superficial ulcers, causing ocular discomfort. Corneal biopsies reveal lymphoplasmacytic inflammation. The only other evidence that it may be immunologic in origin is its rapid positive response to topical antiinflammatory medication. Treatment consists of topical corticosteroids or cyclosporine combined with antibiotics if ulcers are present.

CANINE IDIOPATHIC EPISCLERITIS

Also called nodular granulomatous episcleritis, several proliferative inflammatory diseases affect the sclera and episcleral tissues. While some are secondary to infections, foreign bodies, or trauma, most of these lesions are assumed to be primary and immune mediated because of their characteristic histopathology, lack of any other obvious cause, and a positive response to immunosuppressive treatments. These lesions may be diffuse or nodular, unilateral or bilateral. The nodular lesions typically present as a raised smooth, firm pink or yellowish mass affecting the temporal limbus, cornea, and nictitating membrane in one or both eyes. These inflammatory lesions usually contain proliferating fibroblasts together with T and B cells, macrophages, and occasional plasma cells surrounding necrotic scleral collagen. They also show vascular congestion and edema. The discomfort may be associated with blepharospasm and an ocular discharge.

The lesion appears to originate as a local immune-complex–mediated vasculitis. In humans, it is associated with other inflammatory diseases such as rheumatoid arthritis or systemic lupus, as well as the presence of a vasculitis mediated by antineutrophil cytoplasmic antibodies (ANCA). Susceptible breeds include Collies and Collie crosses, American Cocker Spaniels, and Golden Retrievers. Unilateral cases tend to resolve spontaneously, while bilateral cases require prolonged treatment. The diffuse lesions respond rapidly to topical immunosuppression with corticosteroids, but nodular lesions do not respond as fast. Other immunosuppressants such as cyclosporine, chlorambucil, cyclophosphamide, and azathioprine may also be of benefit.

Canine necrotic scleritis is much less common than episcleritis. It is a serious inflammatory disease also associated with collagen necrosis and collagen lysis. It is also characterized by infiltration with lymphocytes, plasma cells, and macrophages and is assumed to be immune mediated. In humans, this condition is associated with the presence of ANCA. A case has been reported in a Scottish Terrier in which the dog possessed ANCA in the form of antimyeloperoxidase antibodies.

Autoimmune Diseases of the Uvea

The uvea consists of three components: the iris, the ciliary body, and the choroid. It is highly vascularized and thus the part of the eye where the blood-ocular barrier acts to protect these tissues from immune attack.

The autoimmune disease sympathetic ophthalmia has been known since the days of Hippocrates. It is a bilateral granulomatous uveitis of humans that develops following a penetrating injury to one eye. This is followed by destructive inflammation in the nontraumatized eye. It takes from a few days to decades to develop, but about 80% of cases develop within 3 months. It is believed to result from the release of antigens from the traumatized eye that reach a draining lymph node and trigger a systemic autoimmune T-cell response directed against choroidal melanocytes. Immunosuppressive therapy with glucocorticosteroids and/or cyclosporine will control the developing inflammation. This disease has yet to be recorded in domestic animals, but several experimental models exist (see Chapter 22), and (as described later) there are related diseases that occur naturally in animals.

EQUINE RECURRENT UVEITIS

The most common cause of blindness in horses is recurrent uveitis (ERU) (also called periodic ophthalmia, moon blindness, or iridocyclitis). It affects horses worldwide with an estimated prevalence of 10% to 25% (2%–25% have been reported to be affected in the United States, but only 1%–2% of horses suffer serious disease affecting vision). Horses suffer repeated episodes of intraocular inflammation mainly involving the anterior uveal tract, followed by periods of remission. In acute cases, they develop severe ocular pain, blepharospasm, lacrimation, corneal changes such as edema and vascularization, aqueous flare, and photophobia (Fig. 8.3). Some horses develop a persistent low-grade uveitis without overt signs of ocular discomfort, while others develop a posterior uveitis, including vitritis and retinitis, resulting in photoreceptor destruction. After repeated attacks, horses may develop cataracts, intraocular adhesions, retinal detachment, secondary glaucoma, and eventual loss of vision associated with a shrunken nonfunctional eye.

ERU is an immune-mediated disease. The uveal tract has a good blood supply protected by the vascular barriers, as discussed earlier. However, once the blood-ocular barrier has been disrupted, perhaps by infection or trauma, T cells and antibodies may escape into the eye. They may do this repeatedly, causing recurrent inflammatory episodes.

$CD4^+$ T cells in ERU-affected horses lack a cell surface molecule called septin 7. The septins are cytoskeletal proteins involved in regulating cell shape and movement (cytokinesis). A deficiency of septin 7 increases lymphocyte cytoplasmic fluidity so they can efficiently squeeze through small pores. It is possible that the septin 7 deficiency in ERU allows these flexible T cells to penetrate the blood-eye barrier. The ciliary body, choroid, and retina of affected horses are infiltrated with T cells. About half of these are $CD4^+$ Th1 cells and about 20% are $CD8^+$ cytotoxic T cells. Also present are neutrophils together with extensive fibrin and C3 deposition. The $CD4^+$ cells produce both IL2 and IFNγ. Th17 cells. Their stimulating cytokine IL23 are also present and contribute to the chronic inflammatory process.

Affected horses make a diversity of autoantibodies that likely contribute to disease pathogenesis. These are directed against antigens that are normally hidden behind the blood-ocular barrier. Their B cells are considered "ignorant." As a result, peripheral tolerance is weak, and B cells may be activated once they encounter these antigens. The dominant autoantigen in the equine eye is the interphotoreceptor retinoid-binding protein (IRBP) with subsequent epitope spreading to the retinal S-protein (also called arrestin-1). Other autoantibodies detected in ERU horses include those directed against recoverin, cellular retinaldehyde-binding protein, synaptotagmin-1, and malate dehydrogenase. Their significance in the pathogenesis of ERU is probably not great. These autoantibodies may not be detectable in affected horse serum but are present in the vitreous fluid.

ERU commonly develops after infection with *Leptospira interrogans*. Following natural outbreaks of leptospirosis, most surviving horses developed ERU within 18 to 24 months.

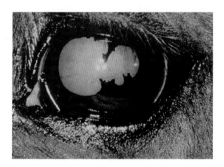

Fig. 8.3 Chronic equine recurrent uveitis (ERU). A horse with secondary late immature cataract formation and posterior synechiae as a result of ERU. (From Keller RL, Hendrix DVH. New Surgical Therapies for the Treatment of Equine Recurrent Uveitis. Clin Tech Equine Pract, 2005; 4:81–86.)

Affected horses develop circulating antibodies to three lipoproteins found on the inner leaflet of the outer membrane of *L. interrogans* called Lru A, B, and C. The titer of these antibodies tends to rise during disease flares and drop while in remission. These leptospiral lipoproteins show strong antigenic cross-reactivity with the equine lens, ciliary body, and retina. If horses are experimentally immunized with either equine cornea or certain serovars of killed *L. interrogans*, they develop corneal opacity 10 days later when antibodies appear in the bloodstream. Partial antigenic cross-reactivity also exists between the equine cornea and the *L. interrogans* lipoproteins. *L interrogans* serovar Pomona is the primary species triggering ERU in North America, whereas *L. kirschneri* serovars Grippotyphosa, Pomona, and Bratislava are most prevalent in Europe.

Many other infections have also been associated with the development of ERU. These include *Brucella abortus, Strep equi, Prescottella equi,* and *Toxoplasma gondii.* Some cases may also be associated with *Borrelia burgdorferi* infection or with the nematode *Onchocerca cervicalis.* In the latter case, dead or dying worms may release cross-reacting antigens. Numerous other environmental antigens have been suggested as the initiating triggers through molecular mimicry. For example, rotaviruses possess an antigen that cross-reacts with retinal S-antigen, as does the dietary component α_{S2}-casein. Both of these can induce experimental autoimmune uveitis when used to immunize Lewis rats.

Three single nucleotide polymorphisms (SNPs) in Appaloosa horses are correlated with the development of ERU. One such SNP is strongly associated with the leopard complex spotting locus on chromosome 1. This determines the size and number of pigmented spots on the animal's coat. Homozygosity at this locus further increases the risk of developing disease. A nearby gene modifier called PATN1 is also associated with increased ERU risk. The other two SNPS are associated with the equine MHC region (ELA) on chromosome 20. In German Warmbloods, the ELA-A9 haplotype is associated with increased susceptibility. Other genes involved include those regulating Th17 activity and a SNP on chromosome 18 associated with cataract formation.

Clinical Disease

Horses may develop ERU at any age, but peak prevalence is between 4 and 6 years of age. The disease is not gender specific. Some breeds appear to be predisposed. These include Appaloosas, Warmbloods, and American Quarter Horses. ERU has been subdivided into three clinical forms: classic, insidious, and posterior.

In the most common, classic disease, horses suffer from recurrent acute inflammatory episodes of uveitis separated by periods of relative remission. The inflammatory process may affect the anterior uveal structures such as the iris and ciliary body and the posterior choroid and retina. Clinical signs include severe photophobia, ocular pain, blepharospasm, increased lacrimation, corneal edema, aqueous flare, hypopyon, a vitreous haze, and a chorioretinitis. These acute episodes last 10 to 21 days. Each attack gets progressively more severe and gradually spreads to involve other eye tissues until complete blindness results.

In the insidious form of the disease, chronic low-grade uveitis over time results in severe damage and blindness. This form is not obviously painful. The most serious chronic type is seen in *Leptospira*-infected Appaloosas. In one series, all such horses lost vision in one eye, and 50% became completely blind. Of noninfected non-Appaloosas, only 34% became blind in one eye and 6% became totally blind.

The posterior form of ERU primarily affects the posterior ocular structures, including the vitreous and the retina. It results in vitreous opacity, retinitis, and eventual degeneration. This form is generally observed in Warmblood and European horses.

Diagnosis and Treatment

Diagnosis of ERU involves exclusion of other causes such as infectious agents (other than leptospirosis), trauma, or neoplasia. The primary acute form should be distinguished from the chronic recurrent form. Hematology and *Leptospira* serology should be performed in endemic areas.

Aggressive systemic, local, and topical corticosteroid therapy using prednisolone or dexamethasone is an effective treatment. Dexamethasone is used most often since it is available as an ointment and relatively inexpensive. In severe cases, placement of a subpalpebral lavage system for more frequent application of ophthalmic suspensions and solutions may be warranted. These steroids will usually bring the ocular inflammation under control, although the disease often recurs. Encouraging results have been obtained by the use of suprachoroidal sustained-release cyclosporine implants.

UVEODERMATOLOGIC SYNDROME

Uveodermatologic syndrome (UDS) affects dogs. It may affect up to 4% of Akitas and is a sporadic disease in related dog breeds such as Samoyeds, Siberian Huskies, and Alaskan Malamutes. However, any breed can be affected. A similar disease, Vogt-Koyanagi-Harada syndrome, occurs in humans. The disease results from autoimmune attack on melanin-containing cells. As a result, cytotoxic T cells attack the melanocytes in pigmented tissues. Affected dogs develop uveitis with iris and choroid depigmentation along with ulcerative skin lesions, whitening of the hair (poliosis), and skin (vitiligo) (Fig. 8.4A). The eye lesions tend to develop first. Most animals present with bilateral panuveitis, often leading to blindness. The early lesions vary from a severe panuveitis to a bilateral anterior uveitis. Some dogs may suffer retinal detachment. There is a diffuse infiltration of the uveal tract with lymphocytes, plasma cells, and pigment-laden macrophages. There may be progressive depigmentation of both choroid and iris.

Depigmentation of the hair and skin gradually follows the onset of eye lesions. Some cases may be generalized, involving the eyelids, nasal planum, lips, scrotum, and footpads. These depigmented areas may become ulcerated and crusted. The skin lesions consist of a mononuclear cell (macrophages, giant cells, lymphocytes, plasma cells) infiltration of the dermal-epidermal junction (see Fig. 8.4B). The amount of melanin in the epidermis and hair follicles is greatly reduced.

In humans, Vogt-Koyanagi-Harada syndrome is believed to result from an autoimmune attack on melanocytes. In dogs, no consistent immunologic abnormalities have been observed. The predisposition in Akitas suggests a significant genetic influence. One such factor is possession of

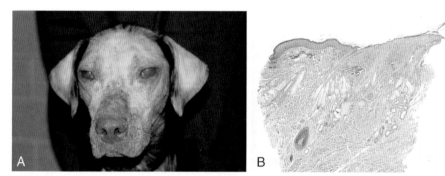

Fig. 8.4 (A) A case of uveodermatologic syndrome. Note the ocular clouding, alopecia, and depigmentation of the nasal planum. (B) Canine uveodermatologic syndrome, showing subepidermal, lichenoid (bandlike) inflammation. There is pigmentary incontinence on the left of the figure. Original magnification 20×. H&E stain. (A. Courtesy of Drs R. Kennis, J. Dziezc and L. Wadsworth.) (B. Courtesy of Dr. Dominique Wiener.)

DLA-DQA1*00201. An experimental disease resembling UDS can be induced in rats, monkeys, and Akitas by immunization against the enzymes involved in melanin synthesis. These are tyrosinase gp100 and tyrosinase-related proteins-1 and -2. In the case of the Akitas, the immunizing antigen was a 30–amino acid peptide derived from tyrosinase-related protein-1. The experimental disease in these dogs took 2 to 3 weeks to develop following immunization. It resulted in severe anterior chamber inflammation, retinal detachment from the pigmented epithelium, and a mild blepharoconjunctivitis. The ocular inflammation subsided after 6 to 8 weeks. Skin lesions, vitiligo, and alopecia did not develop until 8 weeks after immunization. Histopathology confirmed exudative retinal detachment and infiltration of inflammatory cells (mainly lymphocytes) into the subretinal space. The choroid was thin and depigmented. Lymphocytes also infiltrated the ciliary body. Autoantibody titers varied with the disease state, climbing during relapses and falling during remissions.

Clinical Disease

The initial lesions of UDS develop in dogs between 1 and 6 years of age. Ocular signs precede dermatologic signs. Common clinical signs include blepharospasm, epiphora, aqueous flare, posterior synechiae, retinal detachment, and choroidal depigmentation. Many dogs develop secondary glaucoma or are blind when first presented. In untreated dogs, the median time to permanent blindness is about 1 year. The skin lesions are also bilateral and symmetric (see Chapter 10).

Diagnosis and Treatment

Diagnosis is based on clinical signs and the breeds involved. Histopathology should be performed on skin biopsies and eyes that are enucleated due to intractable secondary glaucoma.

Aggressive management of the ocular and skin lesions includes a combination of systemic and ophthalmic corticosteroids, although the disease may recur when therapy stops. Therefore long-term management with immunosuppressive drugs is often required. The cytotoxic drug azathioprine may also be given if corticosteroids are insufficient to stop disease progression. Likewise, cyclosporine has been used with success in humans. Tetracycline plus niacinamide therapy has also been reported to be effective.

Autoimmune Retinal Diseases
SUDDEN ACQUIRED RETINAL DEGENERATION SYNDROME

Sudden acquired retinal degeneration syndrome (SARDS) occurs in dogs. Its etiology is unknown. Dachshunds, Miniature Schnauzers, Pugs, and Brittany Spaniels appear to be most commonly affected, and spayed females are overrepresented. The disease is characterized by sudden irreversible blindness developing over several days. It results from apoptosis of retinal photoreceptors (Fig. 8.5). A lack of activity detected by an electroretinogram confirms this loss of photoreceptor activity. Initially, the animals appear to have a normal fundus and mydriatic pupils that are slowly responsive to white light, responsive to blue, but unresponsive to red light. The retina, however, begins to degenerate over the months following this loss of vision.

The pathogenesis of SARDS is unknown. Many of the clinical signs point to hyperadrenocorticism as an initiating factor since affected animals may demonstrate polydipsia, polyphagia, obesity, and a hepatopathy. Alternatively, it has been proposed that SARDS is an autoimmune disease since it resembles some autoimmune retinopathies in humans. It has been claimed that the disease may be partially reversed by immunosuppressive therapy. Some dogs produce autoantibodies against retinal components.

Human autoimmune retinopathies are also associated with sudden vision loss. Some are primary autoimmune diseases while others are paraneoplastic and associated with cancers such as melanomas. It is believed that these may be a consequence of molecular mimicry.

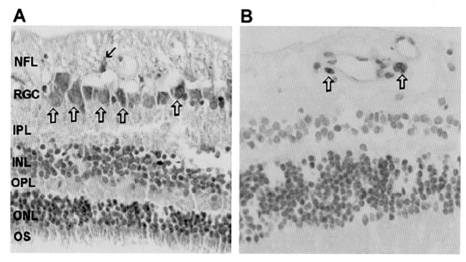

Fig. 8.5 Immunohistochemistry of the retina of a dog with sudden acquired retinal degeneration syndrome (SARDS). (A) Note the presence of T lymphocytes (CD3+ small cells, *small arrow*). Strong CD3 immunoreactivity was detected in all neuronal cells, especially in retinal ganglion cell bodies *(open arrows)*. (B) Note the sporadic presence of CD79+ B cells *(open arrows)* in a SARDS-affected retina. (Grozdanic SD, Harper MM, Kekova H. Antibody-mediated retinopathies in canine patients: mechanism, diagnosis, and treatment modalities. *Vet Clin Small Anim.* 2008;38:361–387.)

Autoantibodies directed against retinal antigens have been detected in both SARDS-affected dogs and humans. The most significant antibodies in dogs are those directed against a neuron-specific enolase. These autoantibodies have been found in about 25% of SARDS-affected dogs but not in normal dogs. Microarray studies on affected dog retinas show a significant increase in gene expression of IgA and complement C3.

It must be pointed out, however, that Witebsky's postulates have not been met in the case of canine SARDS. It is entirely possible that these autoantibodies are a consequence, not a cause of, the retinal damage. It has been reported that long-term treatment with high doses of systemic steroids and other immunomodulatory drugs is beneficial, but this has proved difficult to replicate. For instance, mycophenolate mofetil as a sole agent had no measurable effects on dogs with SARDS. It has also been reported that intravenous immunoglobulin therapy may produce beneficial results, though this treatment remains controversial due to a lack of peer-reviewed reports. A variant of immune-mediated retinitis seen in dogs is related to SARDS but presents with a more gradual onset of blindness developing over months or years. It too is similar to some of the human retinopathies. In these cases, however, affected animals tend to respond rapidly to corticosteroid treatment.

OPTIC NEURITIS

An idiopathic optic neuritis (ON) that is responsive to immunosuppressive medication has been reported to occur in small-breed dogs. Differentiation of optic neuritis from SARDS may be difficult since the clinical presentations overlap significantly. The condition presents as a sudden-onset blindness and dilated unresponsive pupils secondary to inflammation in the optic nerve. The optic neuritis may be bilateral (about 75% of cases) or unilateral. The optic nerve head may show swelling, hyperemia, papilledema, and retinal hemorrhage. Blepharospasm and exophthalmos may also be present. Asymmetric visual defects are more likely to occur in ON dogs than in SARDS dogs. An electroretinogram differentiates between the two conditions. Cerebrospinal fluid (CSF) analysis of affected dogs showed neutrophil pleocytosis and increased protein in about 44% of cases. About a third of cases of ON are associated with the sterile inflammation caused by the ocular form of granulomatous meningoencephalitis (GME) (see Chapter 7). The use of magnetic resonance imaging in these dogs may reveal optic nerve enlargement. GME dogs will also show evidence of inflammatory changes in their CSF.

Treatment consists of systemic corticosteroids, either alone or in combination with other immunosuppressants such as cytosine arabinoside, cyclosporine, or azathioprine. About one-third of the treated dogs recover their vision within 2 to 60 days (median 10 days) after initiation of treatment. In view of the positive response to immunosuppressive therapy the disease is assumed to be immune mediated.

Ancillary Structures

KERATOCONJUNCTIVITIS SICCA

Keratoconjunctivitis sicca (KCS), otherwise known as dry eye, is one of the most common ophthalmic diseases of dogs. It has also been recorded in horses. In this disease, tear film volume or quality is greatly reduced. In the absence of a normal tear film, as a result either of reduced production or excessive evaporation, affected animals develop corneal dryness. The resulting loss of lubrication leads to blepharospasm and chronic inflammation of the conjunctiva and cornea. A mucoid or mucopurulent ocular discharge, blepharitis, conjunctivitis, corneal vascularization and pigmentation, and secondary bacterial infections develop. Corneal ulceration may occur and progress to perforation if untreated. The breeds at highest relative risk include Cavalier King Charles Spaniels, English Bulldogs, West Highland White Terriers, Lhasa Apsos, Shih-Tzu, Pugs, Cocker Spaniels, and Pekingese, suggesting a genetic predisposition.

While the list of possible causes for KCS is extensive (congenital, drug induced, iatrogenic gland removal, neurogenic, infectious, endocrine, etc.), most cases are presumed to be immune mediated. An immunologic basis for disease is supported by histopathologic studies of lacrimal tissue from KCS dogs revealing a lymphoplasmacytic adenitis and acinar atrophy. Glandular tissue may eventually be replaced with fibrous connective tissue. The infiltrating lymphocytes consist of both T and B cells. Presumably, they participate in the destruction of the tear-producing acinar cells (Box 8.1).

Clinical Disease

Dogs with KCS present with a dry cornea and a history of bilateral chronic keratoconjunctivitis and mucoid to mucopurulent ocular discharge. There may also be corneal vascularization, cellular infiltration, and secondary pigmentation. In some cases, corneal ulceration may occur. KCS may also permit bacterial overgrowth, leading to a secondary bacterial conjunctivitis requiring treatment with topical antibiotics.

Diagnosis and Treatment

Quantitative KCS is diagnosed by use of the Schirmer tear test. This is a rapid test that is part of a routine canine eye examination. A 5- × 30-mm strip of filter paper is placed in the ventrolateral conjunctival cul-de-sac for 1 minute. Normal dogs should produce greater than or equal to 15 mm of aqueous tears/min. Dogs that produce less than 15 mm/min in conjunction with clinical signs of keratoconjunctivitis are considered positive for KCS. Other tests, such as the tear film breakup time, may aid in the diagnosis.

KCS has traditionally been treated by use of supplemental artificial tears. These contain high-molecular-weight viscous chemicals such as polyvinyl pyrrolidine, hyaluronic acid, polyvinyl alcohol, or methylcellulose; however, they do not affect the cause of the problem. They evaporate rapidly and have to be administered frequently. Therefore the standard therapy for canine immune-mediated KCS employs topical immunosuppressive agents to suppress the destructive reactions within the lacrimal glands. Ophthalmic solution and ointment formulations of both cyclosporine and tacrolimus have been shown to be effective in most cases of canine KCS, although it may take 4 to 6 weeks before improved lacrimation is seen. Slow-release episcleral cyclosporine implants are available for dogs that respond to topical cyclosporine. A related calcineurin inhibitor, pimecrolimus, has also been reported to be both safe and effective in treating KCS when applied in the form of oil-based eye drops.

EQUINE KCS

KCS has been reported in a horse. The 3-year-old animal presented with bilateral ulcerative keratoconjunctivitis and improved clinically with ophthalmic cyclosporine therapy. The lacrimal glands showed an eosinophil infiltration with lesser numbers of lymphocytes, plasma cells, and macrophages. Although this suggests an immunologic origin for the disease, it must be pointed out that nonimmunologic mechanisms such as facial nerve damage can also result in corneal dryness.

BOX 8.1 ■ Sjögren Syndrome

In 1933, Henrich Sjögren recognized a syndrome consisting of keratoconjunctivitis sicca and xerostomia in association with other systemic inflammatory diseases such as rheumatoid arthritis (RA) and systemic lupus erythematosus (SLE). This is now recognized as one of the commonest autoimmune diseases of humans, especially middle-aged and elderly women. It has been occasionally recorded in dogs and cats.

Affected dogs commonly present with conjunctivitis and keratitis. In addition, however, the mouth is very dry, a necrotizing gingivitis may be present, calculus may accumulate, and the teeth become carious. Other mucous membranes such as the vagina may also be abnormally dry. There may be bilateral enlargement of the lacrimal and submandibular salivary glands. A biopsy will reveal a bilateral lymphoplasmacytic sialadenitis with no evidence of infection (Fig. 8.6). Imaging of the salivary glands by ultrasonography or computed tomography may assist in confirming this. Two major autoantigens have been identified in Sjögren syndrome cases. One is SSA, an RNA-degrading protein; the other is SSB, an RNA-binding phosphoprotein. Both are ubiquitous in vertebrate cells. About 90% of affected animals are also hypergammaglobulinemic, and many have antinuclear antibodies and rheumatoid factors. Immunosuppressive treatment with glucocorticoids is usually effective.

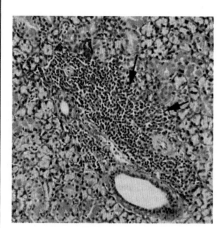

Fig. 8.6 Salivary gland inflammation in an NZB/NZW F1 female mouse, showing a large perivascular and periductal lymphocytic focus extending into the gland parenchyma. A model of Sjögren syndrome in other species. The arrows point to the lymphocyte focus. (Bagavant H. et al. The NZB/W F1 mouse model for Sjögren's syndrome: A historical perspective and lessons learned. Auto Immunity Rev 2020; 19:102686.)

BOX 8.1 ■ Sjögren Syndrome (Continued)

Sjögren syndrome has also been described in a cat with low-grade fever, lethargy, ocular pain, dysphagia, and weight loss. The oral mucosa was described as "dry and tacky."

As a fairly common disease in humans, the immunopathogenesis of Sjögren syndrome has been extensively studied. It results from immunologic attack on the cells of the salivary and lacrimal glands. As a result of this damage, the production of tears and saliva is greatly impaired. Cells contain a multiprotein complex that binds and transports noncoding RNA. This complex consists of three proteins, two of which are forms of SSA and one a form of SSB. (Their full names are Sjögren syndrome [SS] A [or Ro] and SSB [or La].) These ribonucleoproteins are potent autoantigens. They are also classified as extractable nuclear antigens because they can be readily separated from other nuclear components and found in the cytoplasm.

Antibodies to SSA are found in up to 90% of patients with Sjögren syndrome, in 40% to 60% of patients with SLE, and in some RA cases. Antibodies to SSB usually occur in sera together with anti-SSA. They are found in about 60% of patients with Sjögren syndrome and in about 15% of lupus patients. Antibodies to another small nuclear RNP called Sm (Smith) are found in patients with SLE. (The designations Ro, La, and Sm are abbreviations of the patient's names in whom these autoantigens were first identified.)

Nabeta R, Kambe N, Nakagawa M, et al. Sjögren's-like syndrome in a dog. *J Vet Med Sci.* 2019;81: 886-889.

Sources of Additional Information

Assis de Andrade F, Fiorot SHS, Benchimol EI, et al. The autoimmune diseases of the eyes. *Autoimm Revs.* 2016;15:258–271.

Caspi RR. Understanding autoimmunity in the eye: from animal models to novel therapies. *Discov Med.* 2014;17:155–162.

Immune Privilege

Caspi RR. Ocular autoimmunity: the price of privilege? *Immunol Rev.* 2006;213:23–35.

Niederkorn JY, Stein-Streilin J. History and physiology pf immune privilege. *Ocular Immunol Inflamm.* 2010;18:19–23.

Chronic Superficial Keratitis

Andrew SE. Immune mediated canine and feline keratitis. *Vet Clin Small Anim.* 2008;38:269–290.

Chavkin MJ, Roberts SM, Salmon MD, et al. Risk factors for development of chronic superficial keratitis in dogs. *J Am Vet Med Assoc.* 1994;204:1630–1634.

Jokinen P, Rusanen EM, Kennedy LJ, et al. MHC class II risk haplotype associated with canine chronic superficial keratitis in German Shepherd dogs. *Vet Immunol Immunopathol.* 2011;140:37–41.

Williams DL. Histological and immunohistochemical evaluation of canine chronic superficial keratitis. *Res Vet Sci.* 1999;67:189–193.

Williams DL. Immunopathogenesis of keratoconjunctivitis sicca in the dog. *Vet Clin Small Anim.* 2008. doi:10.1016/j.cvsm.2007.12.002.

Equine Immune-Mediated Keratitis

Matthews A, Gilger BC. Equine immune-mediated keratopathies. *Vet Opthalmol.* 2009;12(1):S10–S16.

Pate DO, Clode AB, Olivry T, et al. Immunohistochemical and immunohistologic characterization of superficial stromal immune-mediated keratitis in horses. *Am J Vet Res.* 2012;73:1067–1073.

Equine Recurrent Uveitis

Deeg CA, Kaspers B, Gerhards H, et al. Immune responses to retinal autoantigens and peptides in equine recurrent uveitis. *Invest Ophthalmol Vis Sci.* 2001;42:393–398.

Dwyer AE, Crockett RS, Kalsow CM. Association of Leptospiral seroreactivity and breed with uveitis and blindness in horses: 372 cases (1986-1993). *J Am Vet Med Assoc.* 1995;207:1327–1331.

Gerding JC, Gilger BC. Prognosis and impact of equine recurrent uveitis. *Equine Vet J.* 2016. doi:10.1111/evj.12451.

Malalana F, Stylianides A, McGowan C. Equine recurrent uveitis: human and equine perspectives. *Vet Jour.* 2015;206:22–29.

Rockwell H, Mack M, Famula T, et al. Genetic investigation of equine recurrent uveitis in Appaloosa horses. *Animal Genet.* 2019;51:111–116.

Sudden Acquired Retinal Degeneration Syndrome

Grozdanic SD, Harper MM, Kekova H. Antibody-mediated retinopathies in canine patients: mechanism, diagnosis, and treatment modalities. *Vet Clin Small Anim.* 2008;38:361–387.

Grozdanic SD, Lazic T, Kecova H, et al. Optical coherence tomography and molecular analysis of sudden acquired retinal degeneration syndrome (SARDS) eyes suggests the immune-mediated nature of retinal damage. *Vet Ophthalmol.* 2019;22:305–327.

Keller RL, Kania S, Hendrix DVH, et al. Evaluation of canine serum for the presence of antiretinal autoantibodies in sudden acquired retinal degeneration syndrome. *Vet Opthalmol.* 2006;9:195–200.

Komaromy AM, Abrams KL, Heckenlively JR, et al. Sudden acquired retinal degeneration syndrome (SARDS)—a review and proposed strategies toward a better understanding of pathogenesis, early diagnosis and therapy. *Vet Ophthalmol.* 2016;19:319–331.

Optic Neuritis

Bedos L, Tetas R, Crespo V, et al. Presumed optic neuritis of non-infectious origin in dogs treated with immunosuppressive medication: 28 dogs (2000-2015). *J Small Anim Pract.* 2020;61:676–683.

Smith SM, Westermeyer HD, Mariani CL, et al. Optic neuritis in dogs: 96 cases (1983-2016). *Vet Ophthalmol.* 2018;21:442–451.

Autoimmune Reproductive Diseases

Autoimmune diseases can attack and destroy the reproductive organs. One reason for this is if the reproductive tissues, especially the testes and ovaries, do not develop at birth, when central tolerance pathways are at their most active. The gonads develop much later under hormonal influences at puberty. This is long after central tolerance has become established and at a time coinciding with thymic regression. Thus the reproductive organs must rely exclusively on peripheral tolerance mechanisms or immune privilege for protection against immune attack.

Autoimmunity in Males

AUTOIMMUNE ORCHITIS

Like the interior of the eye, the interior of the testis is an immune privileged site. A blood-testis barrier (BTB) serves to minimize immune responses within the testes, and seminiferous tubules. Immunosuppressive molecules such as transforming growth factor-beta (TGFβ), as well as a population of intratesticular regulatory T (Treg) cells, maintain a tolerant environment. Sertoli cells help support this immunosuppressive environment by serving as a source of indoleamine 2,3-dioxygenase (IDO). Among the late-developing testicular cells are the spermatogonia that are first produced at puberty. They possess their own unique antigens, and if they are to develop successfully within the testes, they must be protected against immune attack. Like the eye, discussed in the previous chapter, the testes are therefore immune-privileged sites from which T cells are normally excluded. The testes have impermeable blood vessels, the BTB, that effectively prevent unwanted immune cell entry and any resulting inflammation or damage. The BTB is formed by tightly linked Sertoli cells (Fig. 9.1). When intact, these cells protect developing spermatozoa from contact with any wandering lymphocytes. The tubuli recti and the rete testis are permeable to antibodies, although the seminiferous tubules are not. If the BTB is breached, then the autoantigens from the developing haploid cells can leak into the circulation and trigger an autoimmune

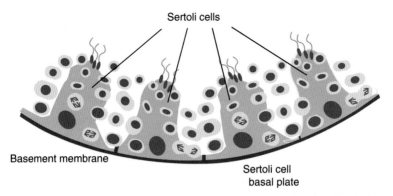

Fig. 9.1 The structure of the blood-testes barrier. It is formed by tightly linked Sertoli cells that serve to exclude inquisitive T cells.

response. It is also clear that damage to the BTB in one testis can induce orchitis in the contralateral testis (Fig. 9.2). This may occur as a result of physical trauma or secondary to an infectious orchitis. Peripheral tolerance to testicular antigens can therefore be readily broken.

Experimental Autoimmune Orchitis

Experimental autoimmune orchitis (EAO) is a classic animal model of an organ-specific autoimmune disease. It can be induced in many experimental species, including rabbits, rats, mice, guinea pigs, and monkeys. Inbred mouse strains differ significantly in their susceptibility to EAO. For example, if a resistant mouse strain such as DBA/2J is crossed with a susceptible strain such as BALB/cByJ, the offspring are orchitis resistant. Further analysis has identified three resistance genes and two susceptibility genes in mice.

When homologous testicular homogenates are injected into guinea pigs together with potent adjuvants such as Freund's complete adjuvant and *Bordetella* toxin (because two adjuvants are needed to break down the BTB), acute orchitis results. This orchitis eventually results in aspermatogenesis. The initial sites of the lesions within the testes depend on the antigens selected for

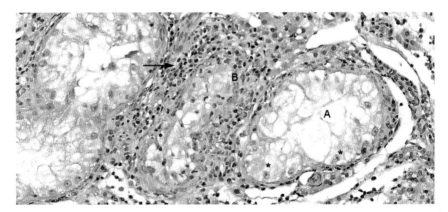

Fig. 9.2 Histology of a testis with autoimmune orchitis. Seminiferous tubules undergoing severe progressive changes with tubular degeneration *(A)* and tubular collapse *(B)* with intense lymphoplasmacytic infiltrates *(arrow)*. Only scattered Sertoli cells *(*)* line the lumen. (Davidson AP et al. Adult-Onset Lymphoplasmacytic Orchitis in a Labrador Retriever Stud Dog. Topics in Compan Anim Med. 2015; 30:31–34.)

immunization. Investigations in rats and other laboratory animals have shown that the initial damage is mediated by both B and T cells acting on the seminiferous epithelium. Once this initial damage has occurred, invading T cells can then spread throughout the testes and attack and destroy Sertoli cells, resulting in sperm developmental arrest. Further analysis suggests that T-cell–mediated responses are responsible for the destructive lesions in the seminiferous tubules, whereas the antibody-mediated responses only interacted with sperm in the rete testis and the epididymis. The T-cell attacks result in the shedding and apoptosis of germ cells.

A similar EAO has been induced in bulls after they had been immunized with testicular extracts or testicular homogenate in Freund's complete adjuvant. Acute inflammatory reactions developed first in the ductus efferens and ampulla but then spread rapidly to the caput epididymis and then to the seminiferous tubules. A chronic interstitial orchitis then followed. Breakdown of the epididymal duct permitted spermatozoa to escape into the tissues, where they formed chronic inflammatory granulomas. Minor inflammatory reactions also occurred in the cauda epididymis, the accessory glands, and the pelvic urethra. Antisperm antibodies and delayed hypersensitivity reactions to sperm antigens were positive in these bulls by 19 days post injection.

Secondary Autoimmune Orchitis

Autoantibodies to sperm may be detected in some animals following injury to the testes or long-standing obstruction of the seminiferous ducts. For example, dogs infected with *Brucella canis* develop serum antibodies that agglutinate spermatozoa. These antibodies can also be detected in seminal plasma. The dogs develop chronic epididymitis and become sensitized by sperm antigens carried to the circulation after phagocytosis by macrophages. These sperm antigens stimulate the production of immunoglobulin G (IgG) or IgA autoantibodies. The autoantibodies agglutinate and immobilize sperm, causing infertility. Some infected dogs may even develop delayed hyper-sensitivity skin responses to sperm antigens.

Primary Autoimmune Orchitis

Dogs can develop a primary autoimmune orchitis. The testes in these animals tend to be small and soft. Animals have a progressive decline in total sperm counts, eventually resulting in azoosper-mia within a few months. Histologic examination shows a lymphocytic orchitis and fibrosis with impaired spermatogenesis, seminiferous tubules with spermatogenic arrest, and Sertoli cell–only syndrome. There may be focal interstitial and intratubular mononuclear cell aggregations as well as tubular degeneration, germ cell apoptosis, and sloughing. In some cases, the primary lesion may develop in one testis, but sympathetic contralateral orchitis may subsequently develop in the other. An autoimmune orchitis may be associated with other systemic autoimmune diseases such as IgG4 vasculitis. In stallions and bulls (and men), antisperm autoantibodies may be associated with reduced fertility or infertility. In certain inbred lines of black mink, males may be infertile as a result of high levels of naturally developing antisperm antibodies (Box 9.1).

Autoimmunity in Females
AUTOIMMUNE OOPHORITIS

As with the testes, autoimmunity to the ovary (autoimmune oophoritis) may be induced experi-mentally or develop spontaneously.

Experimental autoimmune oophoritis (EAO) can be induced by immunization of mice with zona pellucida 3 (ZP3) peptide. Neonatal thymectomy of some mouse strains (BALB/c or A/J) may also result in the development of an autoimmune oophoritis. This appears to be due to an imbalance between Tregs and effector T cells, resulting in Treg depletion. These thymectomized female mice develop ovarian inflammation and autoantibodies, resulting in ovarian atrophy and infertility. The disease develops at puberty and is most severe between 4 and 14 weeks after

---

BOX 9.1 ■ Infertility in Black Mink

When selecting mink for fine black fur, a colony was developed in which 20% to 30% of the males were infertile. On analysis, many were found to suffer from orchitis as a result of the development of antisperm autoantibodies. In one study, 45/77 of the male mink were infertile at their first mating (primary infertility) at 10 months of age. The remaining mink progressively lost fertility over the next 3 years. Antisperm antibodies were present in both fertile and infertile black mink; however, antibody levels were low in those with primary infertility. Half of the infertile mink suffered from an orchitis characterized by an infiltration of lymphocytes, monocytes, plasma cells, and neutrophils. The germinal epithelium was replaced by macrophages. These animals developed a monocytic orchitis, and immune complexes were deposited along the basal lamina of the seminiferous tubules. Aspermatogenesis involving more than 50% of the seminiferous tubules was found in 87% of infertile mink, while 67% had a lymphocytic epididymitis. Thus aspermatogenesis without orchitis was most frequent in mink with primary infertility. Severe orchitis and antisperm antibodies were more prevalent in animals that developed infertility later in life.

Tung KSK, Ellis L, Teuscher C, et al. The black mink *(Mustela vison):* a natural model of immunologic male infertility. *J Exp Med.* 1981;154:1016–1032.

---

thymectomy. The locus that controls this phenotype *(Aod2)* has been mapped to chromosome 3. It colocalizes with *Idd3*, a gene linked to susceptibility to autoimmune type 1 diabetes mellitus (T1DM) in NOD mice. Lymphocytic infiltrates develop, as do autoantibodies against several ovarian proteins, especially those expressed on oocytes. Analysis indicates that one of the most important of these autoantigens is a 125-kDa protein called NLRP5 (NOD-like receptor family pyrin domain containing 5). NLRP5 is also known to be a major autoantigen in humans suffering from autoimmune polyglandular syndrome type 1 (APS-1) as a result of defective autoimmune regulator (AIRE) function. Immunization of mice with inhibin A generates neutralizing antibodies that result in an initial increase in fertility by stimulating follicle-stimulating hormone (FSH) production, followed by ovarian exhaustion and loss of fertility. EAO can also be induced in monkeys such as macaques. Using ZP3, immunized monkeys developed an ovarian lymphocytic infiltrate, but fertility was not impaired. A combination of T cells and autoantibodies appeared to cause the most damage.

Premature ovarian failure (POF) is a disease of women under 40 years of age. An underlying autoimmune response has been identified in about 20% of POF patients. It is often associated with subsequent autoimmune thyroiditis and adrenalitis and is an occasional component of the autoimmune polyglandular syndromes (see Fig. 6.4). POF can result in ovarian atrophy. It is characterized by inflammatory cell infiltration of developing ovarian follicles and the production of autoantibodies against multiple ovarian autoantigens, especially the steroidogenic enzymes, P450 side chain cleavage (a mitochondrial enzyme that converts cholesterol to pregnenolone), 17α-hydroxylase, and 3β-hydroxysteroid dehydrogenase. In addition, some patients may also make antibodies against FSH, gonadotrophin, ZP, NLRP5, α-enolase, or HSP90. Currently, there is no effective treatment for POF.

Autoallergy

The term *autoallergy* describes an autoimmune response that results in type I hypersensitivity. There are examples of this in humans where autoantibodies of the IgE class or self-reactive T cells may contribute to atopic dermatitis. Patients may develop chronic spontaneous urticaria by producing IgG autoantibodies directed against either IgE itself or against the mast cell IgE receptor FcεR1. When these autoantibodies bind, they crosslink the cell surface receptors and so trigger mast cell and basophil degranulation. This results in release of mast cell mediators, especially histamine, and the development of severe urticaria. Likewise, autoantibodies of the IgE class may be produced in diseases such as bullous pemphigoid, systemic lupus erythematosus, and lymphocytic thyroiditis.

AUTOALLERGY TO HORMONES

Autoimmune progesterone dermatitis and estrogen dermatitis are rare diseases that have been reported in women. These skin diseases are generally allergic in nature, with lesions such as intensely pruritic urticaria and papulovesicular eruptions. A similar disease has been reported in intact female dogs. The animals develop a hypersensitivity to endogenous progesterone or estrogen. The disease presents as a bilaterally symmetric, intensely pruritic, erythemic, and papular eruption. Its development usually coincides with estrus or pseudopregnancy. Corticosteroid treatment may have little effect, but testosterone may help.

In another form of autoimmunity to progesterone, Dogs, especially German Shepherd Dogs, may experience shortened estrus cycles, embryonic death, and abortion as a result of insufficient progesterone production by the corpus luteum. Investigations on short-cycling bitches showed that their progesterone levels were abnormally low. Out of 20 short-cycling bitches, 5 had detectable levels of serum IgE directed against progesterone (1 of 18 control bitches also had these antibodies). These autoantibodies may play a role in unexplained pregnancy failure in dogs.

AUTOALLERGY TO MILK PROTEINS

One of the most important examples of autoallergy occurs in dairy cattle when they make IgE autoantibodies against their own milk proteins (Fig. 9.3). This typically happens during the drying-off period at the end of lactation, when cessation of milking with continuing milk production results in a rise in intramammary pressure. As a result, milk proteins are forced into the bloodstream. In response to these self-antigens, some cows mount an IgE response. On subsequent exposure to these milk proteins, they may develop clinically significant allergic responses. Once an animal is sensitized to its own milk, the condition may recur in subsequent lactations. When this happens, these cows develop urticaria and respiratory distress. The urticaria varies in severity,

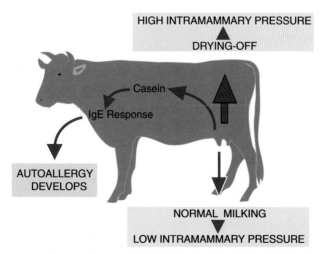

Fig. 9.3 The mechanism of bovine milk allergy. Raised intramammary pressure at drying off results in α-casein being forced into the bloodstream, where it acts as an autoallergen and triggers an allergic response. *IgE,* Immunoglobulin E.

but large, edematous plaques may develop on the skin of the face, perineum, and udder. Affected animals may develop dyspnea with tachypnea and severe coughing. In extreme cases, cows may die as a result of acute anaphylaxis.

In a survey in Upper New York State in 1968, Dr. Gordon Campbell determined that the annual incidence of milk allergy in cows in that region was 0.5%. The disease appeared either when the cows were being dried off at the end of lactation or at calving, when their udders were beginning to fill and become engorged. Campbell's survey indicated that this autoallergic response occurs predominantly in Channel Island breeds. In some Jersey herds, as many as 22% of the cows are affected. The appearance of urticaria coincides with milk letdown prior to milking. Other clinical signs include restlessness, evidence of pruritus with scratching, increased respiratory rate, edema of the eyelids, copious lacrimation, bilateral nasal discharge, excessive salivation, and difficulty swallowing. In terminal cases with severe dyspnea, some animals become obviously cyanotic. As urticaria develops, some cows pass a large volume of fluid feces. Some farmers believed that the allergy also caused cows to abort. Urticaria of the udders results in significant edema and very tender teats so that milking becomes difficult. Skin urticaria is revealed by the hair standing upright over an area of skin thickening. These urticarial areas may be itchy and painful. Angioedema may develop on the ears, muzzle, anus, vulva, and udder. Hemorrhage may also occur at urticarial and angioedematous sites. Some animals develop a generalized lymphadenopathy. Recovery after milking may be rapid, although the condition frequently recurs.

Campbell also demonstrated that affected cows responded to intracutaneous injection of their own diluted defatted milk by the development of large wheals. Thus 0.1 mL of milk diluted to 1:10,000 could elicit a visible reaction. They were equally sensitive to autologous and homologous bovine milk. Hypersensitivity to milk could also be transferred to the skin of an unsensitized cow by means of serum from a milk-allergic cow. Subsequent studies indicated that the allergen that caused this allergy was α-casein. As Campbell noted, the best way to manage this condition is to establish a milking routine that ensures milk is never allowed to engorge the udder and so prevents an excessive rise in intramammary pressure. Some of these affected cows have been successfully treated with antihistamines.

There are reports of women developing allergy-like symptoms associated with the milk ejection reflex during breastfeeding. Some veterinarians have reported encountering a similar condition in lactating mares and bitches.

Immune Contraception

Under some circumstances, it is desirable to reduce the size of animal populations without killing individuals. This may be accomplished by fertility control. Contraceptive vaccination is one technique that can do this. It is easily administered, cost effective, and efficacious in multiple species. Killing is irreversible, while vaccination is not. However, this method of contraception relies on inducing an autoimmune response in a recipient animal.

ZONA PELLUCIDA IMMUNIZATION

While there are many different potential targets for contraceptive vaccines, two have proven most practical. One such vaccine contains ZP3 glycoproteins. These are highly glycosylated proteins that form a matrix around the ovum and whose function is to bind sperm. Anti-ZP vaccines work by binding to these proteins and either blocking sperm-binding sites or causing structural changes that block sperm penetration. Studies have also shown that these antibodies may cause temporary or permanent ovarian destruction. This vaccination approach has the benefit of no hormonal side effects, and consequently, animal behavior is unaffected. The ZP proteins are conserved across different phyla, and one vaccine may be used in multiple species. ZP vaccination has also been studied in species such as horse, deer, rabbit, mice, and feral cats. There are, however, great variations in antibody levels, effectiveness, and duration between species and among individuals. Insofar as the vaccine must induce an autoimmune response, adjuvants are critical to its success.

In captive situations such as zoos, these vaccines have proven very effective. Most ungulates follow a consistent response pattern. After receiving a vaccine booster at 3 to 6 weeks, antibody levels peak at 1 to 3 months and maintain high levels for 8 months to 1 year. Contraception lasts for at least 12 months, so annual revaccination is appropriate.

GONADOTROPIN-RELEASING HORMONE IMMUNIZATION

The second successful type of contraceptive vaccine immunizes animals against gonadotropin-releasing hormone (GnRH). GnRH is a small, poorly immunogenic peptide. To make the vaccine work, multiple GnRH peptides are therefore conjugated to the large immunogenic carrier protein such as hemocyanin. The GnRH-hemocyanin conjugate is adjuvanted with a water-in-mineral oil emulsion.

GnRH secreted by the hypothalamus controls the production of FSH and luteinizing hormone (LH) and as a result, controls gamete production. Immunity to GnRH attenuates gamete production and secondary sexual behavior. GnRH vaccines have an advantage over ZP vaccines in that by reducing sex hormone production, they eliminate estrus and its associated misbehaviors. Several commercial GnRH vaccines are available for use in horses and pigs.

One such vaccine, GonaCon, has been developed as a reproduction inhibitor by the National Wildlife Research Center of the US Department of Agriculture. GonaCon induces antibodies that bind and neutralize GnRH and effectively blocks the release of FSH and LH from the pituitary. This in turn inhibits breeding and its behaviors in both males and females. GonaCon has induced contraception with a single dose for up to 5 years in domestic cats, pigs, wild horses, bison, and white-tailed deer. It is currently registered by the Environmental Protection Agency as a contraceptive for white-tailed deer and wild horses, thus effectively managing overabundant wildlife populations. (The vaccine is classified as a "restricted use pesticide"!) Tests showed that a single dose reduced fertility in urban white-tailed deer by 88% in the first year and 47% in the second. In adult mares and burros, it also inhibited sexual behavior. While working well in domestic species, GnRH vaccines encounter the same delivery difficulties as ZP vaccines when used in free-roaming wildlife.

GonaCon may also be used for the prevention of adrenocortical disease in domestic ferrets. The development of adrenal hyperplasia, adenomas, and adenocarcinomas in spayed ferrets results from continuous overproduction of LH due to a lack of gonadal feedback. Subcutaneous vaccination with a single dose of the GnRH vaccine generates antibodies to endogenous GnRH and suppresses its production. This in turn suppresses production and release of LH. This results in clinical remission of adrenocortical disease and can prevent its recurrence for up to 3 years.

If dogs are immunized with bovine or ovine LH, the autoantibodies produced may neutralize their own LH. As a result, the reproductive cycle is abolished in females, and testicular, epididymal, and prostatic atrophy occurs in males. Other experimental immunocontraceptive vaccines have been directed against prostaglandin F2α, reproductive steroids, and the LH receptor.

Production-Enhancing Vaccines

Many companies have developed vaccines that can enhance animal production. These vaccines commonly interfere with normal hormone production or reproductive behavior by inducing an autoimmune response. Thus the vaccine that neutralizes production of GnRH effectively lowers testosterone levels in males. This results in improved meat quality, faster growth, and reduced aggression by bulls. This vaccine is also used to reduce aggressive behavior in male pigs and block the production of androstenone, the steroid that contributes to boar taint. Similar vaccines may be used to treat benign prostatic hyperplasia in dogs.

Sheep immunized with polyandroalbumin (androstenedione-7-carboxyethyl thioester linked to human serum albumin) produce about 23% more lambs than untreated sheep. These vaccines are marketed under the names Androvax, Fecundin, and Ovastim. Ewes are normally given two doses of this vaccine before mating. These vaccines induce autoantibodies that reduce serum androstenedione levels. This temporarily blocks ovulation so that when the effect wears off, a rebound occurs, and the ewe produces more mature ova. If bred at this time, the number of multiple births will be increased. The vaccine is used in young, healthy ewes of breeds that are capable of raising the increased number of lambs.

Sources of Additional Information

Autoimmune Orchitis

Carmichael LGL. Antisperm responses in male dogs with chronic *Brucella canis* infections. *Am J Vet Res.* 1984;45:274–281.

Naito M, Terayama H, Hirai S, et al. Experimental autoimmune orchitis as a model of immunological male infertility. *Med Mol Morphol.* 2012;45:185–189.

Papa FO, Alvarenga MA, Lopes MD, et al. Infertility of autoimmune origin in a stallion. *Equine Vet J.* 1990;22:145–146.

Parsonson IM, Winter AJ, McEntee K. Allergic epididymo-orchitis in guinea pigs and bulls. *Vet Pathol.* 1971;8:333–351.

Autoimmune Oophoritis

Bagavant H, Sharp C, Kurth B, et al. Induction and immunohistology of autoimmune ovarian disease in Cynomolgus macaques (*Macaca fascicularis*). *Am J Pathol.* 2002;160:141–149.

Domniz N, Meirow D. Premature ovarian insufficiency and autoimmune diseases. *Best Pract Res Clin Obs Gyn.* 2019;60:42–55.

Autoallergy to Milk Proteins

Campbell SG. Milk allergy, an autoallergic disease of cattle. *Cornell Vet.* 1970;60:684–721.

Immune Contraception

Eade JA, Roberston ID, James CM. Contraceptive potential of porcine and feline zona pellucida A, B, and C subunits in domestic cats. *Reproduction.* 2009;137:913–922.

Fayrer-Hoskin R. Controlling animal populations using antifertility vaccines. *Reprod Dom Anim.* 2008;43:179–185.

Fayrer-Hoskin R, Dookwah HD, Brandon CI. Immunocontrol in dogs. *Anim Repro Sci.* 2000:60–61:365-373.

Kirkpatrick JF, Lyda RO, Frank KM. Contraceptive vaccines for wildlife: a review. *Am J Repro Immunol.* 2011;66:40–50.

Krachudel J, Bondzio A, Einspanier R, et al. Luteal insufficiency in bitches as a consequence of an autoimmune response against progesterone? *Theriogenology.* 2013. doi:10.1016/j.theriogenology.2014.02.025.

Autoimmune Skin Diseases

Immune-mediated skin diseases driven by either autoantibodies or self-reactive T cells are among those most commonly encountered by veterinarians. For many of these diseases, the autoantigens have been identified. However, there remain others where the pathogenesis remains unclear. The reader will therefore encounter many skin diseases where Witebsky's postulates have never been met. They are included herein because of circumstantial evidence. This includes a clear inherited predisposition often associated with genes in the major histocompatibility complex (MHC); a histopathologic presentation characterized by infiltration with lymphocytes, especially T cells, B cells, plasma cells, and macrophages; and by a positive clinical response to immunosuppressive therapy.

Like other autoimmune diseases, diverse factors may predispose to these diseases. These can include not only genetic background but also environmental factors, epigenetic modifications, infectious triggers, molecular mimicry, development of neoantigens, and gender predispositions. It is also important to point out that while the autoimmune response itself is the cause of primary disease, there are also many examples of secondary autoimmunity where the autoimmune processes appear to be a consequence of the initial lesions and simply serve to perpetuate existing tissue damage. Some diseases such as cutaneous lupus erythematosus (CLE) may not even be autoimmune in nature, although they are clearly autoinflammatory.

Blistering Diseases

Many important autoimmune diseases result from the destruction of the desmosomes that bind skin cells together. This destruction causes the skin cells to separate from their neighbors, and as a result pustules (blisters or vesicles) form in the epidermis. Cells fall apart, and blisters form within the skin and mucous membranes. This process of cell separation is called acantholysis. Dermatologists use the terms *pemphigus* or *pemphigoid* to describe these diseases, after the Greek word *pemphix* meaning "a blister."

Multiple blistering autoimmune skin diseases have been described in humans, dogs, horses, and cats. Known as the pemphigus complex, they are classified according to the depth of the lesions within the skin. They are primary autoimmune diseases that result from the production of autoantibodies against desmosomal proteins in the epidermis or at the dermal-epidermal junctions. Desmosomes maintain the structural integrity of the skin by binding cells together and anchoring intracellular cytoskeletal filaments. Desmosomes may be disrupted by mutations, by infectious agents, or more commonly, by autoantibodies.

It is unclear just how autoantibodies disrupt desmosomes. Humans with pemphigus make autoantibodies against at least 50 different skin proteins. Among these proteins, the most important are members of the cadherin family called desmogleins. These are major components of the desmosomes. The most important are desmoglein-3 (Dsg-3) and Dsg-1. It has long been assumed that binding of antibodies to Dsg-3 and in some cases Dsg-1 was the critical step in causing acantholysis; however, desmogleins are not the only autoantigens found in desmosomes. Other major antigens include the desmocollins and plakins. Autoantibodies are also made against keratinocyte surface receptors such as the nicotinic acetylcholine receptors. Another theory is that the antibodies trigger keratinocyte apoptosis. The dying cells round up (acantholysis) and in doing so, they pull apart from each other. (Acantholytic cells are characterized by a round shape, eosinophilic cytoplasm, and large dark nuclei surrounded by a light blue halo.)

Antimitochondrial antibodies may also play an important role by releasing damaging oxidants, while other autoantibodies stimulate keratinocyte secretion of cytokines such as tumor necrosis factor-alpha (TNFα), interleukin-1-beta (IL1β), and IL6. These cytokines in turn can activate macrophages that release the enzyme caspase-8 that can then cleave Dsg-3. None of these theories are mutually exclusive, and it is likely that multiple autoantibodies collectively disrupt the desmosomes.

The autoimmune blistering diseases are divided into two major groups. One is the pemphigus group in which autoantibodies target desmosomal proteins and as a result, cause a loss of adhesion between keratinocytes within the epidermis. The second is the pemphigoid group, where the autoantibodies target proteins in the hemidesmosomes located at the dermal-epidermal junction and as a result, separate the epidermis from the underlying dermis.

Pemphigus Group

The pemphigus group of diseases is associated with the development of flaccid vesicles, pustules, and erosions on the skin and mucous membranes (Fig. 10.1). These vesicles may be very superficial and rupture readily, while others form deep within the epidermis, where they remain intact for longer.

SUPERFICIAL PEMPHIGUS

Canine Pemphigus Foliaceus

Pemphigus foliaceus (PF; from the Latin *folium*, "a leaf") is the most common form of pemphigus in dogs and the most common autoimmune disease of dogs. PF has also been described in

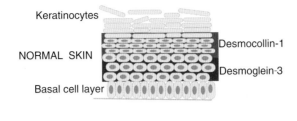

Keratinocytes

NORMAL SKIN

Basal cell layer

Desmocollin-1

Desmoglein-3

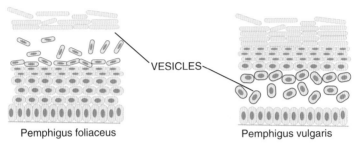

VESICLES

Pemphigus foliaceus

Pemphigus vulgaris

Fig. 10.1 The pemphigus group of autoimmune skin diseases are conveniently divided into two major subgroups based on the depth of the vesicles that form. The diseases that form shallow vesicles are typified by pemphigus foliaceus, while the diseases that form deep vesicles are typified by pemphigus vulgaris.

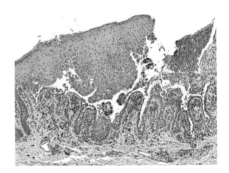

Fig. 10.2 A skin section from a case of canine pemphigus foliaceus. Note the subcorneal location of the cell-filled vesicle (pustule). (Courtesy of Dr J. Mansell.)

humans, cats, sheep, goats, and horses. In dogs, it is a superficial pustular disease in which the lesions develop in the subcorneal epidermis as a result of the actions of immunoglobulin G (IgG) autoantibodies directed against keratinocyte desmosomal proteins. As a result, the desmosomes break down, and the keratinocytes separate. Because they form so close to the surface, PF blisters are very fragile and rupture readily, leaving crusting, shallow erosions rather than ulcers. When they are intact, they fill with inflammatory cells, primarily neutrophils, and are described as pustules (Fig. 10.2). IgG is the dominant serum autoantibody, but in some cases, the subclass may be restricted to IgG2 or IgG4. In humans, the major autoantigens in PF are desmogleins. In dogs, however, the major PF autoantigen is a desmosomal protein called desmocollin-1 (Dsc-1). While usually a primary disease, some cases of canine PF may be secondary to the use of antibiotics such as trimethoprim-sulfadiazine, oxacillin, cephalexin, and ampicillin, as well as to a topical flea control product containing amitraz and metaflumizone. Some of these secondary cases may result from the binding of drug thiol groups to keratinocyte membranes resulting in the generation of neoantigens.

Clinical Disease. The average age of onset of canine PF is 6 years. There is no significant gender predisposition. It is most frequently diagnosed in Bearded Collies, Akitas, Newfoundlands, Schipperkes, Doberman Pinschers, and Finnish Spitz. Other susceptible breeds include English Cocker Spaniels, Chow Chows, Shar-Peis, and Australian Shepherds.

Superficial pustules usually appear first on the dorsum of the nose, nasal planum, periocular skin, and ears (Fig. 10.3A). The pustules tend to be bilateral and symmetric. As they spread, other affected sites may include the trunk, hind limbs, footpads, mucocutaneous junctions, and muzzle. PF lesions rarely develop on mucosal surfaces such as in the oral cavity. PF pustules are fragile and rupture easily. As a result, they rapidly develop into crusting erosions, and alopecia develops on the trunk, inner pinnae, face, and footpads over the next 3 to 12 months. Footpad lesions with hyperkeratosis develop in a high proportion of cases. Pruritus is not usually a feature of canine PF, but secondary bacterial infections, anorexia, fever, and depression may occur in dogs with widespread lesions.

IgA pemphigus (also called panepidermal pustular pemphigus) is a variant of PF. In these cases, the pustules are found in the granular and upper spinous layers of the epidermis. IgA is the primary autoantibody class, and Dsc-1 and Dsc-3 have been identified as the important autoantigens.

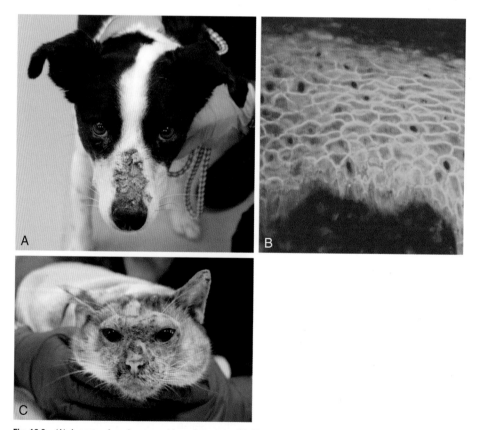

Fig. 10.3 (A) A case of canine pemphigus foliaceus. (B) Direct immunofluorescence of a section of normal dog skin that had been incubated in serum from a dog with pemphigus vulgaris. Note the chicken-wire staining pattern of the intercellular cement. (C) A case of feline pemphigus foliaceus. (A, Courtesy of Dr. Robert Kennis.) (B, Courtesy of Dr. K. Credille.) (C, Courtesy of Dr. Robert Kennis.)

Diagnosis and Treatment. Diagnosis of PF must be confirmed by histopathology. Acantholytic keratinocytes are found in impression smears of the bullae. Neutrophils and occasional eosinophils are also found in large numbers within the blister fluid. Histology in the early stages shows subcorneal vesicles. However, these develop into subcorneal pustules. Direct fluorescent antibody (FA) or immunoperoxidase staining will detect the presence of immunoglobulins in the epidermis, bound to the intercellular cement in a chicken-wire pattern (see Fig. 10.3B). Indirect FA may be used to test the serum of affected animals for its ability to bind to mouse skin sections or to cultured keratinocytes in a similar pattern. Indirect FA is, however, considered unreliable since its sensitivity very much depends on the cell substrate used, and free antibody levels may be very low.

Immunosuppression is the treatment of choice for PF. Oral prednisolone or prednisolone in conjunction with azathioprine is widely used. A prednisolone-cyclosporine combination also appears to be highly effective, and the prognosis is fair to good (Box 10.1).

Pemphigus erythematosus is a mild localized variant of PF that shares many features with CLE (see Chapter 15). Indeed, some dogs with pemphigus erythematosus may have antinuclear antibodies in their serum. This variant is commonly seen in German Shepherd Dogs, Collies, and Shetland Sheepdogs. The pustules, erosions, and crusts are restricted to the face, nose, and ears. Nasal and periocular depigmentation may occur, while erosion and ulceration are obvious. Histopathology of the pustules is similar to PF; however, the presence of a lichenoid interface dermatitis also resembles that seen in CLE. Immunofluorescence assays on biopsies show intercellular immunoglobulins as found in PF plus basement membrane fluorescence as found in CLE.

Feline Pemphigus Foliaceus

Feline PF is similar to the canine disease, although much less common. There is no apparent breed predisposition. The average age of onset is 5 years. Subcorneal acantholytic pustules develop, especially on the footpads and buccal mucosa. Pustules rupture easily so that ulcers, crusts, and erosions primarily affect the pinnae and claw folds. Many affected cats are febrile and anorexic, while some may be pruritic. The lesions are usually mild, localized, bilateral, and symmetric (see Fig. 10.3C). Lesions also commonly develop around the nipples and nailbeds. Cats with PF have detectible antikeratinocyte IgG, but the autoantigens in this species are yet to be characterized. The diagnosis of PF is confirmed by cytology and histology. The prognosis is good under glucocorticoid monotherapy, but treatment may be prolonged, and there is a tendency for these cats to relapse.

BOX 10.1 ■ Fogo Selvagem

Brazilian endemic pemphigus foliaceus, otherwise known as fogo selvagem (Portuguese for "wildfire"), is an autoimmune skin disease resulting from the production of IgG4 autoantibodies against Dsg-1. Its name refers to the severe stinging or burning sensation in affected skin that develops after ultraviolet exposure. It occurs in rural endemic foci, primarily in Brazil, but occasional cases have been reported from other tropical South American countries. The lesions develop primarily on the scalp, face, neck, and upper trunk of its victims. It appears to be associated with the bites of hematophagous insects such as black flies (*Simulium*), mosquitoes, sandflies, and midges. Both IgG4 and IgE autoantibodies from affected patients cross-react with salivary antigens from sandflies. Thus it is believed to result from an initial IgE response to the biting fly salivary proteins that then spreads to become an IgG4 response against skin Dsg-1. Many healthy adults living in the endemic areas have antibodies directed against Dsg-1. It is likely that while many develop these antibodies and an allergic response to sandfly bites, only a genetically predisposed minority go on to develop the autoimmune disease. This susceptibility appears to be primarily associated with genes controlling B-cell responses. Fogo selvagem has not yet been recorded in domestic animals.

Quian Y, Culton DA, Jeong JS, et al. Non-infectious environmental antigens as a trigger for the initiation of autoimmune skin disease. *Autimmun Rev.* 2016;15:923-930.

Equine Pemphigus Foliaceus

PF is also the most common autoimmune disease in horses. It appears that Appaloosas may be predisposed, but this is not consistent. Affected animals cover a very wide age range, from 6 months to 25 years. Animals develop multifocal lesions. Because of the fragility of the pustules, they readily rupture, so that generalized crusting, scaling, and alopecia develop. Lesions usually begin on the face or legs but if left untreated may spread to become generalized over a few months. Sometimes animals develop ventral edema as well as systemic signs such as fever, depression, and lethargy. Some of these lesions may be painful or pruritic. Treatment options include corticosteroids, azathioprine, and pentoxifylline.

DEEP PEMPHIGUS

The most important form of deep pemphigus in domestic species is called pemphigus vulgaris (PV). There is also a very rare variant of PV, pemphigus vegetans, that occurs in dogs.

Canine Pemphigus Vulgaris

The most severe blistering disease in middle-aged dogs is the rare disease PV (Fig. 10.4). PV has also been reported in cats, horses, and a llama.

In PV, deep epidermal bullae develop around the mucocutaneous junctions, especially the nose, lips, eyes, prepuce, and anus, as well as on the inner surface of the ear. Unlike PF, PV also affects the oral mucosa, including the gingiva, palate, and tongue. Discrete, deep, nonhealing ulcers develop on the lips. Histologic examination of intact bullae shows acantholysis in the suprabasal region of the lower epidermis.

In canine and human PV, the major autoantigen is the desmosomal protein Dsg-3. T cells also participate in the pathogenesis of PV, thus helper T type 1 (Th1) cells mediate the proinflammatory immune responses through interferon-gamma (IFNγ). In addition, Th2-derived cytokines such as IL4 promote the proliferation of B cells, antibody production, and immunoglobulin class switching. Th17 cells activated by this cytokine mixture also contribute to the inflammatory process and damage skin cells.

Panepidermal pustular pemphigus (pemphigus vegetans) is a very rare variant of PV reported in dogs. It is characterized by a hyperkeratotic and papillomatous proliferation of the base of the bullae that occurs on healing. The lesions become verrucous, or warty. They tend to affect the perioral and perianal areas as well as large skin folds. They readily become secondarily infected. The prime autoantigen in this form of the disease is Dsg-1.

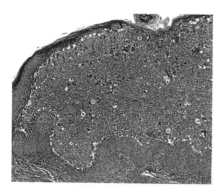

Fig. 10.4 A section of an oral lesion of pemphigus vulgaris in a dog. Note the cleft formation at the base of the epidermis accompanied by extensive cellular infiltration. (Courtesy of Dr J. Mansell.)

OTHER TYPES OF PEMPHIGUS

A topical ectoparasiticide containing metaflumizone and amitraz has been associated with the development of an acantholytic pustular dermatitis resembling PF in treated dogs. One or two applications were sufficient to induce the disease. Some dogs developed the disease at the application site, while others developed generalized lesions. Antikeratinocyte IgG was detected in the epidermis of 8 of 19 cases, while serum antikeratinocyte IgG was detected in 10 of 14 cases; 11 of 14 dogs had detectable antibodies to Dsc-1. Thus the lesions closely resembled naturally occurring PF (Box 10.2).

A reliable diagnosis of pemphigus can only be made by histopathology. Direct immunofluorescence assays on pemphigus lesions reveal immunoglobulins deposited on the intercellular cement in a typical chicken-wire pattern (see Fig. 10.3B). It is important to differentiate among the forms of pemphigus for prognostic reasons. PV has a poor prognosis; treatment tends to be unsatisfactory, and the lesions are persistent. In contrast, PF is milder, and the results of treatment are usually more satisfactory. Treatment primarily involves the use of corticosteroids. In refractory cases, azathioprine, cyclophosphamide, chlorambucil, or cyclosporine may be of benefit. As with other autoimmune diseases, skin lesions often recur when treatment is stopped.

Paraneoplastic Pemphigus

Paraneoplastic pemphigus occurs in humans and has been recorded in three dogs, a cat, and possibly in a horse. It is not related to either PF or PV. Instead, it is a manifestation of an autoimmune syndrome called paraneoplastic autoimmune multiorgan syndrome (PAMS) that develops in association with lymphoid or solid tumors. PAMS targets not only the skin but also many other body surfaces, including the bronchial epithelium and the oral mucosa. Some cases resemble PV, and autoantibodies against skin antigens such as Dsg-3 and plakins may be present. Treatment must be directed toward removal of the tumor.

Pemphigoid Group

This group of blistering diseases results from the development of autoantibodies against structural proteins and subepidermal adherence molecules found deep within the skin at the dermal-epidermal junction. The epidermis and the mucosal epithelia are attached to the underlying basement membrane by structures called hemidesmosomes. Hemidesmosomes consist of a complex of intra- and extracellular proteins (Fig. 10.5). Mutations in the genes encoding these proteins can result in defective hemidesmosomes and result in hereditary epidermolysis bullosa. These proteins are also the targets of autoantibodies. As a result, several distinct subepidermal blistering diseases develop

---

BOX 10.2 ■ Walnut Antigens and Pemphigus Vulgaris: A Case of Hit-and-Run?

One possible mechanism of inducing autoimmunity is that an inciting environmental antigen may trigger an autoantibody response and then leave. When monoclonal antibodies directed against Dsg-3, the autoantigen of pemphigus vulgaris, were tested against a panel of possible allergens (including insects, foods, fungi, and pollens), they were found to cross-react with the major allergens of walnut (Jug r 2). Sera from patients with pemphigus vulgaris contained low levels of walnut-specific antibodies. It has been suggested that some human patients may be initiated by sensitization to walnuts but that the subsequent antibody response may then be sustained by Dsg-3.

Lin ML, Moran TP, Peng B, et al. Walnut antigens can trigger autoantibody development in patients with pemphigus vulgaris through a "hit-and-run" mechanism. *J Allergy Clin Immunol.* 2019;144. doi. org/10.1016/j.jaci.2019.04.020

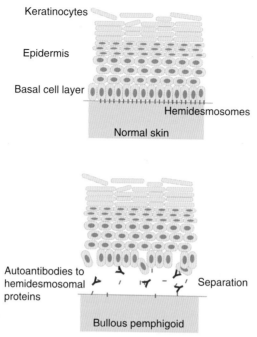

Keratinocytes

Epidermis

Basal cell layer

Hemidesmosomes

Normal skin

Autoantibodies to hemidesmosomal proteins

Separation

Bullous pemphigoid

Fig. 10.5 The pathogenesis of the pemphigoid group of diseases. Autoantibodies directed against the hemidesmosomes that bind basal epidermal cells to the basement membrane result in their separation and vesicle formation in the subepidermis.

in dogs and other domestic species. They include bullous pemphigoid (BP), linear IgA dermatosis, and epidermolysis bullosa acquisita (EBA). All are rare.

CANINE BULLOUS PEMPHIGOID

BP is a blistering skin disease of dogs that clinically resembles PV. Collies, Shetland Sheepdogs, and Doberman Pinschers appear to be predisposed to it. It has also been described in humans, pigs, horses, and cats. Affected dogs develop tense subepidermal blisters and erosions that may also involve the mucous membranes. Oral lesions are present in about 80% of cases, especially in Collies. The lesions develop on the lips, oral mucosa, axillae, inguinal regions, footpads, and concave surfaces of the pinnae. However, the disease differs from PV in that the bullae develop in the subepidermis (and are therefore much less likely to rupture) (Fig. 10.6). They tend to be filled with fibrin as well as mononuclear cells or eosinophils, and they heal spontaneously. BP results from the production of IgG and IgE autoantibodies directed against two glycoproteins called BP180 and BP230. These are components of the hemidesmosome attachment plaques on basal cells. BP180 (BP antigen 2) is a transmembrane type XVII collagen. BP230 or dystonin (also called BP antigen 1) is a protein of the plakin family. The presence of IgG bound to these basement membrane antigens may be demonstrated by a direct immunofluorescence assay. This characteristically shows intense linear staining along the basement membrane. T cells also participate in the disease processes. For example, local Th17 cells activate neutrophils resulting in inflammation and tissue damage. Likewise, regulatory T (Treg) cells are dysregulated in BP permitting Th2 cells to produce IL4 and so further promote autoantibody formation. The prognosis of BP is usually poor, but mild cases may recover after treatment with corticosteroids. More commonly, aggressive treatment such as high doses of prednisolone, supplemented if necessary with cyclophosphamide, azathioprine, or

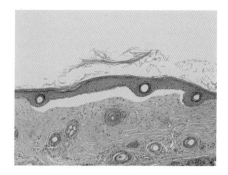

Fig. 10.6 Histology of an extensive subepidermal vesicle in a cat. This may be a case of bullous pemphigoid. 10 × magnification. H&E stain. (Courtesy of Dr. Dominique Wiener.)

chlorambucil, may be needed. Some dogs may develop a BP-like disease in response to autoantibodies against the basement membrane protein laminin-5.

LINEAR IGA DERMATOSIS

A variant of BP is characterized by the deposition of IgA in the lamina lucida of the skin basement membrane. Linear IgA dermatosis has been recorded in Dachshunds. The disease presents with pruritic pustular and papular lesions, resembling pyoderma, with eosinophil-filled subepidermal bullae. They develop around the mouth, nose, ears, and paws. The target autoantigen is a form of collagen XVII. The drug dapsone has been recommended as the specific treatment for this disease.

EPIDERMOLYSIS BULLOSA ACQUISITA

Epidermolysis bullosa describes a family of inherited diseases that result from mutations encoding the genes for the structural proteins in the hemidesmosomes that link basal keratinocytes to the epithelial basement membrane. EBA, as its name implies, is an acquired version of the same lesion caused by autoimmune attack. EBA is a generalized skin disease characterized by severe blistering and ulcerative lesions. The skin layers separate at the dermal epidermal junction. This is accompanied by a neutrophil infiltration in the superficial dermis. This may eventually result in microabscess formation. The bullae rapidly rupture and ulcerate. Dogs develop generalized urticaria, oral ulceration, and eventually cutaneous sloughing, especially of the footpads. Secondary changes include deep ulceration, necrosis, and bacterial infections.

Affected animals make IgA and IgG autoantibodies against the distal end of the anchoring fibrils of the lower basement membrane (lamina densa). These autoantibodies are specific for the amino terminal globular noncollagenous NC1 domain of type VII collagen and are distinctly different from those responsible for BP. Minor epitopes have been detected on other collagen domains such as NC2 or the central collagenous domain.

Clinical Disease, Diagnosis, and Treatment

Most dogs with EBA are young (median 1.2 years of age), and there is a clear preponderance of males. Great Danes appear to be predisposed. Lesions may begin as urticarial erythematous patches that develop into vesicles and ulcerate. Tense vesicles, deep erosions, and ulcers are common. Epidermal sloughing occurs in areas where the skin is under tension or friction, such as external pressure points. Lesions may also be present in the oral cavity, nasal planum, pinnae, axillae, and footpads. A localized variant of the disease has been observed in a German Short haired Pointer.

Histopathology shows a neutrophilic perivascular dermatitis, but eosinophils or monocytes are also present. Lymphocyte and plasma cell numbers are highly variable. The subepidermal vesicles may be empty of cells but can contain small numbers of neutrophils, eosinophils, fibrin, or blood.

Glucocorticoid therapy, either alone or in conjunction with azathioprine or dapsone is the recommended treatment. Secondary bacterial infection may cause complications, and the disease may recur.

MUCOUS MEMBRANE PEMPHIGOID

Yet another variant of BP targets mucous membranes. Mucous membrane pemphigoid is a chronic subepidermal blistering disease of dogs, cats, and humans. In humans, it is also known as cicatricial pemphigoid because of its tendency to cause scarring when the lesions heal. It is characterized by a combination of vesicles, ulcers, and scarring that primarily affects mucous membranes and mucocutaneous junctions, especially the mouth, nose, eyes, genitalia, or anus. It is associated with the development of autoantibodies directed against multiple autoantigens located in the basement membrane region. The major autoantigen is found on the NC16A domain of collagen XVII (BP180). Some dogs may have antibodies that bind to the carboxy terminus of collagen XVII. Minor autoantigens include laminin-332, integrin $\alpha6/\beta4$, BP230, and sometimes collagen VII. The mechanisms of blister formation remain unclear. Mucous membrane pemphigoid has also been recorded in cats. In this species, the autoantibodies appear to target laminin-5.

Clinical Disease, Diagnosis, and Treatment

German Shepherd Dogs are overrepresented in canine mucous membrane pemphigoid cases. The average age of onset is about 6 years. Animals present with symmetric skin lesions (i.e., erosions and ulcers associated with mucocutaneous junctions). The disease is nonpruritic and slowly progressive, with crusting vesicles and scarring. The lesions are primarily found around the mouth, but others are periocular, nasal, genital, and within the pinnae. Lesions develop on the lips, gingiva, hard and soft palate, oral mucosa, and tongue. Nasal planum, eyelids, genitalia (prepuce, scrotum, vulval margin), and perianal sites are also involved.

Histopathology shows the presence of subepidermal vesicles as a result of dermal-epidermal separation. The blister fluid may contain no cells or small numbers of eosinophils, neutrophils, or mononuclear cells. There is variable dermal inflammation. Mucosal hyperplasia is common. Immunofluorescence assays on skin biopsies show the presence of IgG (and in some cases IgM or IgA) or C3 at the dermal-epidermal junction.

Treatment depends on disease severity and location of the lesions. Thus oral disease tends to be less severe than disease in dogs with eye, genital, respiratory, or upper gastrointestinal tract lesions. Low-risk dogs may receive topical glucocorticoids, perhaps together with oral glucocorticoids as well as doxycycline and niacinamide or dapsone. It is important to avoid the scarring caused by this disease, so the high-risk group should also receive more potent immunosuppressives such as azathioprine or cyclophosphamide. The prognosis is not good, and relapses are common.

ACQUIRED JUNCTIONAL EPIDERMOLYSIS BULLOSA

A subepidermal blistering dermatosis has been described in humans, dogs, and cats in which autoantibodies are directed against laminin-332 in the basement membrane. Laminin-332 is an important component of the epithelial basement membrane, since it plays a role not only in adhesion but also in wound healing and tumor invasion. It consists of a polymeric protein complex, and its components can serve as target antigens in mucous membrane pemphigoid as well as bullous systemic lupus erythematosus. The skin blistering and ulceration in these cases is associated with microscopic subepidermal vesiculation. The canine disease is complex, since it can present as one of at least three phenotypes, One resembles EBA, one resembles mucous membrane pemphigoid, and the third resembles BP.

Melanocyte Diseases

Melanocytes are the pigment cells found in the skin, oral mucosa, eye, and sometimes the meninges. Under some circumstances, they are subjected to autoimmune attack by cytotoxic T cells. As a result of their destruction, tissues become pale and unpigmented.

VITILIGO

Vitiligo is a chronic condition that manifests itself as a patchy whitening of the skin and hair. (The origins of the term vitiligo are unclear but are most likely from the Latin *vitium,* "a blemish.") Vitiligo occurs in dogs, cats, and horses in addition to humans. It appears to be an autoimmune disease resulting from the production of antibodies to melanin and related pigments. Autoantibodies to melanin are commonly present in humans and dogs with vitiligo; however, natural killer (NK) cells and cytotoxic CD8+ cells have also been implicated in its pathogenesis.

　　While uncommon in dogs, Rottweilers, Doberman Pinschers, and Collies appear to be predisposed to vitiligo. It is rarely seen in cats, in which Siamese appear to be predisposed. In horses, it has been reported in multiple breeds, including Gelderlands, Spanish Thoroughbreds, and Belgians. In Arabians it is sufficiently common to be called Arabian fading syndrome or pinky syndrome.

　　Vitiligo develops in young adult dogs. Multifocal lesions appear first on the face, especially the gingiva and lips. They may then spread to involve the nasal planum, oral cavity, pinnae, and muzzle (Fig. 10.7). Depigmentation may also occur in the footpads, scrotum, trunk, and limbs. Generalized depigmentation has also been reported. In cats, the nasal planum, periocular area, and footpads are usually affected. In horses too, depigmentation first occurs on the muzzle, lips, and periocular areas.

　　The autoantibodies are directed primarily against the melanocyte-specific enzyme tyrosinase as well as two tyrosinase-related proteins (TRP) 1 and 2 and several minor proteins. Antibodies to a melanocyte-specific 85-kDa protein have also been described in dogs, cats, and horses. These antibodies damage melanocytes in vitro either through complement-mediated lysis or by antibody-dependent cellular cytotoxicity (ADCC). Cytotoxic T cells are directed against a melanocyte cell-surface 22-kDa antigen called Melan A, suggesting that this too may be a key target in the cytotoxic process.

　　Histopathology shows a loss of melanocytes in the epidermis and/or hair follicles, although the epithelial architecture remains normal. There may be pigmentary incontinence, with the escape of

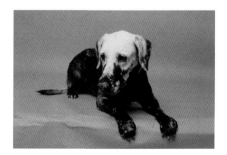

Fig. 10.7　A case of leukotrichia and vitiligo. (Courtesy of Dr Robert Kennis.)

melanin granules into the intercellular spaces. In active cases, there may also be local infiltration with mononuclear cells.

Vitiligo is a cosmetic disease. Severe immunosuppression such as glucocorticoid therapy is rarely justified. Milder treatments that have been applied with some success include the use of psoralens and careful irradiation with ultraviolet light.

UVEODERMATOLOGIC SYNDROME

This is an uncommon depigmenting syndrome that occurs in young to middle-aged dogs. It has been discussed previously in connection with the development of inflammatory lesions in the uvea of the eye (see Fig. 8.4). Normally, the eye lesions and visual impairment develop first. Eventually, however, skin lesions also develop. The disease results from a T-cell attack on the tyrosinase and glycoprotein gp100 in melanocytes. As a result, affected dogs develop skin and hair abnormalities. These include leukoderma and leukotrichia. Lesions commonly develop first on the face and head. They tend to be bilaterally symmetric. They often involve the eyelids, nasal planum, periorbital skin, lips, scrotum, vulva, and footpads. Alopecia may also develop on the dorsal muzzle. Erythema develops and then progresses to crusting and ulceration in the depigmented areas. The lesions are both painful and pruritic.

Skin biopsies show a lichenoid dermatitis and a mononuclear cell infiltration consisting mainly of macrophages (Fig. 10.8). This results in a partial or complete loss of melanocytes. Pigmentary incontinence (melanophagia) may be obvious when melanin granules initially escape into the tissues. Systemic treatment with glucocorticoids may reduce the inflammation. Additional immunosuppression with cyclosporine and/or azathioprine is also beneficial. The disease should be treated aggressively since the eye lesions can cause blindness. Short-term remissions may occur, but so do relapses.

In Akitas experimentally immunized with the antigen tyrosinase, vitiligo and alopecia developed after about 8 weeks and persisted for several months. After 3 months, the degree of hair loss decreased, while the areas of vitiligo enlarged. The disease in Akitas is associated with an increased frequency of the MHC allele DLA-DQA1*00201.

Hair Follicle Diseases

Hair follicles house many of the skin commensals since they provide a sheltered, lipid-rich environment. The presence of these organisms together with local immune privilege make follicles susceptible to autoimmune attack should this immune privilege collapse. Three canine autoimmune skin diseases target hair follicles, resulting in their destruction and consequent alopecia. These three diseases are alopecia areata (AA), sebaceous adenitis (SA), and pseudopelade (Fig. 10.9).

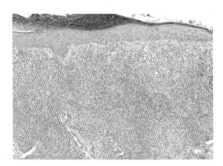

Fig. 10.8 A lichenoid infiltration in a case of uveodermatologic syndrome. Note the band of densely packed lymphocytes in the subepidermis. Subepidermal lichenoid (bandlike) inflammation of lymphocytes, plasma cells, and histiocytes. There is moderate epidermal hyperplasia and a serocellular crust on the surface. 20 × magnification. H&E stain. (Courtesy of Dr Dominique Wiener.)

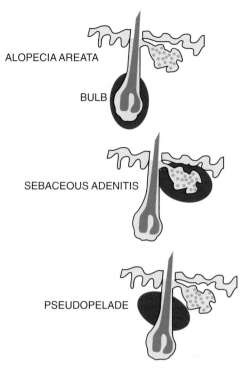

Fig. 10.9 The three major forms of hair follicle diseases differ in the location of autoimmune attack within the follicle.

ALOPECIA AREATA

AA is an uncommon T-cell–mediated disease characterized by gross noninflammatory hair loss. It has been reported in humans, other primates, dogs, cats, horses, mice, rats, and cattle. It is usually patchy and localized and can occur on any haired skin. Some cases may involve the loss of all body hair (alopecia universalis).

Anagen hair follicles normally possesses immunologic privilege in the region between the bulge and the bulb. Active suppressive mechanisms limit local MHC class Ia expression as well as NK cell and macrophage activity in this region. The low expression of MHC molecules appears to be linked to local production of transforming growth factor-beta 1 (TGFβ1) and α-melanocyte-stimulating hormone. These two cytokines suppress IFNγ production. This in turn downregulates MHC class Ia expression and antigen presentation. As pointed out earlier, hair follicles are home to much of the skin microbiota. It is possible that immune privilege within hair follicles may be initiated in part by the immunosuppressive effects of these commensals.

Immunologic privilege is, however, somewhat relative and can collapse. Once privilege collapses, the hair follicles are rapidly invaded by cytotoxic T cells as well as NK cells that proceed to destroy the bulb and hence stop hair growth. These diseases may be self-limiting, and it is possible that the eventual restoration of hair growth may be due to a gradual recovery of this immune privilege.

AA is a chronic, nonscarring skin disease that affects anagen (actively growing) hair follicles. Hair growth normally cycles through different stages, while AA interferes with these cycles. While clinically noninflammatory, affected hair follicles are infiltrated with cytotoxic CD8+ T cells as well as dendritic cells (Langerhans cells) (Fig. 10.10). Local mast cells may also be activated. There are

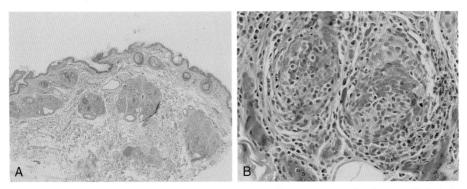

Fig. 10.10 Alopecia areata in a dog. (A) Low-power (4 ×) view of the skin showing the absence of hair shafts in almost all the follicles. (B) High-power (40 ×) view of the hair bulbs showing the lymphocytic infiltration. H&E stain. (Courtesy of Dr. Dominique Wiener.)

few eosinophils and fewer neutrophils in the lesions. Animals also produce IgG directed against antigens in the lower hair follicles. C3 and IgM may accumulate in this region. The immune attack is primarily directed against a protein called trichohyalin located in the inner root sheath of the follicles. Keratins and root matrix proteins may also be targets. The T cells and some plasma cells form an infiltrate that surrounds the hair bulb and the follicular isthmus. Some CD8+ T cells may also enter the hair bulbs. As a result, hair shafts become dysplastic and unpigmented. Pigmentary incontinence occurs. There may also be peri- and intrabulbar infiltration, peribulbar fibrosis, and degenerate matrix cells with clumped melanosomes.

Clinical Disease, Diagnosis, and Treatment

AA is a rare condition in dogs without any apparent age, breed, or sex predisposition. The alopecia starts locally but may spread to involve the entire body. It is often symmetric. It normally presents as patchy, isolated, circular areas of hair loss. The initial lesions are often restricted to the face (muzzle, chin, ears, periocular region) but then expand progressively. Vibrissae and eyelashes may be lost. Black or dark brown hair may be affected first. Some dogs may lose hair pigment (leukotrichia). The disease may also be associated with nail dysplasia. The regrowing hair is often white, and this may persist through multiple growth cycles. Diagnosis is based on histopathology. Biopsies taken from the periphery of developing lesions are preferable.

Many dogs with AA may self-cure. Thus, in one study, 60% of 20 affected dogs regrew their hair completely and so did not require treatment. The hair regrowth often begins in the center of the lesions and is initially thin and only lightly pigmented. In severe or generalized cases, glucocorticoid and/or cyclosporine immunosuppressive therapy appears to be beneficial.

SEBACEOUS ADENITIS

SA in dogs results from an autoimmune attack on and total destruction of the sebaceous glands. These glands connect to hair follicles and produce sebum, the oily secretion that spreads over the skin thus retaining moisture and proper hydration. There is a genetic predisposition to the disease, which is autosomal recessive disease in Akitas and Standard Poodles. In Standard Poodles one dog leukocyte antigen (DLA) class 1 haplotype, 1003, has been associated with a slightly increased risk of developing SA. This haplotype is not common in the overall dog population. SA is most common in Standard Poodles, Springer Spaniels, Akitas, Samoyeds, Chow Chows, and Vizslas, but it can also occur in many other breeds as well as in cats and rabbits. The disease in Springer Spaniels appears to be most severe, and it may be local or generalized. As dogs lose sebum there is increased skin dryness and scaling. In the absence of sebum's antibacterial properties, secondary staphylococcal folliculitis may develop.

Clinical Disease, Diagnosis, and Treatment

SA tends to affect young to middle-aged dogs (mean age at diagnosis 4.8 years), and there is no sex predisposition. Animals show alopecia, hyperkeratosis, and seborrhea, and follicular casts are a feature of the disease. The clinical presentation depends on the length of the hair coat. Thus in short-coated breeds, symmetric multifocal erythematous papules or plaques develop. They progress to lesions that are annular and irregular in shape. The lesions can coalesce into areas of alopecia and scaling. The alopecia is often associated with broken hair shafts.

In long-haired breeds, hyperkeratosis, local scaling, dryness, and brittle hairs with a dark brown tint develop. Silvery-white or yellowish-brown epidermal scales and scales adhering to hair shafts (follicular casts) are present. Eventually, patchy alopecia develops. The lesions often begin on the head, neck, and pinnae, then spread progressively to the trunk and extremities. Pruritus is not present initially but may develop in response to bacterial infections.

Diagnosis of SA is based on history and clinical presentation. Definitive diagnosis is by biopsy and histopathology. This shows a focal inflammatory reaction centered at the sites where sebaceous glands are normally found in the perifollicular region. Remnants of the sebaceous glands are infiltrated with lymphocytes, plasma cells, macrophages, and neutrophils. Many of these infiltrating lymphocytes have been shown to be T cells. In advanced cases, there may be follicular atrophy or dysplasia, and the sebaceous glands are absent.

Treatment tends to be unsatisfactory once the sebaceous glands are destroyed. As a result, SA is unresponsive to steroid therapy. Nutritional supplementation, synthetic retinoids, shampoos, humectants, and oral fatty acids have all been used as treatments. If there is active inflammation, then prednisolone plus cyclosporine therapy is appropriate. Once the inflammation has subsided, then the disease can be controlled by a combination of low-dose cyclosporine and topical therapy.

PSEUDOPELADE

Pelade is French for "baldness, hair loss." A form of alopecia in dogs and cats has been reported in which mononuclear cells, mainly CD8+ cytotoxic lymphocytes, invade the hair follicle isthmus. Pseudopelade differs from AA in the precise location of the inflammatory infiltrate within the hair follicles, since the hair follicle bulb is unaffected. The damage results in atrophy of both the hair follicle and the sebaceous gland. Affected animals produce autoantibodies against hair keratins and trichohyalin. The disease results in a focal persistent alopecia that is unresponsive to immunosuppressive therapy. The hair loss is permanent.

Other Immune-Mediated Diseases

ERYTHEMA MULTIFORME

Erythema multiforme (EM) is an uncommon disease of dogs that affects the skin, mucous membranes, or mucocutaneous junctions. It is characterized by sudden-onset raised patchy eruptions, skin loss affecting less than 10% of the body surface, and low morbidity. Animals develop flat or raised macular or patchy eruptions, mucocutaneous vesicles, and urticarial plaques. EM may be triggered by drugs and by allergies to certain foods. In dogs and cats, it has been caused by diverse medications, including antibiotics, sulfonamides, aurothioglucose, propylthiouracil, and griseofulvin. It may disappear without sequelae within a few days once the drug is discontinued. It is subclassified into two forms, EM-minor and EM-major. EM-minor cases generally involve no more than one mucosal surface. EM-major involves two or more.

The skin lesions are infiltrated mainly by CD8$^+$ T cells. These cytotoxic T cells infiltrate the lesions and release large amounts of their cytotoxic protein granulysin. Intradermal inoculation of granulysin solutions in mice at a concentration found in blister fluid results in the development of similar lesions.

Treatment of EM involves immediate withdrawal of the offending drug followed by symptomatic treatment, including fluid replacement and wound management. Corticosteroids should be avoided since they increase the animal's susceptibility to skin infections and worsen the prognosis. Antibiotics should only be administered if skin infections occur.

STERILE GRANULOMATOUS DERMATITIS

Also called juvenile sterile granulomatous dermatitis and lymphadenitis or juvenile cellulitis, this is an uncommon skin disease seen in dogs of all ages, although puppies ranging in age from 1 month to about 4 months are regarded as most susceptible. Animals develop facial swelling with a nodular granulomatous pustular dermatitis that affects the muzzle, periocular skin, and ears. In many cases, lesions first appear on the lips and eyelids. In some cases, it may spread to the thorax, abdomen, feet, and perianal skin. A generalized lymphadenopathy develops in about 20% of cases. In some cases there is very marked submandibular and prescapular lymphadenopathy (hence the term "puppy strangles"). The lesions commonly form draining fistulae. Additionally, affected puppies develop a fever, lethargy, and lameness. Golden and Labrador Retrievers, Dachshunds, and Gordon Setters appear to be predisposed. Histology shows dermal granulomas and pyogranulomas that consist of a central core of neutrophils surrounded by a layer of epithelioid macrophages. The cause is unknown, but since it is responsive to therapy with systemic glucocorticoids, it is believed to be immune mediated. The prognosis is good, but scarring and permanent alopecia may result from the severe cellulitis.

PLASMA CELL PODODERMATITIS

In cats, a rare ulcerative condition affecting the central footpads of the metacarpus has been recorded and metatarsus. Its etiology is unknown. The initial lesion is a nonpainful swelling, purple discoloration, and softening of footpads on more than one foot, perhaps all four, hence the colloquial name pillow feet. They change their appearance and appear thin and scaly (Fig. 10.11). The footpads may eventually ulcerate and as a result, secondary bacterial infections are common. Some cats may also develop lesions on the nasal planum. The dermis and the underlying adipose tissue are infiltrated with large numbers of mature plasma cells together with much smaller numbers of lymphocytes and neutrophils. IgG is deposited along the basement membrane, and some cats may be hypergammaglobulinemic. The plasma cells are not monoclonal and hence not neoplastic. The disease is assumed to be immune mediated. It has only been described in cats and no age or breed predilections have been reported, but it does appear to be more common in males. It may

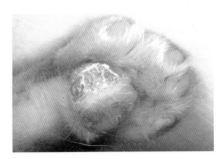

Fig. 10.11 A case of plasma cell pododermatitis in a cat. Note the footpad swelling (hence the name pillow foot) and scaling. (Courtesy of Dr Robert Kennis.)

BOX 10.3 ■ Stiff Skin Syndrome

Otherwise known as scleroderma, stiff skin syndrome is an inherited disease seen in children and very rarely reported in dogs. As its name suggests, affected individuals develop a stony, hard, inelastic skin, often associated with contracture-like joint restrictions, loss of joint mobility, and thoracic and postural abnormalities. Eventually the entire body is enclosed in a rigid shell. It results from the excessive deposition of coarse type IV collagen fibers in the dermis and subcutis by skin fibroblasts, leading to thickening and fibrosis of the skin. Victims have a fibroproliferative vasculopathy and develop autoantibodies and T cells directed against DNA topoisomerase and RNA polymerase. These enzymes stimulate the molecular processes used during wound healing. Thus their stimulation induces fibroblast chemotaxis, migration, and collagen synthesis. It may be generalized (systemic sclerosis) or localized to the skin (morphea). The disease has been reported in a Dachshund, Beagles, and in West Highland White Terriers. It may be inherited as an autosomal recessive condition. Morphea has also been recorded in cats. It usually resolves spontaneously.

Doelle M, Linder KE, Boche J, et al. Initial characterization of stiff skin-like syndrome in West Highland white terriers. *Vet Dermatol.* 2016;27:210-e53.

---

be associated with some underlying infections such as feline leukemia virus or immunodeficiency virus. (Cats experimentally infected with feline immunodeficiency virus have developed an ulcerative pododermatitis.) The disease is responsive to glucocorticoid therapy together with appropriate antibiotics. Doxycycline treatment has also been reported to be effective (see Chapter 21) (Box 10.3).

of Additional Information

Superficial Pemphigus

Bizikova P, Burrows A. Feline pemphigus foliaceus: original case series and comprehensive literature review. *BMC Vet Res.* 2019. doi:10.1186/s12917-018-1739-y.

Levy BJ, Mamo LB, Bizikova P. Detection of circulating anti-keratinocyte autoantibodies in feline pemphigus foliaceus. *Vet Dermatol.* 2020;31:378-e100.

Mueller RS, Krebs I, Power HT, et al. Pemphigus foliaceus in 91 dogs. *J Am Anim Hosp Assoc.* 2006;42:189–196.

Olivry T. A review of autoimmune skin diseases in domestic animals: 1 superficial pemphigus. *Vet Dermatol.* 2006;17:291–305.

Spindler V, Eming R, Schmidt E, et al. Mechanisms causing loss of keratinocyte cohesion in pemphigus. *J Invest Derm.* 2018;138:32–37.

Deep Pemphigus

Olivry T, Joubeh S, Dunston SM, et al. Desmoglein-3 is a target autoantigen in spontaneous canine pemphigus vulgaris. *Exp Dermatol.* 2003;12:198–203.

Tham HL, Linder KE, Olivry T. Deep pemphigus (pemphigus vulgaris, pemphigus vegetans, and paraneoplastic pemphigus) in dogs, cats, and horses: a comprehensive review. *BMC Vet Res.* 2020. doi:10.1186/s12917-020-02677-w.

Pemphigoid Group

Bizikova P, Linder KE, Wofford JA, et al. Canine epidermolysis bullosa acquisita: a retrospective study of 20 cases. *Vet Dermatol.* 2015;26:441-e103.

Favrot C, Dunston SM, Paradis M, et al. Isotype determination of circulating autoantibodies in canine autoimmune subepidermal blistering dermatoses. *Vet Dermatol.* 2003;14:23–30.

Medeiros GX, Riet-Correa F. Epidermolysis bullosa in animals: a review. *Vet Dermatol.* 2015;26:3-e2.

Olivry T, Dunston SM, Schachter M, et al. A spontaneous canine model of mucous membrane (cicatricial) pemphigoid, an autoimmune blistering disease affecting mucosae and mucocutaneous junctions. *J Autoimm.* 2001;16:411–421.

Olivry T, Fine J-D, Dunston SM, et al. Canine epidermolysis bullosa acquisita: circulating autoantibodies target the amino terminal non-collagenous (NC1) domain of collagen VII in anchoring fibrils. *Vet Dermatol.* 1998;9:19–31.

Acquired Junctional Epidermolysis Bullosa

Olivry T, Bizikova P, Dunston SM, et al. Clinical and immunological heterogeneity of canine subepidermal blistering dermatoses with anti-laminin-332 (laminin 5) auto-antibodies. *Vet Dermatol.* 2009. doi:10.1111/j.1365-1364.2010.00870.x.

Feline Polychondritis

Gerber B, Crottaz M, von Tscharner C, et al. Feline relapsing polychondritis: two cases and a review of the literature. *J Fel Med Surg.* 2002;4:189–194.

Hair Follicle Diseases

Ginel PJ, Blanco B, Pérez-Aranda M, et al. Alopecia areata universalis in a dog. *Vet Dermatol.* 2015;26:379-e87.

Paus R, Ito N, Takigawa M, et al. The hair follicle and immune privilege. *J Invest Dermatol.* 2003;8:188–194.

Tham HL, Linder KE, Olivrey T. Autoimmune diseases affecting skin melanocytes in dogs, cats, and horses: vitiligo and uveodermatological syndrome: a comprehensive review. *BMC Vet Res.* 2019. doi:10.1186/s12917-019-2003-9.

Sebaceous Adenitis

Pedersen NC, Brucker L, Green Tessier N, et al. The effect of genetic bottlenecks on two major autoimmune diseases in standard poodles, sebaceous adenitis and Addison's disease. *Canine Genet Epidemiol.* 2015. doi:10.1186/s40575-015-0026-5.

Sousa CA. Sebaceous adenitis. *Vet Clin Small Anim.* 2006;36:243–249.

Tevell EH, Bergvall K, Egenvall A. Sebaceous adenitis in Swedish dogs, a retrospective study of 104 cases. *Acta Vet Scand.* 2008. doi:10.1186/1751-0147-50-11.

Sterile Granulomatous Dermatitis

Inga A, Griffeth GC, Drobatz KJ, et al. Sterile granulomatous dermatitis and lymphadenitis (juvenile cellulitis) in adult dogs: a retrospective analysis of 90 cases (2004-2018). *Vet Dermatol.* 2019;31:219-e47.

Autoimmune Blood Diseases

Among the many possible targets of autoimmune attack are the cells of the blood and bone marrow. Any or all types of red cells, white cells, and stem cells may be prematurely destroyed by immune mechanisms. Some may be targeted by autoantibodies. Other blood cells may bind foreign antigens and then be passively destroyed by conventional immune responses. In some animals, these responses may result in bone marrow suppression, leading to anemia, leukopenia, or thrombocytopenia, or some combination of all three. All the diseases described in this chapter may either be primary (i.e., caused directly by an autoimmune attack) or secondary consequences of some other disease process or drug treatment.

Immune-Mediated Hemolytic Anemias

Immune-mediated hemolytic anemias (IMHA) are a well -recognized, heterogeneous group of diseases in humans and dogs, and have been recorded in cattle, horses, cats, mice, rabbits, and raccoons as well as in birds. Many cases of IMHA are known to be secondary to underlying diseases and are not necessarily mediated by autoimmune processes. Chronic bacterial and viral infections are among the most common causes of these secondary anemias. Acute immune-mediated anemias occur in horses following infection with *Clostridium perfringens* and *Streptococcus faecalis*, in sheep following leptospirosis, in cats with hemobartonellosis, in dogs with babesiosis, and in pigs with eperythrozoonosis. Paraneoplastic IMHA may develop in response to some lymphomas and hemangiosarcomas. Drugs are among the most common causes of secondary IMHA. Examples include penicillins, cephalosporins, and trimethoprim-sulfa.

CANINE IMHA

Canine primary IMHA takes several different forms, as described in the chapter. It tends to be more common in females. The average age of onset is about 4 to 6 years. By definition, the causes of primary IMHA are unknown. The autoantibodies produced in affected dogs are primarily directed against red cell glycophorins, the cytoskeletal protein spectrin, and the membrane anion exchange protein CD233 (band 3). About one-third of canine IMHA cases are secondary to other autoimmune diseases such as systemic lupus erythematosus or autoimmune thrombocytopenia, or are paraneoplastic. The onset of IMHA may be associated with obvious stress such as vaccination, viral disease, or hormonal imbalances as in pregnancy or pyometra.

There is a clear genetic influence on susceptibility to IMHA as shown by their breed and haplotype associations. For example, there is a predisposition to develop IMHA in American and English Cocker Spaniels, Old English Sheepdogs, Miniature and Toy Poodles, Irish Setters, English Springer Spaniels, German Shepherd Dogs, Vizslas, Miniature Dachshunds, and Miniature Schnauzers. In dogs with warm-reactive immunoglobulin G (IgG) hemagglutinins (class III IMHA), the haplotype DLA-DRB1*00601/DQA1*00101/DQB1*00701 is significantly overrepresented. In contrast, a different haplotype, DLA-DRB1*01501/DQA1*00601/DQB1*00301, is associated with class III or class IV IMHA but more so in dogs with cold-reactive IgM hemagglutinins. Two haplotypes, DLA-DRB1*001/DQA1*00101/ DQB1*00201 and DRB1*015/ DQA1*00601/DQB1*02301, are associated with a decreased prevalence of IMHA.

IMHA CLASSIFICATION

IMHAs in dogs clearly result from B cell dysfunction. They are subdivided into five classes based on the immunoglobulin involved, the optimal temperature at which the autoantibodies react, and the nature of the hemolytic process (Fig. 11.1).

Class I IMHA: This is caused by IgG autoantibodies that can agglutinate red cells in saline at body temperature. The agglutination may be seen when a drop of EDTA (ethylenediaminetetraacetic acid) blood is placed on a glass slide followed by multiple drops of saline. After mixing, the red cells may disperse or remain agglutinated. Since IgG does not activate complement efficiently, these antibody-coated red cells are mainly removed from the bloodstream by phagocytosis in the spleen. In some cases, a blood smear may also show erythrophagocytosis by neutrophils and monocytes.

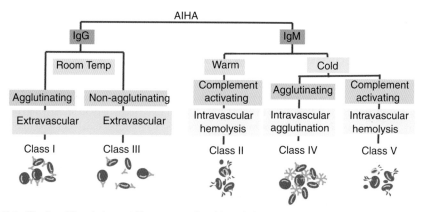

Fig. 11.1 The five different classes of immune-mediated hemolytic anemia that occur in dogs. *AIHA,* Autoimmune hemolytic anemia.

Class II IMHA: IgM autoantibodies activate the classical complement pathway and as a result, can destroy circulating red cells by intravascular hemolysis. This hemolysis results in hemoglobinemia, hemoglobinuria, and icterus. Affected dogs are therefore anemic, weak, and possibly jaundiced. Kupffer cells in the liver or macrophages in lymph nodes effectively capture and remove complement-coated red cells, so these animals may also develop hepatomegaly or lymphadenopathy.

Class III IMHA: Most cases of IMHA in dogs and cats are mediated by IgG1 or IgG4 autoantibodies that bind to red cells at 37°C but neither activate complement nor agglutinate the red cells. Because of their size, surface-bound IgG antibodies can only form short bridges (15–25 nm) between cells. As a result, they cannot counteract the repellent effect of the cell's negative zeta (ζ) potential and will not cause direct agglutination. (In contrast, IgM antibodies are large pentamers, and their antigen-binding sites are sufficiently far apart that they form long bridges [30–50 nm] and can agglutinate cells despite their negative charge.) The antibody-coated red cells are opsonized and effectively removed by splenic macrophages. Splenomegaly is a consistent feature of class III disease.

Class IV IMHA: Some IgM antibodies cannot agglutinate red cells at body temperature but do so when the blood is chilled. These antibodies are called cold agglutinins. They can be detected by cooling a blood sample to between 10°C and 4°C, at which point red cell clumping occurs. The agglutination is reversed on rewarming. Cold agglutinins rely on weak intermolecular interactions such as hydrogen bonds and van der Waal forces to bind red cell antigens. As a result, they cannot form stable complexes at body temperature. Once cooled, however, they can bind with low affinity.

As blood circulates through the extremities (tail, toes, ears, etc.) of affected dogs, it may be cooled sufficiently to permit intravascular agglutination. This may lead to blood stasis, blockage, tissue ischemia, and possibly necrosis. Affected animals may therefore present with erythema, purpura, skin ulcers, and areas of necrosis at their extremities. Anemia may not be a significant feature. As might be anticipated, this form of IMHA is most severe in cold winters.

Class V IMHA: This is mediated by IgM antibodies that bind red cells when chilled to 4°C but do not agglutinate them. These antibodies can only be identified by an antiglobulin test conducted at low temperature. They do not induce necrosis of extremities, but when the red cells return to body core temperature, the antibodies will elute, but activated complement will remain on the cell surface. This activated complement can then cause intravascular hemolysis.

While the evidence points to autoantibodies as being the primary mediators of IMHA and it is assumed that this is a result of rogue B cells that have escaped peripheral tolerance, T cells also play their part. Thus in mouse models of IMHA, follicular helper T (Th) cells play a key role in permitting the B cells to respond to red cell antigens.

CLINICAL DISEASE

The most common presentation of IMHA in dogs is a slowly developing anemia with accompanying evidence of anoxia. Pallor, weakness, lethargy, depression, and eventual collapse may be accompanied by fever, icterus, and hepatosplenomegaly. The anemia may be associated with tachycardia, anorexia, vomiting, or diarrhea. These signs depend on the speed of onset of the disease, its severity, and the precise mechanism of red cell destruction. Red blood cells may be destroyed by intravascular hemolysis in class II disease. More commonly, however, they are removed by extravascular hemolysis (i.e., phagocytosis of antibody-coated red cells by the macrophages lining the sinusoids of the spleen and liver). An acute-onset disease developing within a few days is associated with severe intravascular hemolysis.

Canine IMHA has a 30% to 50% mortality, even with aggressive therapy. Many dogs do not survive the initial hemolytic crisis. About 20% to 30% of IMHA dogs may also suffer from autoimmune thrombocytopenia. Additionally, dogs suffering from IMHA often generate excessive neutrophil extracellular traps (NETs) and so have significant levels of free DNA in their bloodstream. This DNA has the potential to activate platelets and promote thrombosis. In fact, mortality from IMHA tends to be in large part a result of these thromboembolic complications, including pulmonary embolism.

Diagnosis

In cases of primary IMHA, animals usually present with a significant anemia, with a packed cell volume of less than 30% in dogs and less than 20% in cats. The anemia will be hemolytic (although this is not always obvious), and affected dogs are often hypoalbuminemic with evidence of an acute phase response and elevated globulins. Hematology reflects the severe anemia and in most cases, a regenerative response by the bone marrow. Spherocytes are seen in about 67% of cases. Spherocytes are small, round red cells that lack a central pale area (Fig. 11.2). These are erythrocytes that have lost part of their membrane due to partial phagocytosis of antibody-coated red cells. Part of the red cell is pinched off so that what remains is small and rounded. The number of spherocytes seen on blood smears is a measure of the intensity of red cell destruction. Some cases will show hemoglobinemia or hemoglobinuria. Some very severe cases may also show spontaneous autoagglutination of red cells. In some animals, the anemia may be accompanied by a leukocytosis (a leukemoid response) especially involving neutrophils and thrombocytes. Not all cases of IMHA are icteric or develop hyperbilirubinemia.

To diagnose IMHA associated with the presence of nonagglutinating or incomplete antibodies (classes II, III, V), it is necessary to use a direct antiglobulin test (also called the Coombs test, named after Dr. Robin Coombs, the veterinarian who invented it). The red cells of the affected animal are collected in anticoagulant, washed free of serum, and incubated in an antiglobulin serum. The best antiglobulin for this purpose is a polyclonal one with activity against IgM, IgG, and complement. Red cells coated with autoantibody or complement will be crosslinked and visibly agglutinated by the antiglobulin. Occasionally the IgM may have a low affinity for the red cells and it elutes, leaving only complement on their surface—a feature of class V disease. Other new diagnostic technologies such as gel agglutination and flow cytometry are also available (see Chapter 20). Blood samples for immunologic testing should be collected if possible before immunosuppressive therapy begins to reduce the possibility of false-negative results.

Dogs with IMHA may have increased levels of C-reactive protein and α1-acid glycoprotein, and decreased serum albumin. This acute phase response is not predictive of survival, duration of hospitalization, or number of transfusions required, but it normalizes rapidly with disease stabilization.

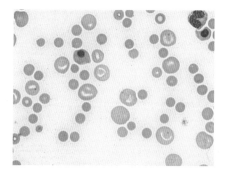

Fig. 11.2 Spherocytosis in a blood smear from a male Schnauzer suffering from immune-mediated hemolytic anemia. Note the small round cells without a central pale area (spherocytes). Original magnification ×100. (Courtesy of Dr. Karen Russell.)

Treatment

The American College of Veterinary Internal Medicine (ACVIM) has issued a consensus statement on the treatment of IMHA. Refer to Garden et al. in Sources of Additional Information at the end of this chapter for complete information.

The consensus statement suggests that most dogs with IMHA will show evidence of erythroid regeneration within about 5 days of becoming anemic. Unfortunately, as many as 30% to 55% of affected dogs may fail to show this regeneration, presumably as a result of destruction of erythroid precursors by phagocytes within the bone marrow. This has been called precursor-targeted immune-mediated anemia. This condition probably represents a severe form of IMHA and is not a different disease. Nevertheless, Whippets, Lurchers, and Miniature Dachshunds appear to be predisposed to this nonregenerative disease—a very different breed predisposition to that noted earlier. It is also clear that lack of a regenerative erythroid response is associated with a poorer prognosis. Pregnancy-associated IMHA in dogs may resolve spontaneously after parturition.

Treatment of IMHA involves prevention of further hemolysis, treatment of hypoxia, prevention of thromboembolism, and aggressive supportive care. Blood transfusions, especially fresh packed red blood cells, may be required to support some very anemic animals until immunosuppressive therapy can take effect. Fluid therapy may also be required. Administration of high doses of glucocorticosteroids reduces erythrophagocytosis by mononuclear cells and is the most effective treatment for IgG-mediated disease. Treated animals may respond within 24 to 48 hours. Corticosteroid treatment may be replaced by other immunosuppressive drugs such as azathioprine, cyclosporine, mycophenolate mofetil, or leflunomide to minimize adverse effects. Thromboprophylaxis such as low-dose aspirin or heparin may reduce the risk of thromboembolism. Splenectomy should only be considered when more conservative therapy has failed and may help cases of refractory class III disease. Most mortality occurs within 30 days after onset. Intravenous immunoglobulin is used in humans but is not recommended for routine treatment in dogs. In humans, the main methods of treatment of IMHAs involve the suppression of autoantibody formation by glucocorticosteroids, often in association with a monoclonal antibody directed against CD20 expressed on B cells (rituximab).

FELINE IMHA

IMHA is uncommon in cats. It mainly occurs in young Domestic Shorthairs. Both primary and secondary diseases have been reported. In the primary disease, the cats develop a regenerative anemia. Spherocytosis may be difficult to see in cats with IMHA (since normal cat red cells do not have a central pallor). Autoagglutination commonly occurs, but false-positive reactions due to increased fibrinogen or immunoglobulin levels are also common. There is a significant association between IMHA and pancreatitis in cats. The reasons for this are unknown. One disease may cause the other, or they may share a similar pathogenesis. An IgM-mediated cold-agglutinin disease has also been described in cats. It can cause ischemic necrosis of the extremities.

Primary IMHA is more common than secondary in cats, and for cats with suspected secondary IMHA, cancers such as lymphomas, drugs, or inflammatory disease are the most common triggers. Feline leukemia virus and *Mycoplasma*-induced diseases are now uncommon. Remember, too, that primary diseases have an unknown cause, so that the diagnosis must be made by exclusion. The primary disease is treated with immunosuppressive corticosteroids. IMHA in cats has a more favorable prognosis than in dogs.

EQUINE IMHA

Both primary and secondary IMHAs have been described in horses. Secondary IMHA is much more common. For example, secondary disease occurs in horses with lymphosarcomas and melanomas as well as with infections such as *C. perfringens, Streptococci,* and *Rhodococcus,* and of course equine infectious anemia virus. IMHA may also be triggered by drugs such as penicillins, sulfonamides, and organophosphates.

Horses with primary disease are depressed and febrile. They exhibit weight loss, splenomegaly, jaundice, and hemoglobinuria. They may be weak, with significant tachycardia and tachypnea. Their serum autoantibodies are usually of the IgG class but sometimes may be IgM. Some cases show red cell autoagglutination, and both warm and cold agglutinins have been reported. Icterus is common, especially in chronic cases. These horses have IgG-coated red cells, so the direct Coombs test is used for diagnosis. Treatment involves removal of the causes of secondary disease and immunosuppression of primary disease. Animals may require immediate support with transfusions. Immunosuppressive drugs are the treatment of choice of primary IMHA. Glucocorticoids such as dexamethasone can induce remission, especially in primary disease. This may be supplemented with cyclosporine and/or azathioprine if necessary. Treatment should last for at least for a minimum of 2 weeks. The prognosis depends on the underlying cause.

BOVINE IMHA

Cold agglutinin disease has been described in Friesian calves infected with *Salmonella* serotype Dublin. A nonregenerative IMHA has also been reported in cattle.

IMMUNE SUPPRESSION OF HEMATOPOIESIS

In humans, dogs, and cats, autoantibodies to erythroid stem cells may cause a precursor-targeted immune-mediated anemia (PIMA). In dogs, PIMA is associated with lack of a bone marrow erythroid regenerative response. Affected bone marrow may show dysmyelopoiesis, myelonecrosis, severe collagen myelofibrosis, interstitial edema, acute inflammation, and stage-selective phagocytosis of myeloid precursors. PIMA has been associated with an IgG autoantibody that inhibits erythroid stem cell differentiation. These animals are often neutropenic and thrombocytopenic.

Diagnosis is based on excluding secondary causes together with a favorable response to immunosuppressive therapy. These diseases can only be diagnosed by careful hematologic analysis and by demonstration of autoantibodies by immunofluorescence on bone marrow smears. These tests are not easy and may not have been validated in domestic species. Affected animals may benefit from high doses of corticosteroids or prolonged immunosuppressive therapy.

Immune-mediated bone marrow aplasia is rare in cats and usually only affects erythrocyte progenitors. It has also been recorded in a ferret. An immune-mediated vaccine-induced neonatal pancytopenia has occurred in cattle in Europe. It is caused by antibodies directed against bovine major histocompatibility complex antigens. (Box 11-1)

AUTOANTIBODIES TO HEMOGLOBIN

While rarely reported, IgM autoantibodies to hemoglobin have been found in the serum of cattle severely infected with *Trueperella pyogenes*. These autoantibodies react not only with hemoglobin but also with lysed red blood cells. This bacterium produces a hemolytic toxin that not only releases hemoglobin but may also act as an adjuvant. Autoantibodies to hemoglobin have also been detected in humans with systemic lupus erythematosus, leishmaniasis, and malaria.

Immune-Mediated Thrombocytopenia

Primary immune-mediated thrombocytopenia (ITP) is characterized by antibody-mediated destruction of blood platelets, resulting in an increased bleeding tendency. It has been reported to occur in humans, dogs, and rarely, horses and cats. Antibodies against platelet antigens cause accelerated clearance due to extravascular destruction of opsonized platelets in the spleen. As a result, platelet lifespan may drop from a normal 4 to 8 days to 1 hour or less. This may be accompanied by decreased platelet production in the bone marrow.

Antiplatelet autoantibodies promote platelet phagocytosis and activate complement. They also inhibit the production of platelets by triggering apoptosis of bone marrow megakaryocytes. Platelets may also be destroyed through direct lysis mediated by cytotoxic T cells. In humans, platelet autoantibodies are initially directed against three glycoproteins expressed on platelet surfaces: glycoprotein 1b-IX that binds to selectins on endothelial cells, glycoprotein IIb-IIIa that is a fibrinogen receptor and so participates in platelet aggregation, and glycoprotein V1 that mediates the interaction of platelets with collagen in the extracellular matrix. Other autoantibodies may also develop as a result of epitope spreading.

In humans with primary ITP, Th1-mediated immunity appears to be enhanced, while Th2 and regulatory T (Treg) responses are suppressed (interferon-gamma [IFNγ] and interleukin-2 [IL2] levels are high). The platelet count correlates inversely with the increased Th1:Th2 ratio. Successful therapy returns this ratio to normal. In about 40% of human patients, CD8+ cytotoxic T cells rather than antibodies may be responsible for platelet destruction. They appear to be specific for glycoprotein IIIa. Interestingly, some individuals vaccinated against Covid-19 develop autoantibodies against platelet factor 4 and so trigger extensive thrombosis.

CANINE ITP

In dogs, the average age of onset of ITP is 4 to 8 years. Predisposed breeds include Airedales, Doberman Pinschers, Old English Sheepdogs, Cocker Spaniels, and both Miniature and Toy Poodles. The disease appears to affect spayed females predominantly. Affected animals usually present with excessive bleeding, including multiple petechiae in the skin, gingiva, other mucous membranes, and conjunctiva. Epistaxis, melena, and hematuria may also occur. Bleeding within the eye is common. Dogs may also bleed for an unusually long time following venipuncture or other minor procedures. Some dogs may develop fever, lethargy, anorexia, or splenomegaly. Melena and a high blood urea nitrogen are associated with a poor prognosis. The predominant cause of death in these dogs is severe gastrointestinal hemorrhage. Primary ITP can occur in cats but is less common.

Diagnosis

The diagnosis of primary ITP is one of exclusion of all secondary causes. Affected animals have unusually low platelet counts of less than 30,000/microL. Variations in platelet size may be obvious on blood smears. Anemia may result from blood loss. Antibodies to platelets may either be measured by direct immunofluorescence or bone marrow aspirates, looking for positive staining on megakaryocytes. Alternatively, it is possible to measure the release of factor III from platelets after exposure to autoantibodies (see Chapter 20). Unfortunately, these tests have relatively poor sensitivity and specificity and do not distinguish between primary and secondary thrombocytopenia.

Treatment

Immunosuppressive doses of a glucocorticosteroid such as prednisolone are used to treat ITP. In most cases, a positive response is seen within a few days. Vincristine also works. It may reduce phagocytosis and it may bind to platelets and kill macrophages when they ingest them. There is limited experience with other drugs such as cyclosporine, cyclophosphamide, azathioprine, mycophenolate mofetil, or leflunomide, although positive clinical results have been reported. Splenectomy may help when other forms of therapy have failed. Short-term survival rates range from 74% to 97%, but recurrence is not uncommon.

EQUINE ITP

Primary ITP in horses is characterized by epistaxis, petechiae, and ecchymoses on mucous membranes and the conjunctiva. Horses may develop swollen joints, hematomas, and gastrointestinal bleeding. Neurologic signs may result from bleeding into the central nervous system. Affected horses have low platelet counts in the order of 20,000 to 30,000/microliter. Diagnosis is based on exclusion of other causes. Secondary thrombocytopenia in horses may be due to infections, drugs, or neoplasia. There is a lack of satisfactory diagnostic tests in this species. Flow cytometry, if available, may be useful in identifying the presence of platelets with increased surface-bound IgG. Platelets from affected horses showed much greater size variation than normal horses. Likewise, in one study, about 5% of platelets had IgG on their surface as compared to 0.15% of the platelets from healthy horses. Horses have been treated successfully with dexamethasone supplemented with azathioprine. Administration of platelet-rich plasma may be helpful in a bleeding emergency.

EVANS SYNDROME

Evans syndrome is the term given to a combination of IMHA and ITP. These diseases may occur simultaneously or sequentially. In humans and dogs, about 20% to 30% of IMHA patients also have ITP, but it is important to remember that thrombotic problems are a common feature of IMHA alone. Evans syndrome may be either primary or secondary to other diseases.

Antiphospholipid Syndrome

Antiphospholipid syndrome is an autoimmune disease of humans characterized by the occurrence of multiple intravascular thromboses. It results from the production of autoantibodies against circulating phospholipids and their binding proteins. The autoantibodies are directed against cardiolipin, β2-glycoprotein-1, and prothrombin. These autoantibodies activate cell surface receptors such as those for endothelial protein C. This results in activation of the NF-κB pathway, the release of inflammatory cytokines, immunothrombosis, and the production of yet more antibodies. The clinical course of this syndrome is highly variable. Some individuals with antiphospholipid antibodies are minimally affected, while others develop recurrent thromboses, resulting in multi-organ failure and death. Many also suffer from systemic lupus.

Autoantibodies against cardiolipin and β2-glycoprotein-1 are present in about 10% of cases of myocardial infarction in humans as compared to less than 1% of normal healthy controls. Thus these autoantibodies may be an important risk factor in some patients. Antiphospholipid antibodies can also be generated during some acute viral infections, including Covid-19.

A similar antiphospholipid syndrome has been described in dogs suffering from ITP. These animals made autoantibodies against multiple phospholipids, including cardiolipin, phosphatidylserine, β2-glycoprotein-1 (that binds phospholipids), phosphatidyl inositol, and phosphatidyl choline. The most significant were those directed against cardiolipin, since these were closely associated with an increased risk of developing severe thrombocytopenia. Autoantibodies to phosphatidylserine were moderately associated with severe disease. These autoantibodies were not associated with the development of thromboembolic episodes in dogs with IMHA. Interestingly, a high proportion (15/22) of healthy Bernese Mountain Dogs have been shown to possess high levels of antibodies against the phospholipid cardiolipin and other phospholipids. The significance of this is unknown.

The term *lupus anticoagulant* is used to describe heterogenous IgG and IgM autoantibodies to the phospholipid-binding proteins. They were first described in patients with systemic lupus where they appear to slow blood clotting in vitro. They are, however, misnamed since, as described earlier, they actually predispose to thrombosis formation.

Immune-Mediated Lymphopenia

The production of autoantibodies against IFNγ results in an adult-onset immunodeficiency in humans. As with other immunodeficiencies, it is associated with increased susceptibility to opportunistic pathogens. It appears to be restricted to people of Southeast and East Asian origin and generally develops around 30 to 50 years of age. Common pathogens associated with this immunodeficiency include nontuberculous *Mycobacteria* such as *M. avium,* salmonellosis, histoplasmosis, cytomegalovirus, and varicella zoster. Given its prevalence in a single ethnic group, it is considered primarily genetic in origin and related to possession of two specific human leukocyte antigen alleles. It appears to be triggered by infections. It has not yet been recorded in domestic animals.

Immune-Mediated Neutropenia

Primary immune-mediated neutropenia (IMN) has been recorded in dogs. It develops most often in spayed females with a median age at diagnosis of 5 years. Its reported prevalence ranges from 0.35% to 7% of neutropenic cases.

Affected dogs present with variable lethargy, anorexia, fever, vomiting, and lameness. Many of these dogs may also have other autoimmune disorders, such as IMHA. Up to 25% of dogs with IMN also have concurrent ITP. Dogs make antibodies against neutrophils located either in the circulation or in the bone marrow. It is believed that these antibodies bind to the neutrophils and opsonize them, resulting in their rapid removal from the circulation by macrophages in the liver, spleen, and bone marrow. In affected dogs, IgG and C3 have been shown to bind to promyelocytes and immature neutrophils within the bone marrow. Both IgG and C3 can also be detected on circulating neutrophils by flow cytometry. Most affected dogs respond by developing myeloid hyperplasia, but many have hypoplasia, and aplasia has been reported. Secondary neutropenia may be due to infections, drugs, or neoplasia. A similar primary disease has been reported in horses in association with anemia and thrombocytopenia.

DIAGNOSIS AND TREATMENT

The diagnosis of primary IMN is based on a disproportionately low blood neutrophil count ($<1.5 \times 10^3$ cells/mL) in the absence of a degenerative left shift and no other identifiable cause. Bone marrow aspirates may show a left-shifted myeloid series. This, together with exclusion of secondary causes of the neutropenia, is required for diagnosis. It is especially important to exclude infectious causes. The presence of antineutrophil autoantibodies can be detected by an indirect fluorescence assay and by counting the fluorescent neutrophils by flow cytometry. The neutropenia may resolve within 2 weeks following corticosteroid therapy, but relapses are not uncommon.

ANTINEUTROPHIL CYTOPLASMIC ANTIBODIES

Antineutrophil cytoplasmic antibodies (ANCA) are a feature of many inflammatory and autoimmune diseases, especially various forms of vasculitis. Their contribution to disease pathogenesis is unclear since they participate in diverse inflammatory conditions.

These autoantibodies are directed against multiple granule and perinuclear antigens in neutrophils as well as in monocytes. The most important of these ANCAs are IgG antibodies directed against neutrophil myeloperoxidase (MPO) and proteinase-3 (PR3). ANCAs are usually detected by an indirect fluorescent antibody test on ethanol-fixed neutrophils (Fig. 11.3). The two major types of ANCA are readily distinguished by their fluorescence pattern. The reactions that stain most intensely around the cell nucleus are called perinuclear ANCAs (pANCA) and are mediated by anti-MPO antibodies. Other antibodies stain the neutrophil granules diffusely. These are called cytoplasmic ANCAs (cANCA) and generally recognize PR3. A few animals may have atypical antibodies that bind and stain both the perinuclear and granule antigens.

Neutrophils are full of granules that are rich in the enzymes needed to kill invading microorganisms. One major antigen, PR3, is a serine protease that plays a role in killing microorganisms

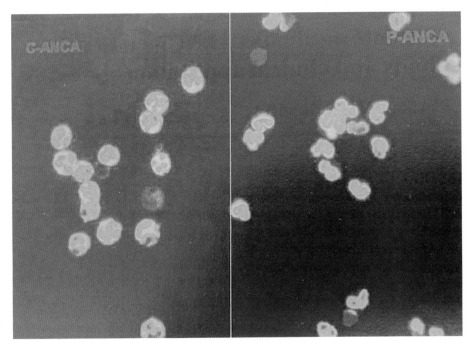

Fig. 11.3 Antineutrophil cytoplasmic antibody (ANCA) staining patterns. The two main patterns of ANCA staining using indirect fluorescence staining on ethanol-fixed neutrophils: (1) P-ANCA staining is characterized by perinuclear staining with or without nuclear involvement since the myeloperoxidase antigen binds to the nucleus during ethanol fixation; (2) C-ANCA staining shows cytoplasmic fluorescence due to staining of the cytoplasmic granules; There is a third, atypical form where both the perinuclear area and the granules stain. (Ramponi G, Folci M, De Santis M, et al. The biology, pathogenic role, clinical implications, and open issues of serum anti-neutrophil cytoplasmic antibodies. *Autoimmun Rev.* 2021;20.)

and degrading the extracellular matrix. Some PR3 is also membrane bound. Its blood level is increased in granulomatous diseases. A second major antigen, MPO, is required for the oxidative killing of microbes since it generates hypochloride in the respiratory burst. Both PR3 and MPO are released in inflamed tissues by activated and apoptotic neutrophils.

It is not clear how ANCAs are generated. Genetic predisposition and molecular mimicry have been proposed. For example, there is cross-reactivity between some epitopes found on *Staphylococcus aureus* and PR3. ANCAs may also develop as a result of impaired apoptosis or even impaired clearance of neutrophil NETs. ANCA titers are often elevated in autoimmune diseases, especially in cases of vasculitis. It is believed that ANCAs potentiate neutrophil MPO and PR3 release and thus exacerbate inflammation in vessel walls. NETs are generated in ANCA-associated small vessel vasculitis. This is a systemic disease causing inflammation of small blood vessels (see Chapter 18). It also occurs in some bacterial infections. ANCAs are also generated in many patients with inflammatory diseases such as rheumatoid arthritis, systemic lupus erythematosus, and autoimmune hepatitis. pANCAs are present in dogs with inflammatory bowel disease and chronic enteropathies, especially lymphoplasmacytic enteritis. They have been detected as early as 2 years before disease onset. Most pANCA-positive dogs are not antinuclear antibody positive. Nor are antibody titers linked to the severity of the disease. Almost half of the dogs with IMHA are positive for pANCA. They are also present in vectorborne diseases such as those caused by Rickettsia, Bartonella, Leishmania, and Ehrlichia. They have been associated with sterile panniculitis, pyometras, idiopathic polyarthritis, and sulfonamide hypersensitivity.

A survey of the serums from healthy Soft -Coated Wheaten Terriers in the United Kingdom demonstrated that 39 of 188 (20.7%) contained detectable pANCAs. These dogs had a greater chance of being positive if they had at least one positive littermate or full sibling with protein-losing enteropathy or protein-losing nephropathy. There was also a significant association between positive pANCA serology and the occurrence of protein-losing diseases in this breed.

Immune-Mediated Hemophagocytic Syndrome

Hemophagocytic syndrome is a proliferative disorder of dogs, cats, and humans that results from the production of activated macrophages (Fig. 11.4). As a result of their aggressive phagocytic activity, these activated macrophages ingest many other cell types, resulting in the development of multiple cytopenias. Hemophagocytic syndromes commonly develop in association with neoplasia or with some infectious diseases. Others appear to be primarily immune mediated. Familial forms of the syndrome have also been identified in humans. An investigation of canine bone marrow specimens submitted to the University of Minnesota found evidence of hemophagocytic syndrome in 24 of 617 (3.9%) blood samples. Tibetan Terriers were overrepresented. Of these dogs, nine had immune-mediated diseases. These included five cases of concomitant IMHA, three of systemic lupus, and a single case of ITP. Affected dogs suffered from weight loss, icterus, anemia, splenomegaly and hepatomegaly, heart murmurs, and collapse, as well as diarrhea. All nine

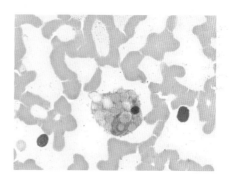

Fig. 11.4 A splenic aspirate from a 5-year-old German Shepherd Dog with immune-mediated hemolytic anemia. Note the macrophage full of ingested erythrocytes. Original magnification ×100. (Courtesy of Dr. Karen Russell.)

BOX 11.1 ■ Pernicious Anemia

Pernicious anemia is a disease of humans that results from a deficiency of vitamin B12 (cyanocobalamin). Vitamin B12 is provided in the diet. When released in the intestine, it binds to a glycoprotein called intrinsic factor produced by gastric parietal cells. The B12 intrinsic factor complex first binds to epithelial cells in the small intestine and is then absorbed into the body. Vitamin B12 is absolutely required for the production of hemoglobin. In its absence, pernicious anemia results. In some cases of pernicious anemia, the body makes autoantibodies directed against intrinsic factor and activated CD4+ Th1 cells directed against gastric parietal cells. The autoantigen in parietal cells is a gastric proton pump enzyme. As a result of this autoimmune attack, the parietal cells are destroyed, intrinsic factor is not produced, and vitamin B12 cannot be absorbed. The subsequent vitamin B12 deficiency results in pernicious anemia. A pernicious anemia has been reported to occur in dogs. It is, however, not an autoimmune disease but results from a *Helicobacter pylori*–induced gastritis. This may, however, be relevant to the human disease since it is believed that the autoimmune gastritis is a result of molecular mimicry between *H. pylori* and the parietal cell proton pump. Pernicious anemia often occurs in association with other human autoimmune diseases such as type 1 diabetes, hypoparathyroidism, Addison disease, and thyrotoxicosis.

Rojas Hernandez CM, Oo TH, Advances in mechanisms, diagnosis and treatment of pernicious anemia. Discover Med 2015; 19:159-168.

suffered from anemia and thrombocytopenia, and three were neutropenic. Their bone marrow was hypercellular, and hemophagocytic macrophages ranged from 7% to 22% of all nucleated cells. They also had high numbers of plasma cells in the bone marrow. None of the dogs survived for longer than 10 days after diagnosis. Necropsies failed to show any additional causes of the disease.

Sources of Additional Information

Immune-Mediated Hemolytic Anemias

Assenmacher TD, Jutkowitz LA, Koenigshof AM, et al. Clinical features of precursor-targeted immune-mediated anemia in digs: 66 cases (2004-2013). *J Amer Vet Med Assoc.* 2019;255:366–376.

Garden OA, Kidd L, Mexas AM, et al. ACVIM consensus statement on the diagnosis of immune-mediated hemolytic anemias in dogs and cats. *J Vet Intern Med.* 2019. doi:10.1111/jvim.15441.

Kennedy LJ, Barnes A, Ollier WER, et al. Association of a common dog leukocyte antigen class II haplotype with canine primary immune-mediated hemolytic anemia. *Tissue Antigens.* 2006. doi:10.1111/j.1399-0039.2006.00715.x.

Lawson C, Smith SA, O'Brien M, et al. Neutrophil extracellular traps in plasma from dogs with immune-mediated hemolytic anemia. *J Vet Intern Med.* 2018;32:128–134.

Piek CJ, Junius G, Dekker A, et al. Idiopathic immune-mediated hemolytic anemia: treatment outcome and prognostic factors in 149 dogs. *J Vet Intern Med.* 2008;22:366–373.

Swann JW, Skelly BJ. Canine autoimmune hemolytic anemia: management challenges. *Vet Med Res Rep.* 2016;7:101–112.

Wilkerson MJ, Davis E, Shuman W, et al. Isotype-specific antibodies in horses and dogs with immune-mediated hemolytic anemia. *J Vet Intern Med.* 2000;14:190–196.

Autoantibodies to Hemoglobin

Spooner RL. Autoantibodies to haemoglobin in cattle. *Clin Exp Immunol.* 1969;5:299–310.

Immune-Mediated Thrombocytopenia

Chen Y-C, Chi L-M, Chow K-C, et al. Association of anticardiolipin, antiphosphatidylserine, anti-b$_2$ glycoprotein 1 and antiphosphatidylcholine autoantibodies with canine thrombocytopenia. *BMC Vet Res.* 2016. doi:10.1186/s12917-016-0727-3.

Kimberly M, McGurrin J, Arroyo LG, et al. Flow cytometric detection of platelet-bound antibody in three horses with immune-mediated thrombocytopenia. *J Amer Vet Med Assoc.* 2004;224:83–87.

Kistangari G, McRae KR. Immune thrombocytopenia. *Hematol Oncol Clin N Am.* 2013;27:495–520.

Miller AG, Dow S, Olver CS. Antiphospholipid antibodies in dogs with immune-mediated hemolytic anemia, spontaneous thrombosis, and hyperadrenocorticism. *J Vet Intern Med.* 2012;26:614–623.

Immune-Mediated Neutropenia

Devine L, Armstrong PJ, Whittemore JC, et al. Presumed primary immune-mediated neutropenia in 35 dogs: a retrospective study. *J Small Anim Pract.* 2017;58:307–313.

Antineutrophil Cytoplasmic Antibodies

Karagianni AF, Solano-Gallego L, Breitschwerdt EB, et al. Perinuclear antineutrophil cytoplasmic autoantibodies in dogs infected with various vector-borne pathogens and in dogs with immune-mediated hemolytic anemia. *Am J Vet Res.* 2012;73:1403–1409.

Ramponi G, Folci M, De Santis M, et al. The biology, pathogenic role, clinical implications, and open issues of serum anti-neutrophil cytoplasmic antibodies. *Autoimmun Rev.* 2021;20. doi:10.1016/j.autorev.2021.102759.

Sundqvist M, Gibson KM, Bowers SM, et al. Anti-neutrophil cytoplasmic antibodies (ANCA): antigen interactions and downstream effects. *J Leukoc Biol.* 2020;108:617–626.

Wieland B, Summers JE, Hasler B, et al. Prevalence of perinuclear antineutrophilic antibodies in serum of healthy Soft Coated Wheaten Terriers in the United Kingdom. *Am J Vet Res.* 2012;73:404–408.

Immune-Mediated Hemophagocytic Syndrome

Weiss DJ. Hemophagocytic syndrome in dogs: 24 cases (1996-2005). *J Amer Vet Med Assn.* 2007;230:697–701.

Autoimmune Muscle Diseases

Domestic animals suffer from immune-mediated muscle and neuromuscular diseases. Many of these are a result of neuropathies such as Guillain-Barré syndrome, and some are paraneoplastic in origin. In this chapter, however, we focus on autoimmune diseases that directly attack muscle fibers and neuromuscular junctions.

Muscle cells may be attacked by autoantibodies and activated T cells. As a result, a consistent feature of immune-mediated myositis (IMM) is the development of a mononuclear cell infiltrate within the affected muscles. T cells, B cells, natural killer (NK) cells, and macrophages may all be engaged in attacking their targets, the myocytes. Thus muscle cell atrophy, necrosis, and apoptosis are consistent features.

Skeletal muscles do not normally participate in adaptive immune responses, and healthy muscle cells do not express major histocompatibility complex (MHC) molecules; however, under some situations, they may activate the necessary genes and express both class I and II MHC molecules. These activated myocytes can then act as antigen-presenting cells and actively participate in local immune responses. In the case of autoimmune myositis in humans, it appears that the responsible autoantibodies are not directed against muscle-specific antigens but against intracellular antigens generated during inflammation, bound to MHC molecules, and presented by the myocytes to T cells. Thus the myocytes themselves may drive the autoimmune process. This is accompanied by increased MHC expression, which plays a key role both in sensitizing the animal and providing a target for cytotoxic T cells. CD8$^+$ cytotoxic T cells clearly have the ability to target and kill autologous myocytes. The usual complex mix of inflammatory and costimulatory cytokines such as interleukin-1β (IL1β), IL2, IL4, interferon-gamma (IFNγ), and tumor necrosis factor-alpha (TNFα) plays a role in these inflammatory responses.

Polymyositis

In humans, the two major autoimmune diseases of muscle, polymyositis and dermatomyositis, both present with muscle weakness and systemic inflammatory disease. Dermatomyositis also presents with a skin rash on the neck and upper back. They differ in their pathogenesis. Thus polymyositis lesions tend to be dominated by CD8+ T cells that infiltrate muscle fascicles; conversely, dermatomyositis lesions contain both CD4+ T cells and B cells and tend to infiltrate the perivascular regions and result in perifascicular atrophy.

Autoantibodies are found in 60% to 80% of human patients with myositis. Some are myositis specific, while others are myositis-associated antibodies. The myositis-specific antibodies include those directed against aminoacyl tRNA synthetases and Mi-2 nuclear antigen (a nucleosome protein that is involved in chromatin modification). Autoantibodies directed against Mi-2 are more than 90% specific for dermatomyositis.

Myositis-associated autoantibodies, in contrast, can include diverse specificities such as anti- Ro/SSA, the RNA-binding protein, anti-DNA-dependent protein kinase, and an anti-RNA-binding protein complex that is also found in scleroderma. Most of these autoantibodies thus target ubiquitous intracellular antigens. These antigens are usually expressed at low levels in normal muscle cells, but their levels increase in inflamed muscles, especially in regenerating muscle cells. As a result, the repair process may sustain and amplify the autoimmune process. These autoantigens can also interact with dendritic cells, the interferon pathway, and immune effector pathways to promote local inflammation.

CANINE POLYMYOSITIS

Immune-mediated polymyositis occurs in dogs and cats. It may either affect specific muscle groups such as the periocular or laryngeal muscles or it may be generalized. A generalized autoimmune myositis occurs in old, large-breed dogs such as German Shepherd Dogs, Greyhounds, Boxers, and Retrievers. Hungarian Vizslas suffer from a breed-specific inflammatory myopathy.

Affected animals may develop either a progressive symmetric muscle weakness associated with increased exercise intolerance or an acute sudden-onset weakness. The dogs may also develop a fever, reflecting excessive cytokine production and their generalized inflammatory state. Changes in laryngeal muscle activity can lead to alterations in their voice and possibly dyspnea and dysphagia. Megaesophagus may also result in dysphagia and, if severe, can lead to chronic vomiting and aspiration pneumonia. Affected animals may also develop a shifting lameness characterized by extreme stiffness. The disease is painful, and affected dogs show evidence of pain on muscle palpation. This is especially the case when larger muscle masses and epaxial muscles are affected.

Diagnosis and Treatment

Because of the extensive skeletal muscle damage, serum creatine kinase (CK) is very much elevated—perhaps as much as 10-fold. There are also increases in alanine aminotransferase (ALT), lactic dehydrogenase (LDH), and creatine phosphokinase (CPK). Biopsies of the most severely affected muscles show a mononuclear cell infiltrate consisting of CD8+ lymphocytes and plasma cells. Eosinophils may also be present. Biopsies will also show muscle fiber degeneration, necrosis, and vacuolation (Fig. 12.1). Animals commonly develop a leukocytosis and eosinophilia. About half of affected dogs have antinuclear antibodies or antibodies to sarcolemma, or both.

Immunosuppressive doses of glucocorticosteroids are the treatment of choice. It may also be necessary to provide affected dogs with additional initial pain relief. The prognosis in these cases is good provided megaesophagus has not developed.

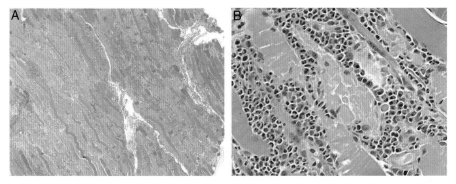

Fig. 12.1 Canine polymyositis. (A) Multifocal-coalescing, subacute to chronic, severe eosinophilic, neutrophilic, and lymphoplasmacytic myositis. There is severe multifocal myofiber necrosis. 4×magnification. (B) Note loss of cross striation in the myofiber to the left (myofiber necrosis) compared to presence of cross striation in the myofiber to the right. H&E, 60×magnification. (Courtesy of Dr. Dominique Wiener.)

EQUINE IMMUNE-MEDIATED MYOSITIS

Some Quarter Horses and related breeds such as Paints and Appaloosas may develop an IMM characterized by rapid-onset muscle wasting. The disease usually targets the gluteal and epaxial muscles, leaving other muscle groups such as the semimembranosus and semitendinosus relatively unaffected (Fig. 12.2). The reason for this localized atrophy is unclear since the affected muscles are not known to express any unique antigens. There is no evidence of immunoglobulin G (IgG) binding specifically to gluteal muscle fibers. As pointed out earlier, normal healthy muscle cells do not normally express MHC molecules; however, in IMM horses, some muscle fibers begin to express MHC and therefore acquire the ability to act as antigen-presenting cells and serve as targets for cytotoxic T cells.

Affected muscles are infiltrated with mononuclear cells. In about half of these cases, the predominant lymphocytes are CD4$^+$ T cells; however, in about a quarter, CD8$^+$ T cells predominate. B cells, macrophages, and multinucleated giant cells may also be present in the infiltrate. These cells are found within or surrounding myofibers, especially around those myofibers that contain the myosin 2X heavy chain (2X fibers account for about 40%–80% of muscle fibers, while 2A fibers account for about 30%–40%) (Box 12.1). There is no evidence of specific binding of

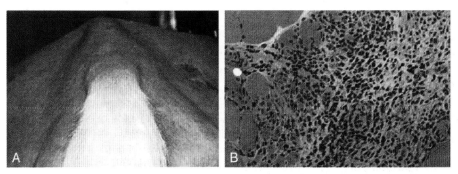

Fig. 12.2 Equine immune-mediated myositis. (A) An affected horse with profound muscle loss. (B) Muscle biopsy showing endomysial, perimysial, and perivascular lymphocytic and histiocytic infiltration. H&E, 40 ×magnification. (Aleman M. A review of equine muscle disorders. Neuromusc Disord. 2008; 18:277–287.)

BOX 12.1 ■ Myosins

Myosins are motor proteins that play a key role in muscle contraction. There are many different myosins, so that in effect they form a superfamily of related isoforms. Each myosin contains two heavy chains, each of about 220 kDa, plus 4 light chains of 20 kDa and 17 kDa. Some myosins are widespread and found in multiple cell types, while others are restricted to a single cell type such as myocytes, or even to subpopulations of cells within these types. The three main striated muscle fiber types contain myosin 1, 2A, or 2B. Type 1 myosin fibers respond to slow contracting motor units. Myosin 2, the most conventional myosin, is responsible for the contraction of most skeletal muscles. Two forms exist. One form, 2A fibers, responds to fast responding, fatigue-resistant motor units, while the other form, 2B fibers, responds to fast responding, fatigue-sensitive motor units. Both are responsible for producing muscle contraction. A third form of myosin 2 has been designated 2X. Myosin 2X fibers have a shortening velocity intermediate between type 2 and type 1 myosins.

---

immunoglobulins to affected myofibers, confirming the suspicion that this is a T-cell–mediated disease.

While the causes of equine IMM are unclear, it is probable that, as usual, environmental triggers combined with a genetic predisposition play an important role. Environmental factors likely include an infectious trigger, thus as many as 40% of affected horses may have a history of recent infection. For example, IMM may be triggered by infection with bacteria such as *Streptococcus equi* subsp. *equi* or *Corynebacterium pseudotuberculosis*, or by prior vaccination against a respiratory virus such as equine herpesvirus-1 or influenza.

Given its predisposition in Quarter Horses, it is clear that IMM has a major genetic component. Certain stallions are overrepresented in the bloodlines of affected Quarter Horses. Genome-wide association studies (GWAS) on Quarter Horses and related breeds clearly indicate an autosomal mode of inheritance. GWAS have identified a close association between IMM and a 6.3-Mb region of chromosome 11. Subsequent analysis identified a mutation located in the MYH1 globular head where a glutamic acid has been exchanged for a normal glycine at position 321. This gene variant is called E321G *MYH1*. It encodes the heavy chain of myosin 2X. It is variably penetrant, thus explaining variations in disease susceptibility. It occurs with a high frequency in some susceptible lines of Quarter Horses but not in nonsusceptible lines or in Arabians.

Interestingly, the M protein of *S. equi* shows considerable homology to myosin heavy chain 2X, and thus molecular mimicry likely plays a role in the induction of IMM. It has been suggested that in the presence of certain environmental triggers, the mutated *MYH1* gene can initiate the development of IMM. For example, an innate immune response could be triggered in IMM by the release of myosin 2X from muscle fibers by microtrauma such as that caused by vaccination. Similar mutations in mice predispose them to develop myocarditis.

Clinical Disease, Diagnosis, and Treatment

IMM has a bimodal distribution. Affected Quarter Horses tend to be under 4 years of age, while affected other breeds tend to be older, with average onset around 17 years. There is no gender predisposition. The disease presents as rapidly progressive, localized symmetric muscle atrophy affecting predominantly the epaxial and gluteal muscles. The cervical muscles may atrophy as well. The onset of atrophy is rapid and can develop within 48 hours. It may persist for several months. Animals show stiffness, weakness, and malaise, while many are febrile.

Hematology may be normal or show a leukocytosis. Serum chemistry may show marked increases in serum CK and aspartate aminotransferase, especially in the acute phase of the disease. The most useful diagnostic procedure is a transcutaneous biopsy. This shows a lymphocytic infiltration into the myocytes and perivascular cuffing. Myocytes show evidence of atrophy and myonecrosis, and there may be signs of myofiber regeneration. Biopsies taken later in the disease process may show fewer lymphocytes.

The prognosis for IMM is good, although horses with a fever or concurrent infections tend to have a somewhat poorer outcome. Antiinflammatory doses of glucocorticoids administered for about 1 month are usually effective. The muscle mass will eventually recover, but this may take 2 to 3 months, and there may be some residual muscle atrophy. About half of apparently recovered horses may undergo recurrent episodes.

CANINE MASTICATORY MUSCLE MYOSITIS

Dogs can develop a focal myositis confined to the muscles of mastication. This masticatory muscle myositis is the second most frequent myopathy diagnosed in dogs after polymyositis. The disease primarily affects large-breed dogs such as German Shepherd Dogs, Labrador Retrievers, Golden Retrievers, and Dobermans. Cavalier King Charles Spaniels are also susceptible, suggesting a specific breed predisposition.

Two types of masticatory myositis have been recognized, an acute and painful eosinophilic form and a chronic form associated with muscle atrophy. They are both characterized by inflammation, atrophy, and necrosis of the masticatory muscles, specifically the temporal, masseter, and pterygoid muscles. These muscles are unique in carnivores since they contain M2 fibers with a myosin isoform that differs from the isoforms found in limb muscles (see Box 12.1). They also contain a variant type 1 muscle fiber not found in other muscle groups. Affected animals make autoantibodies against these M2 myofibrils. Immunoglobulin deposits may be detected by immunohistochemistry in about 80% of biopsy specimens from affected muscles. These autoantibodies recognize masticatory muscle-specific myosin heavy and light chains, and an isoform of myosin-binding protein C that is also restricted to the muscles of mastication.

Histology of the affected muscles shows inflammatory or degenerative lesions affecting the M2 myofibrils. Perimysial or endomysial fibrosis and muscle fiber necrosis are also consistent features. There is a mononuclear cell perivascular infiltrate in affected muscles that consists mainly of CD4+ γ/δ+ T cells. Macrophages and dendritic cells are also present (Fig. 12.3). There are also multifocal clusters of B cells. MHC class I and class II expression is upregulated on the muscle fibers. In some cases, the myositis may be eosinophilic, the muscles may contain large numbers of eosinophils, and affected dogs also have an eosinophilia. Presumably, this reflects the occurrence of a type 2 immune response. The reason for this variation is unknown.

Clinical Disease

An acute eosinophilic form of masticatory myositis tends to occur in young German Shepherd Dogs and Doberman Pinschers. It presents with lethargy, anorexia, fever, pain on opening or closing the mouth (trismus), and swelling or atrophy of the masticatory muscles. There may be a voice change. In some cases, the myositis may affect the extraocular muscles, resulting in exophthalmos, secondary conjunctivitis, and blindness, probably as a result of optic nerve compression. Disease episodes may last 2 to 3 weeks and then go into remission, but there may be frequent recurrences.

In the chronic disease, dogs suffer a single acute attack followed by progressive muscle atrophy. Masticatory muscle fibers may be replaced by fibrous tissue. This chronic muscle fibrosis may result in an inability to open the jaw, even under general anesthesia. Eosinophils are not a prominent feature of the chronic disease.

Diagnosis and Treatment

Infectious causes of the myositis should be ruled out first. Antibodies to 2M fibers may be detected in serum or immune complexes detected on muscle biopsy. Biopsies will also reveal the degree of

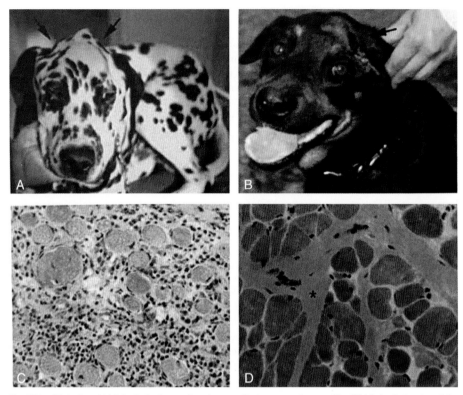

Fig. 12.3 Clinical and histologic features of canine masticatory muscle myositis. (A) Marked atrophy of the temporalis muscles. (B) A dog unable to open its jaw (trismus). (C) Diffuse infiltration of mixed mononuclear cells into the masticatory muscles and myonecrosis. (D) A chronic case with perimysial (*) fibrosis in the temporalis muscle in the absence of detectable inflammation. H&E, 20×. (H&E. 20×. From Paciello O. et al. Expression of major histocompatibility complex class I and class II antigens in canine masticatory muscle myositis. Neuromusc Disorders 2007; 17: 313–320.)

fibrosis that has developed, reflecting on the prognosis. Imaging either by computed tomography scanning or by magnetic resonance imaging may show areas of altered intensity within the masticatory muscles.

Glucocorticoid immunosuppressive therapy will permit jaw function to return, provided the disease is diagnosed and treated before extensive fibrosis sets in. Relapses occur in about a quarter of affected dogs. Some animals may never regain their ability to open the mouth widely.

CANINE DERMATOMYOSITIS

A familial disease of dogs that resembles dermatomyositis in humans has been described in young Collies and Shetland Sheepdogs. It is a microangiopathy in which complement-mediated vascular damage leads to muscle ischemia. The disease is inherited as an autosomal dominant condition involving a gene locus on chromosome 35, although its expression is highly variable. A similar dermatomyositis-like disease has been described in other breeds such as Pembroke Welsh Corgis, Lakeland Terriers, Chow Chows, Russell Terriers, German Shepherd Dogs, and Rottweilers.

Dermatomyositis in dogs has a strong genetic component; thus there is a significant association with the MHC class II haplotype DLA-DRB1*00201/DQA1*00901/DQB1*00101. This association is especially strong in homozygous animals. However, this haplotype is also found in many healthy dogs, suggesting that other risk factors are also involved. These include polymorphisms in conserved regions of the *PAN2* locus on chromosome 10. This encodes the catalytic subunit of a poly (A) nuclease deadenylation complex and plays a role in the regulation of the inflammatory response. The other important canine susceptibility locus is called *MAP3K7CL*, located on chromosome 31. This encodes a kinase gene whose function is unclear but is expressed in blood leukocytes.

Affected dogs develop a dermatitis with a less-obvious myositis. Puppies appear normal at birth, but skin lesions usually develop between 7 and 11 weeks of age. The myositis develops somewhat later, between 12 and 23 weeks. In some cases, the dermatitis developed at 3 to 6 months of age, and the myositis was detected after the dermatitis was investigated. The dermatitis first develops on the face, ears, and tail tip. Subsequently, lesions spread to the limbs and trunk, especially over bony prominences. They are not pruritic. These early skin lesions are erythematous and eventually lead to intraepidermal and subepidermal vesicle and pustule formation. There is diffuse hair follicle atrophy and keratinocyte degeneration that can lead to ulceration. Once the skin vesicles rupture, they ulcerate and crust. Lesions may be found on the bridge of the nose and around the eyes. They show hair loss and changes in pigmentation. There may be local lymph node enlargement. The clinical course and severity are variable, but the skin lesions usually resolve by 1 year of age.

Muscle disease follows the onset of skin disease, but there is poor correlation between the severity of the two. The most common sign of myositis is masseter and temporal muscle atrophy. Some severely affected puppies may have difficulty chewing and swallowing as a result of the myositis. They are weak and lethargic and grow poorly. If the muscles of the esophagus are affected, megaesophagus may develop, and secondary aspiration pneumonia can result. Generalized lymphoid hyperplasia may also occur in these dogs. Many dogs outgrow the disease and are left with moderate hyperpigmentation, some hypopigmentation, and alopecia, plus atrophy of the muscles of mastication. Leg muscles may also atrophy, affecting the animal's gait. Other dogs develop a progressive disease with severe dermatitis and myositis. Dogs with progressive disease may also develop signs of immunodeficiency, especially pyoderma and septicemia, as well as demodicosis. On necropsy, myositis may be detected in the esophagus and arteritis in the skin, muscle, and bladder.

The key immune target in dermatomyositis is capillary endothelium. The skin and muscle lesions are a result of ischemic vasculopathy. Thus skin blood vessels have swollen endothelial cells, vacuolization, capillary necrosis, inflammation, and ischemia (Fig. 12.4). The onset and progression of the disease correlates with a rise in circulating immune complexes and serum IgG, but the reason for these increases is unclear. Immune complexes and IgG levels return to normal as the disease resolves, suggesting a causal association. Muscle biopsy, especially of the temporal muscle, shows multifocal accumulations of lymphocytes, plasma cells, and macrophages as well as a few

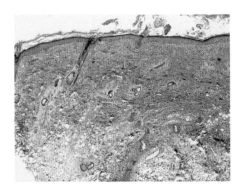

Fig. 12.4 A skin lesion from a case of canine dermatomyositis. Note the diffuse ischemic hair follicle atrophy and multifocal basal keratinocyte degradation in the epidermis. (Courtesy of Dr. J. Mansell.) (Tizard, IR. Veterinary Immunology. 2016; 10 edition, Elsevier.)

neutrophils and eosinophils. The myofibers are atrophied and may show fragmentation and vacu-olation. Symptomatic and corticosteroid treatment may be of benefit in severely affected cases. Pentoxifylline is also beneficial because of its ability to counteract the vasculopathy.

Autoimmune Heart Failure

Autoimmunity is increasingly recognized as a significant contributory factor to heart failure in humans. Some autoantibodies are directed against contractile muscle proteins such as troponin or myosin. Other autoantibodies bind to G protein–coupled receptors. As a result, they can act as agonists and effectively stimulate receptor signaling and are termed functional auto-antibodies. Thus autoantibodies against the β1-adrenergic receptor (β1-AAB) and against the muscarinic receptor 2 (M2-AAB) have been detected in humans. In patients suffering from arrhythmias, one study showed that 40% had autoantibodies to M2. More significantly, autoantibodies directed against β1-AAB appear to be the major drivers of left ventricular dysfunction and dilated cardiomyopathy in humans. They also appear to be associated with the development of atrial arrhythmias and the development of hypertensive heart disease. They are also present in the serum of humans and dogs affected by Chagas disease due to *Trypanosoma cruzi* (Box 12.2).

Immune checkpoint mediators have revolutionized the immunotherapy of some human cancers by inhibiting the immunosuppressive effects of cytotoxic T-lymphocyte–associated antigen 4 (CTLA-4) and programmed death 1 (PD-1). Unfortunately, by removing these con-straints on the immune system, specifically T cells, tolerance may be lost and autoimmunity result. T-cell clones reactive with the tumor as well as skeletal and cardiac muscle may develop in some patients. One such consequence is the development of a lethal lymphocytic myocar-ditis. This may result in the acute onset of hemodynamic compromise leading to cardiogenic shock and death.

CANINE CARDIOMYOPATHY

English Cocker Spaniels can develop a cardiomyopathy with antinuclear and antimitochon-drial autoantibodies and reduced serum IgA levels. It is associated with possession of a specific

---

BOX 12.2 ■ Autoimmunity in Chagas Disease

Trypanosoma cruzi is a protozoan parasitic disease of humans and dogs that occurs in Latin America and the southern United States. In the chronic form of the disease, infected individuals develop an in-tense immune response against the parasite. As a result of bystander activation and molecular mimicry, they also develop diverse autoimmune responses. These are directed against many different autoantigens in the nervous system, the immune system, and the heart. As a result, autoantibodies against cardiac myosin, β1-adrenoceptors, and acetylcholine receptors cause patients to develop a chronic, and often lethal, cardiomyopathy.

Dogs experimentally infected with a pathogenic strain of *T. cruzi* also developed autoantibodies against cardiac tissue. Antibody titers peaked during the acute disease (~30 days) but progressively declined thereafter and were almost undetectable by ~240 days, when the dogs developed dilated car-diomyopathy. The autoantigens in the heart tissue were probably β-adrenoceptors.

DeBona E, Lidani KCF, Bavia L, et al. Autoimmunity in chronic Chagas disease: a road of multiple pathways to cardiomyopathy? *Front Immunol.* 2018. doi:10.3389/fimmu.2018.01842.
Barr SC. Anti-heart tissue antibodies during experimental infections with pathogenic and non-patho-genic *Trypanosoma cruzi* isolates in dogs. *Int J Parasitol.* 1993;23:961–967.

complement component 4 allotype (C4-4). The autoantigen has not been identified, but in humans, similar cardiomyopathies are due to autoantibodies directed against the adenine nucleotide translocator of mitochondria.

DOBERMAN PINSCHER DILATED CARDIOMYOPATHY

Doberman Pinschers also suffer from a dilated cardiomyopathy. Affected dogs develop clinical signs that are very similar to those in humans, such as congestive heart failure, arrhythmias, syncope, and exercise intolerance. Many of these dogs also make autoantibodies against the β1-AAB. These autoantibodies bind a specific epitope on the extracellular part of the receptor. This is the same epitope that is targeted in humans. In one study, about 70% of Dobermans both with and without dilated cardiomyopathy possessed autoantibodies to β1-AAB. The levels of these antibodies were slightly but not significantly higher in the cardiomyopathy group. However, when the dogs were followed, sudden death in the antibody-positive dogs (79%) was significantly greater than in the negative dogs (20.4%) with a median survival time of 130 days. The majority of affected dogs survived for less than 2 years after diagnosis.

Neuromuscular Junction Disorders

CANINE MYASTHENIA GRAVIS

Myasthenia gravis (MG) is a syndrome of neuromuscular transmission failure characterized by abnormal fatigue and weakness in skeletal muscles following mild exercise. It has been reported in humans, ferrets, dogs, and cats. MG results from a failure of transmission of nerve impulses across the motor endplate of striated muscle as a result of a deficiency of acetylcholine receptors on the postsynaptic membrane.

MG is either a rare congenital disease or an acquired autoimmune disease in dogs. Thus in Jack Russell Terriers, Springer Spaniels, and Fox Terriers, inherited deficiencies occur in the acetylcholine receptor. These defects result in the development of a congenital myasthenic syndrome. They can result from mutations at many points in the neuromuscular signaling pathway. (In humans, at least 60 such mutations have been identified.) Congenital MG is therefore a disease of very young dogs occurring in the first weeks or months of life.

In adult dogs, however, acetylcholine receptor deficiency is primarily due to the activities of autoantibodies directed against the receptor (AChR). Motor endplate receptors are pentameric complexes with five subunits ($\alpha1$, ε, $\alpha1$, δ, and $\beta1$) surrounding a central ion channel. IgG autoantibodies accelerate degradation of the receptors by binding to extracellular sites on the receptor $\alpha1$ subunits. They can impair signaling in three ways. First, antibodies can directly block AChR signaling. Second, they can crosslink multiple receptors. This results in receptor aggregation and internalization, thus reducing the receptor half-life from 10 days to 3 days. Third, the antibodies may trigger complement-mediated damage to the postsynaptic membrane. As a result, the number of functional acetylcholine receptors drops significantly, and signal transmission between the nerve and muscle is severely impaired.

In about 10% of human cases, there is a second form of MG associated with the production of autoantibodies against an enzyme called muscle-specific receptor tyrosine kinase (MuSK). MuSK normally induces AChR clustering in the postsynaptic membrane, while the autoantibodies prevent this. MuSK-mediated MG differs in some respects from anti-AChR-mediated MG in that it tends to be more focal. It also appears to be specifically associated with IgG4 autoantibodies rather than IgG1 and IgG3 that are associated with conventional MG. It has been suggested that MuSK antibodies act by triggering Th17 responses as opposed to AChR antibodies that trigger Th1 responses. MuSK-mediated MG has been recorded in a dog.

Some dogs and people with MG also make autoantibodies against other striated muscle proteins. These other antigens include titin, a giant intracellular muscle protein, the ryanodine receptor, and a Ca⁺⁺ release channel found in the sarcoplasmic reticulum. Other reported strial antigens include actin, myosin, tropomyosin, α-actinin, and cortactin. The occurrence of antibodies to these strial proteins is associated with the presence of a thymoma in humans and dogs, and their detection may therefore be a useful diagnostic test.

The mechanisms of the loss of peripheral tolerance in MG are unclear. It is probable that the problem lies with the CD4⁺ helper T cells that permit autoreactive B-cell clones to develop. Like most of the autoimmune diseases described in this book, there is a breed predisposition to the acquired disease. Thus Great Danes, Labrador Retrievers, Scottish Terriers, Golden Retrievers, German Shepherd Dogs, and Dachshunds appear to develop more severe disease. Rottweilers appear to be at low risk. There is a form of early onset MG that occurs in Newfoundlands that also appears to be familial. Genotyping of affected Newfoundlands indicates that susceptibility is associated with possession of the class II allele DLA-DQB1*00301. This association is not found in other susceptible breeds.

In normal muscles, the binding of acetylcholine to its receptor opens a sodium channel to generate a localized endplate potential. Provided the amplitude of the endplate potential is sufficient, this will generate an action potential and trigger muscle contraction. The endplate potential from a normal neuromuscular junction is usually more than sufficient to generate a muscle action potential. Only after this surplus capacity is eroded will signal transduction impairment begin to result in loss of function. In myasthenic junctions, although there is sufficient acetylcholine, the number of available receptors eventually becomes limiting. As a result, the endplate potentials fail to trigger action potentials (Fig. 12.5). This is manifested as muscle weakness. Since the amount of acetylcholine released from a nerve terminal usually declines after the first few impulses, repeating the stimulus leads to a progressive increase in weakness as transmission failure occurs at more and more neuromuscular junctions.

Clinical Disease

Immune-mediated MG may develop at any time after 6 months of age. The disease may present focally or in a generalized manner, or even as an acute fulminating disease. Animals may present with a history of difficulty swallowing, regurgitation, labored breathing, eyelid and

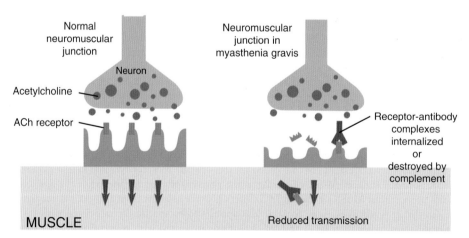

Fig. 12.5   The pathogenesis of myasthenia gravis. *(Left)* Normal neuromuscular signaling. *(Right)* The interference with acetylcholine signaling caused by antireceptor antibodies.

head droop, and generalized muscle weakness. Focal MG occurs in about 40% of canine cases and is characterized by weakness in one or more muscle groups such as facial, esophageal, laryngeal, and pharyngeal muscles. Megaesophagus and facial paralysis can develop without any involvement of limb muscles. Generalized MG cases show a wide range of clinical signs. The dogs develop muscle weakness, especially in the pelvic limbs. This may also be associated with facial paralysis and megaesophagus. Generalized MG accounts for about 60% of canine cases. Acute fulminating MG can lead to quadriplegia and respiratory difficulty. Usually less than 5% of canine cases are considered fulminating. Aspiration pneumonia is the main cause of death in myasthenic dogs.

A paraneoplastic form of MG is associated with the presence of a thymoma and some other cancers. In 3% to 4% of dogs, the thymus may show medullary hyperplasia, germinal center formation, or even a thymic carcinoma (Box 12.3). Surgical thymectomy may result in clinical improvement.

Diagnosis

MG should be considered in dogs with extreme weakness that worsens rapidly with exercise. Megaesophagus and dysphagia are also presenting signs. Other conditions such as thyroid disease should be ruled out. A chest radiograph is needed to exclude the presence of a thymoma. A presumptive diagnosis of MG may be based on the effects of intravenous administration of a short-acting anticholinesterase drug such as edrophonium chloride (Tensilon, Roche) 0.1 to 0.2 mg/kg. This can lead to a rapid but temporary gain in muscle strength in many MG dogs. This

---

BOX 12.3 ■ Autoimmune Paraneoplastic Diseases

Among the many factors that can trigger autoimmune diseases are cancers. As they develop, the cancer cells often synthesize neoantigens (i.e., antigens new to the body or not previously encountered by the immune system). These arise as a result of mutations or abnormal gene expression, and they may trigger autoimmune responses.

While cancers can develop anywhere within the body and autoimmunity may be directed against any organ, most paraneoplastic autoimmune diseases in humans develop in the skin. Thus paraneoplastic pemphigus has been known for many years, commonly developing in response to lymphoid tumors. This form of pemphigus differs from the conventional form in that patients develop a wide diversity of autoantibodies directed against multiple cutaneous antigens rather than just desmoglein in "normal" pemphigus. Other recognized paraneoplastic diseases include paraneoplastic autoimmune blood disorders such as hemolytic anemia, thrombocytopenia, and red cell aplasia.

A well-recognized example of a paraneoplastic autoimmune disease is myasthenia gravis. There is a close association between the presence of a thymoma and the development of MG. In humans, about 30% of thymoma patients develop MG, while 10% to 20% of patients with MG have a thymoma. In dogs, this figure is about 3% to 4%, while in cats, it has been reported to be as high as 50%! In many cases, thymectomy may decrease the titer of anti-AChR antibodies suggesting that the tumor is the source of the problem. Recent studies suggest that these MG-associated thymomas may secrete IL6 and IL21 and thus promote Th17 production while suppressing Tregs.

Other human paraneoplastic autoimmune syndromes include retinopathy, cerebellar degeneration, and encephalitis. The pathogenesis of most of these paraneoplastic autoimmune diseases is unclear. Patients may develop autoantibodies and/or autoreactive T cells. Many are associated with responses to cancer cell exoantigens (i.e., neoantigens released in immunizing quantities by the tumor cells themselves). These may be structurally modified so that they are sufficiently different to trigger an immune response but sufficiently similar to cross-react with normal self-antigens. Less commonly, the paraneoplastic autoimmune response is directed against intracellular antigens. In this case, cytotoxic T cells are probably responsible for disease development.

anticholinesterase, by permitting the acetylcholine to accumulate at the neuromuscular junction, enables the remaining receptors to be stimulated more effectively. Definitive diagnosis requires the measurement of autoantibodies by radioimmunoassay.

Treatment

Without treatment, about half of MG-affected dogs will soon die, whereas the others may show spontaneous remissions. Unlike human MG, some canine cases may go into spontaneous remission within about 6 months. Dogs with transient or mild MG may be supported temporarily with long-acting cholinesterase inhibitors such as pyridostigmine bromide or neostigmine bromide. The former is preferred because it can be given orally in syrup, and it has a longer duration of action. If the animal has difficulty in swallowing, then injectable neostigmine may be given. These drugs inhibit the hydrolysis of ACh and prolong its activities. This provides only symptomatic treatment for the disease and does not alter its immunopathology. Dogs with progressive disease that show no signs of remission may also benefit from immunosuppression. This is especially the case in animals that require long-term treatment. Positive clinical responses have been reported in dogs treated with prednisone or azathioprine or both. However, corticosteroid treatment may result in transient exacerbation of weakness—a myasthenic crisis—so it should not be used for initial therapy. Other drugs that may be used in refractory cases include cyclosporine, leflunomide, or mycophenolate mofetil. Plasmapheresis has been used for short-term therapy to stabilize patients before thymectomy. Thymectomy is required in cases with a thymoma. Supportive care is critical since aspiration pneumonia is a common cause of death, especially in cases of megaesophagus and pharyngeal dysfunction.

FELINE MYASTHENIA GRAVIS

A congenital myasthenic syndrome has been reported to occur in the Devon Rex and Sphynx breeds. Acquired MG is uncommon in cats. However, Abyssinian and Somali cats appear to have a higher prevalence of the disease. It is often associated with polymyositis. Animals present with generalized weakness and a floppy head, easy fatigability, and regurgitation (Fig. 12.6). As many as 25% to 50% of affected cats may also have an anterior mediastinal mass, usually a thymoma. Affected animals are seropositive for antibodies to AChR. Spontaneous remission is not common, and long-term treatment may be required.

Methimazole is a thioureylene antithyroid agent used to treat hypothyroidism in cats. MG is a well-recognized adverse effect of methimazole therapy. The disease is, however, reversible and usually resolves when this medication is discontinued.

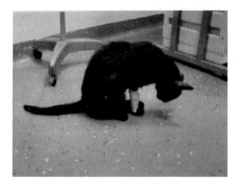

Fig. 12.6 A myasthenic cat showing the dropped head sign, reflecting a generalized muscle weakness and an inability to hold up its head. (Shelton DG, Myasthenia gravis and congenital myasthenic syndromes in dogs and cats: A history and mini-review. Neuromuscular disorders 2016; 26(6), 331–334.)

Sources of Additional Information

Canine Polymyositis

Pumarola M, Moore PF, Shelton GD. Canine inflammatory myopathy: analysis of cellular infiltrates. *Muscle Nerve.* 2004. doi:10.1002/mus.20043.

Shelton GD, Hoffman EP, Ghimbovschi S, et al. Immunopathogenic pathways in canine inflammatory myopathies resembling human myositis. *Vet Immunol Immunopathol.* 2006;113:200–214.

Tauro A, Addicott D, Foale RD, et al. Clinical features of idiopathic inflammatory polymyopathy in the Hungarian Vizsla. *BMC Vet Res.* 2015. doi:10.1186/s12917-015-0408-7.

Equine Immune-Mediated Myositis

Durward-Akhurst SA, Valberg SJ. Immune-mediated muscle disease in the horse. *Vet Pathol.* 2018;55:68–75.

Hunyadi L, Sundman EA, Kass PH, et al. Clinical implications and hospital outcomes of immune-mediated myositis in horses. *J Vet Intern Med.* 2017;31:170–175.

Canine Masticatory Muscle Myositis

Castejon-Gonzalez AC, Soltero-Rivera M, Brown DC, et al. Treatment outcome of 22 dogs with masticatory muscle myositis (1999-2015). *J Vet Dent.* 2018;35:281–289.

Wu X, Li Z-F, Brooks R, et al. Autoantibodies in canine masticatory muscle myositis recognize a novel myosin binding protein-C family member. *J Immunol.* 2007;179:4939–4944.

Canine Dermatomyositis

Evans JM, Noorai RE, Tsai K, et al. Beyond the MHC: a canine model of dermatomyositis shows a complex pattern of genetic risk involving novel loci. *Plos Genetics.* 2017. doi:10.1371/journal.pgen.1006604.

Haupt KH, Prieur DJ, Moore MP, et al. Familial canine dermatomyositis: clinical, electrodiagnostic, and genetic studies. *Amer J Vet Res.* 1985;46:1861–1869.

Doberman Pinscher Dilated Cardiomyopathy

Wess G, Wallukat G, Fritscher A, et al. Doberman Pinschers present autoimmunity associated with functional autoantibodies. A model to study the autoimmune background of human dilated cardiomyopathy. *PlosOne.* 2019. doi:10.1371/journal.pone.0214263.

Myasthenia Gravis

Gomez AM, Van den Broeck J, Vrolix K, et al. Antibody effector mechanisms in myasthenia gravis—pathogenesis at the neuromuscular junction. *Autoimmunity.* 2010;43:353–370.

Hague DW, Humphries HD, Mitchell MA, et al. Risk factors and outcomes in cats with acquired myasthenia gravis (2001-2012). *J Vet Intern Med.* 2015;29:1307–1312.

Lascano AM, Lalive PH. Update in immunosuppressive therapy of myasthenia gravis. *Autoimm Rev.* 2021. doi:10.1016/j.autrev.2020.102712.

Mignan T, Targett M, Lowrie M. Classification of myasthenia gravis and congenital myasthenic syndrome in dogs and cats. *J Vet Intern Med.* 2020. doi:10.1111/jvim.15855.

Wolf Z, Vernau K, Safra N, et al. Association of early onset myasthenia gravis in Newfoundland dogs with the canine major histocompatibility complex class I. *Neuromusc Disorders.* 2017;27:409–416.

Wu Y, Chang Y-M, Lawson BS, et al. Myeloid-derived suppressor cell and regulatory T cell frequencies in canine myasthenia gravis: a pilot study. *Vet J.* 2021. doi:10.1016/j.tvjl.2020.105581.

CHAPTER 13

Autoimmune and Immune-Mediated Liver and Kidney Diseases

No organ of the body is free from the risk of autoimmune attack, and this includes the major abdominal organs such as the liver and kidneys. As pointed out previously, a consistent feature of many autoimmune diseases is that animals may possess autoantibodies and suffer from gradual organ failure for months or years before the disease becomes clinically obvious. This is especially the case when organs have much spare capacity that must first be eroded before defects become apparent. This insidious onset applies to immune-mediated diseases of the liver and kidneys.

In addition to being a potential target of autoimmune attack, the kidney is vulnerable to other forms of immune-mediated disease. Most importantly, it is tasked with cleaning the blood. As a result, the glomeruli filter out immune complexes from the bloodstream. The deposition of these complexes in glomeruli results in immune-mediated renal disease. In many cases, these complexes are generated as a result of autoimmunity. They include systemic lupus erythematosus, rheumatoid arthritis, and immunoglobulin A (IgA) nephropathy. On the other hand, many such cases of immune complex–mediated disease are of unknown origin.

The liver receives most of its blood supply directly from the intestine via the portal vein. As a result, it is the first organ to trap any commensal organisms that may penetrate a leaky gut. These organisms and their metabolites can trigger innate responses and drive inflammation. Immune cross-reactivity may also serve as a trigger of autoimmunity. Likewise, the liver will also be the first organ to encounter any released mucosal lymphocytes. These primed cells may trigger autoimmune responses by cross-reactions with commensal antigens. Thus autoimmune liver disease may be secondary to disturbances in the intestinal microbiota and the development of a "leaky gut".

Autoimmune Liver Diseases

CHRONIC ACTIVE HEPATITIS

The large mass of the liver means that it contains an enormous quantity of potentially antigenic material and so plays an important role in maintaining peripheral tolerance. As a result, for

161

example, large liver allografts are well tolerated in both humans and dogs. Their mass is sufficient to maintain tolerance. However, when the liver is damaged and intracellular antigens escape, then autoimmune responses may develop rapidly. In humans and domestic animals, numerous autoantibodies are produced in response to liver destruction. These autoantibodies may not necessarily be clinically significant but can be useful in diagnosing disease or determining prognosis. These autoantibodies fall into two distinct categories. In the first category are nonliver-specific autoantibodies such as antinuclear antibodies (ANA), smooth muscle antibodies, antimitochondrial antibodies, and antibodies to microsomal proteins. For example, smooth muscle antibodies are directed against components of the cellular cytoskeleton such as microfilaments found in many different cell types and tissues. The second category of antiliver autoantibodies are directed against liver-specific antigens. Examples include antibodies against liver-specific enzymes such as cytochrome P450 2D6, UDP-glucuronosyltransferases, and the hepatocyte asialoglycoprotein receptor.

CANINE HEPATITIS

Canine immune-mediated hepatitis may be primary or secondary to other disease entities. Thus most cases of canine hepatitis are secondary to infections caused by viruses such as canine adenoviruses and toxicities due to drugs or toxins. However, in some cases, chronic hepatitis cannot be linked to any of these causes, and they are probably autoimmune in nature.

Dogs, especially middle-aged female Doberman Pinschers and English Springer Spaniels, can develop a chronic progressive autoimmune liver disease (chronic active hepatitis). In Dobermans, the disease is associated with homozygosity for the major histocompatibility complex (MHC) haplotype DLA-DRB1*00601/DQA1*00401/DQB1*01303. Conversely, the MHC-DQ alleles DLA-DQA1*00901/DQB1*00101 appear to confer resistance.

Chronic active hepatitis commonly presents in dogs around 8 years of age but may have been present subclinically for years previously. In the early disease, the most prominent feature is a mononuclear cell infiltration of the parenchymal and portal regions of the liver. There is intense inflammation and fibrosis around small hepatic veins. The centrilobular lesions contain lymphocytes, plasma cells, and macrophages. There is an increased ratio of CD4+ to CD8+ cells and a pan-T-cell infiltration mainly in these centrilobular areas. The disease eventually results in progressive destruction of hepatocytes and hepatic fibrosis (Fig. 13.1).

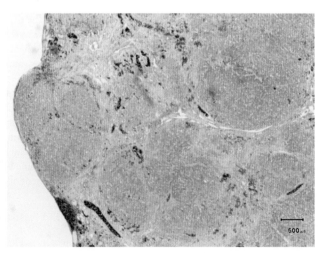

Fig. 13.1 Low-power photomicrograph of liver tissue from a Doberman Pinscher with idiopathic chronic hepatitis demonstrating marked fibrosis (light green staining). Masson trichrome. Original magnification 40 ×. (Bexfield N. Canine idiopathic chronic hepatitis. *Vet Clin Small Anim.* 2017;47:645–663.)

About 60% to 75% of affected dogs develop antibodies to hepatocyte membrane proteins. These antibody-positive dogs have more severe disease than dogs that do not develop antibodies. In addition, lymphocytes from about 75% of affected dogs respond to liver membrane proteins by proliferating in vitro. Hepatocytes from affected dogs, but not from normal dogs, aberrantly express MHC class II antigens either in their cytoplasm or on their surface. This MHC expression correlates with the presence of lymphocytes as well as the severity of the disease, whereas corticosteroid treatment reduces both MHC expression and disease severity. Such aberrant expression of MHC molecules is commonly triggered by exposure to interferon-gamma (IFNγ). It may permit the hepatocytes to act as antigen-presenting cells. It has been suggested therefore that the disease results from a T-cell–mediated attack on hepatocytes with abnormally expressed MHC molecules or on antigens presented by them.

The autoantibodies produced by these dogs include ANA, antismooth muscle, and antiliver membrane proteins. Measurement of ANA and antihistone antibodies (AHA) in affected Dobermans showed the presence of AHA in 23 of 25 (92%) Dobermans with subclinical hepatitis, in 11 of 13 clinically affected dogs, and in 0 of 17 healthy control dogs. Further studies also detected IgG autoantibodies against glyceraldehyde-3-phosphate dehydrogenase (GADPH) and alcohol dehydrogenase in both subclinically and chronically affected Dobermans. Interestingly, anti-GADPH antibodies have also been found in Dobermans with dilated cardiomyopathy.

Clinical Disease

As in so many autoimmune diseases, dogs may suffer from subclinical hepatitis for many years prior to developing clinical signs. Eventually, affected dogs develop a variety of nonspecific signs such as weight loss, lethargy, and vomiting. Biochemical evidence is obtained by liver enzyme studies, especially aspartate transaminase and alkaline phosphatase levels and histopathology from a liver biopsy. The signs are typical of liver disease with anorexia, depression, weight loss, diarrhea, polydipsia, polyuria, icterus, and eventually ascites. The loss of hepatocytes will eventually result in chronic inflammatory disease with fibrosis, leading to liver failure and death. The prognosis is poor once liver failure develops. Many affected dogs may also suffer from other immune-mediated diseases at the same time such as autoimmune hypothyroidism or immune-mediated hemolytic anemia.

Diagnosis and Treatment

Chronic active hepatitis in dogs is diagnosed by the usual criteria for hepatitis and the elimination of other possible causes. In the early subclinical stage, dogs initially show an increase in scrum alanine transferase followed by an increase in alkaline phosphatase. Hepatic copper levels are also increased in subclinical cases. If the alanine transferase remains persistently high, then a liver biopsy is warranted. Bilirubin levels increase last, and this is associated with the development of clinical disease. The hepatitis is characterized by the presence of lymphocytic infiltrates within the liver, the presence of serum autoantibodies against one of the major autoantigens, and (most obviously) a strong predisposition toward Dobermans, English Springer Spaniels, and female dogs.

The prognosis is not good. Immunosuppressive treatments reported to be effective include prednisone/prednisolone, azathioprine, cyclosporine, and mycophenolate. Corticosteroid treatment has been shown to significantly reduce MHC class II expression on hepatocytes. Glucocorticoids should be used cautiously in dogs with cirrhosis, portal hypertension, or bridging fibrosis.

Autoimmune Kidney Diseases

Autoimmune kidney disease has rarely been reported in domestic animal species. When cases do occur, they appear to be directed mainly against one specific autoantigenic component, the glomerular basement membrane (GBM). It is also clear that these kidney lesions usually develop in conjunction with other autoimmune diseases originating elsewhere in the body.

ANTIGLOMERULAR BASEMENT MEMBRANE DISEASE

Anti-GBM disease, formerly known as Goodpasture syndrome, is a rare autoimmune disease of humans associated with the development of autoantibodies against basement membrane antigens in the kidneys and lungs. On electron microscopy, there are no obvious electron-dense deposits since the autoantibodies simply bind directly to the GBM. The specific autoantigen is believed to be the M2 subunit of the globular domain of type IV collagen. Patients develop pulmonary hemorrhage and kidney failure.

Repeated immunization of experimental sheep with human GBM M2 resulted not only in the production of autoantibodies against human GBM but also antibodies to sheep GBM. Their appearance coincided with the development of acute nephritis in the sheep. The sheep did not develop lung lesions.

A somewhat similar disease has been reported in horses and dogs in which the kidneys alone appear to be affected (Fig. 13.2). For example, horses may develop autoantibodies to GBM resulting in glomerulonephritis and renal failure. In one study, glomerulonephritis was detected in 7 of 45 horses examined. Three of these horses showed deposits of IgG and complement on their GBM. Immunofluorescence studies showed that the basement membrane of affected animals was coated with a smooth, linear deposit of immunoglobulin. These anti-GBM autoantibodies provoke proliferation of the glomerular epithelial cells and the formation of epithelial crescents containing fibrin, neutrophils, and macrophages. It proved possible to elute the antibodies from the kidney of one horse, a 6-year old Thoroughbred mare, and demonstrate that they were directed against the GBM.

An anti-GBM disease has also been reported in a West Highland White Terrier with necrotizing encephalitis. At necropsy, in addition to the brain lesions, there was strong, smooth, linear fluorescent labeling of IgG antibodies bound to the GBM. There was weaker linear staining with IgM. There was also diffuse damage throughout the renal cortex, accompanied by infiltration of lymphocytes and plasma cells.

IgA NEPHROPATHY

The most common cause of chronic kidney disease and renal failure in humans is IgA nephropathy. This is an autoimmune disease in which large amounts of IgA in the form of immune complexes are deposited on the GBM and so cause kidney failure. It has been reported to occur in dogs.

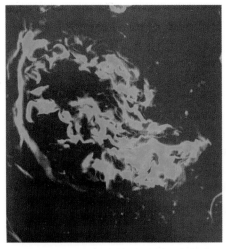

Fig. 13.2 Antiglomerular basement membrane disease in a West Highland White Terrier with a necrotizing encephalitis. A glomerulus labeled with fluorescent anti-canine immunoglobulin G showing linear labeling along the capillary walls. 400 ×. (Aresu A, et al. Canine necrotizing encephalitis associated with anti-glomerular basement membrane glomerulonephritis. J Comp Path. 2007; 136:279–282.)

Like other autoimmune diseases, IgA nephropathy appears to be triggered by a combination of environmental and genetic factors. As a result, patients make autoantibodies against a galactose-deficient form of IgA. The O-glycans in the IgA hinge region lack galactose residues (Gd-IgA). This Gd-IgA acts as an autoantigen and triggers an IgG autoantibody response. The autoantibodies form IgG-Gd-IgA immune complexes in the circulation. These immune complexes are filtered out and accumulate in the mesangium of the GBM. Here, they trigger mesangial cell proliferation. The deposited immune complexes cause local inflammation with cytokine and growth factor production. These in turn activate mesangial cells and provoke their production of extracellular matrix. As a result, the glomeruli eventually become sclerotic and nonfunctional.

IgA nephropathy patients have greatly elevated serum IgA levels. Gd-IgA–containing immune complexes can be found in the glomeruli of up to 35% of some human populations and up to 47% of dogs. In these dogs, the IgG-IgA complexes are deposited in the mesangial and paramesangial areas resulting in membranoproliferative glomerulonephritis (MPGN). A slightly different condition has also been described in dogs aged 4 to 7 years. These animals developed MPGN with mild hematuria, proteinuria, and hypertension. IgA-containing immune complexes were present in both the subepithelial and subendothelial locations in these animals (Fig. 13.3).

Surveys of dog kidneys have reported finding IgA deposits in the glomeruli of dogs over 10 years of age. The IgA is located primarily in the glomerular mesangial areas, in association with IgG, IgM, and small amounts of C3. It is associated with a moderate increase in mesangial cell numbers and glomerular sclerosis, fibrosis, and epithelial crescent formation. IgA deposits are most often observed in dogs suffering from enteritis or liver diseases. IgA deposition has also been detected in dogs suffering from persistent proteinuria due to an MPGN.

Other immunoglobulin-induced nephropathies have been reported to occur in animals. Thus a case of a severe protein-losing nephropathy due to an IgM-specific glomerulopathy has been reported in a Quarter Horse. Likewise, nephritis occurs in dogs in association with IgG4 disease (see Chapter 14). The most common form of IgG4 disease is a tubulointerstitial nephritis, although a membranous glomerulonephropathy may also develop.

LUPUS NEPHRITIS

The kidneys are affected in more than half of human patients with systemic lupus erythematosus. Among the many autoantibodies produced by these patients are some that react with autoantigens in the kidneys. These appear to be antibodies against double-stranded DNA that cross-react with nucleosomes and annexin II in the glomerular mesangial cells. Again, immune complexes form and eventually lead to glomerular sclerosis. The cellular infiltrates within lupus kidneys also contain increased numbers of helper T type 17 (Th17) cells, dendritic cells, and activated macrophages. These contribute significantly to the proinflammatory local type 1 IFN response.

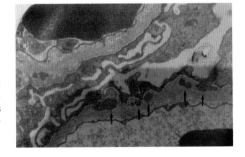

Fig. 13.3 Electron micrograph of a section of kidney from a dog with immunoglobulin A nephropathy. Note the basement membrane thickening and subepithelial electron-dense deposits *(arrows)*. (Harris CH, Krawic DR, Gelberg HB, et al. Canine IgA glomerulonephropathy. *Vet Immunol Immunopathol.* 1993;36:1–16.)

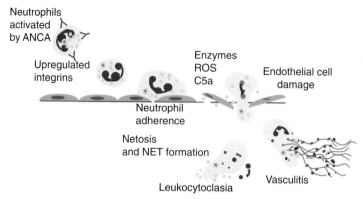

Fig. 13.4 The pathogenesis of antineutrophil cytoplasmic antibodies *(ANCA)*–associated vasculitis. Neutrophils activated by the antineutrophil autoantibodies bind to vascular endothelial cells. The neutrophils then release their contents, including their extracellular traps *(NET)*, which collectively cause severe endothelial damage and trigger blood clotting and thrombus formation.

SJÖGREN SYNDROME

Kidney involvement is a common complication of Sjögren syndrome. Patients develop an interstitial nephritis and/or a glomerulonephritis. This presumably reflects autoimmune attack on the ubiquitous autoantigens in this disease.

ANTINEUTROPHIL CYTOPLASMIC ANTIBODIES (ANCA)–ASSOCIATED VASCULITIS

Antibodies against ANCA, the neutrophil cytoplasmic antigens (myeloperoxidase and proteinase 3), are associated with the development of a systemic vasculitis. These antibodies can activate and alter the flow characteristics of neutrophils so that they adhere to vessel walls. Additionally, the activated neutrophils produce increased amounts of oxidants and extracellular traps (NETs). As a result, they can cause a focal necrotizing vasculitis and glomerulonephritis (Fig. 13.4). Immune complexes are not present on the GBM in this form of glomerulonephritis. Although dogs with inflammatory bowel disease can develop positive ANCA serology, this form of kidney disease has yet to be reported in them.

ANTIPHOSPHOLIPID SYNDROME

As described in Chapter 11, antiphospholipid syndrome is a complex autoimmune disease defined by the occurrence of multiple vascular thromboses as a result of the production of autoantibodies against key phospholipids such as cardiolipin. It has been recorded in dogs. Antiphospholipid syndrome nephropathy is a thrombotic microangiopathy that affects the glomeruli and other renal vessels. It results in infarction, necrosis, and fibrosis.

Immune Complex–Mediated Glomerulopathies

Immune complex–mediated glomerular lesions are of much greater significance than autoimmunity as a cause of chronic kidney disease in dogs. Surveys have suggested that the prevalence of these glomerular lesions in canine populations may be as high as 90%, most of which are clinically insignificant. Immune complexes circulating in the bloodstream are filtered out in the glomeruli, where they cause basement membrane thickening and stimulate glomerular cells to proliferate.

Practically speaking, immune complex glomerulonephritis can be classified as either membranous or membranoproliferative. Membranous glomerulopathy is characterized by basement membrane thickening. Electron microscopy shows the presence of subepithelial and mesangial electron-dense deposits on GBM. There may also be limited mesangial cell proliferation. The capillary loops in such cases are also coated with IgG and C3, detectable by immunofluorescence assays. As a result, the capillary basement membrane in this membranous disease appears grossly thickened when stained with specialized stains such as periodic acid–Schiff, a so-called wire-loop lesion.

The membranoproliferative form (MPGN) of immune complex disease, in contrast, is defined by obvious hypercellularity within the glomerulus. The GBM is coated with either subendothelial or subepithelial electron-dense deposits that are presumably immune complexes. Any or all of the three glomerular cell populations—epithelial cells, endothelial cells, and mesangial cells—can proliferate in response to these complexes. This may eventually result in glomerular sclerosis.

There are two major types of MPGN lesions based on the site of deposition of the immune complexes. The most common form of MPGN is caused by immune complex deposition in the walls of glomerular blood vessels. The complexes are trapped on the vascular side of the basement membrane, where they stimulate endothelial cell proliferation (Fig. 13.5). Continued activation of the endothelial cells by immune complexes leads to production of transforming growth factor-beta (TGFβ) (see Fig. 2.9). This stimulates nearby cells to produce fibronectin, collagen, and proteoglycans, which eventually results in further thickening of the basement membrane. The second major type of MPGN is characterized by the presence of immune complexes on both the endothelial and epithelial sides of the basement membrane. It is believed that very small immune complexes can penetrate the basement membrane and are therefore deposited on the external surface where they stimulate epithelial and mesangial cell proliferation. Mesangial cells are modified smooth muscle cells. As such, they can produce cytokines and prostaglandins, and ingest immune complexes. They respond to immune complex deposition by proliferating and producing

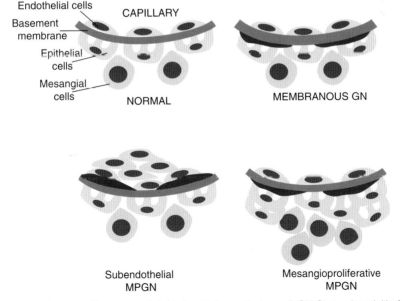

Fig. 13.5 The major types of immune-mediated lesions that occur in glomeruli. *GN,* Glomerulonephritis; *MPGN,* membranoproliferative glomerulonephritis.

interleukin-6 (IL6) and TGFβ. The IL6 stimulates mesangial cell growth, while the TGFβ stimulates production of extracellular matrix. If excessive, these proliferating cells may fill the glomerular space to form epithelial crescents.

A rare third type of MPGN (dense deposit disease) is characterized by the presence of homogeneous dense deposits within the lamina densa of the GBM rather than on its surface. These deposits contain C3 but not immunoglobulin. This type of MPGN results from uncontrolled complement activation and develops in complement factor H deficiency in pigs.

Clinical Features of Glomerulonephritis

MPGN develops when prolonged antigenemia persists in the presence of antibodies. It is therefore secondary to chronic viral diseases such as equine infectious anemia, infectious canine hepatitis, feline leukemia, feline coronavirus, bovine virus diarrhea, Aleutian disease of mink, and African swine fever; parasitic diseases such as leishmaniasis and demodicosis; and chronic bacterial infections such as Lyme disease, recurrent staphylococcal pyoderma, and ehrlichiosis. MPGN has also been reported in dogs with pyometra, chronic pneumonia, distemper encephalitis, acute pancreatic necrosis, and bacterial endocarditis. In some animals with tumors, large amounts of antigen may be shed into the bloodstream and result in a MPGN. This paraneoplastic MPGN is associated with lymphosarcomas, osteosarcomas, and mastocytomas. Some cases may be due to complement deficiencies in which removal of immune complexes is impaired so that they accumulate in glomeruli. Many cases of MPGN develop in the absence of an obvious predisposing cause.

Clinically, it should be suspected in an animal with a high proteinuria without evidence of infection, although definitive diagnosis requires a renal biopsy and histologic evaluation. The presence of immune complex lesions within the glomeruli stimulates neutrophils, mesangial cells, macrophages, and platelets to release thromboxanes, nitric oxide, and platelet-activating factor. These molecules increase basement membrane permeability so that plasma proteins, especially albumin, are lost in the urine. This loss can be severe and exceed the ability of the body to replace the protein. As a result, serum albumin levels drop, the plasma colloid osmotic pressure falls, fluid passes from blood into tissue spaces, and the animal may become edematous and ascitic. This loss of fluid into tissues results in a reduction of blood volume, a compensatory increase in secretion of antidiuretic hormone, increased sodium retention, and accentuation of the edema. The decreased blood volume also results in a drop in renal blood flow, reduction in glomerular filtration, retention of urea and creatinine, azotemia, and hypercholesterolemia. Although all these may occur as a result of immune complex deposition in glomeruli, the development of this nephrotic syndrome is not inevitable. In fact, the clinical course of these conditions is unpredictable, with some animals showing a progressive deterioration in renal function while others show spontaneous remissions. Many animals may be clinically normal despite the presence of immune complexes in their glomeruli, and immune complexes are commonly observed in old, apparently healthy dogs, horses, and sheep.

The most common initial signs are anorexia, weight loss, and vomiting. Polyuria and polydipsia occur when about two-thirds of the glomeruli are destroyed. Azotemia occurs when 75% are destroyed. Development of nephrotic syndrome (proteinuria, hypoproteinemia, edema, or ascites) only occurs in about 15% of affected dogs but in up to 75% of affected cats. Some dogs become hypertensive. Thromboembolic disease may also develop. Because of the unpredictable occurrence of spontaneous remissions, it is difficult to judge the effects of treatment. It has been usual to treat affected animals with corticosteroids and immunosuppressive drugs, but the rationale and effectiveness of this treatment is unclear except when the glomerulonephritis is associated with a concurrent autoimmune disease such as systemic lupus erythematosus. Encouraging clinical responses have also been obtained with angiotensin-converting enzyme inhibitors (captopril) and thromboxane synthase inhibitors. Protein restriction may help reduce the clinical signs of renal failure. If the glomerulopathy is secondary to infection as in Lyme-associated glomerular disease or leishmaniasis, the underlying cause should be treated. The glomerular lesion is not inflammatory, and although the lesion contains immunoglobulins, there is no evidence to suggest that it is caused by hyperactivity of the immune system. For disease associated with a profound proteinuria, nephrotic syndrome, or progressive azotemia, mycophenolate alone or in combination with prednisolone has been recommended. For stable or slowly progressive disease, mycophenolate or chlorambucil alone, or in combination with azathioprine on alternate days, is appropriate. Therapeutic effectiveness should be assessed serially by changes in proteinuria, renal function, or serum albumin concentrations. In the absence of adverse side effects, at least 8 to 12 weeks of therapy should be provided before altering or abandoning a treatment.

SWINE GLOMERULOPATHY

Spontaneous MPGN is observed in pigs. It is especially common in Japan, where it appears to be due to deposition of immune complexes containing IgG and IgA antibodies against *Actinobacillus pleuropneumoniae*. In other countries, it may be secondary to chronic virus infections such as hog cholera or African swine fever. Occasionally, however, proliferative glomerulonephritis appears to develop spontaneously. In most cases, epithelial crescent formation suggests that the proliferating cells are epithelial in origin. However, occasional membranoproliferative lesions are observed as well. There is usually strong staining for C3 and weaker staining for IgM using immunofluorescence assays. Pigs rarely have IgG or IgA deposits. Affected pigs are relatively young (<1 year). There is a high prevalence of gastric ulcers in affected animals, but whether this is related is unclear.

FINNISH-LANDRACE GLOMERULOPATHY

Some lambs of the Finnish-Landrace breed die within a few weeks of age as a result of renal failure due to MPGN. The lesions develop in utero and are present at birth. The glomerular lesions are similar to those seen in experimental serum sickness, with mesangial cell proliferation and basement membrane thickening. In extreme cases, epithelial cell proliferation may result in epithelial crescent formation. Neutrophils may be present in small numbers within glomeruli, and the rest of the kidney may exhibit diffuse interstitial lymphoid infiltration and necrotizing vasculitis. Deposits containing IgM, IgG, and C3 are found in the glomeruli and choroid plexus, and serum C3 levels are low (Figs. 13.6 and 13.7). The lesions are therefore probably a result of immune complex deposition, although the nature of the inducing antigen is unknown.

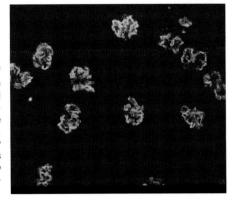

Fig. 13.6 A fluorescent micrograph of a section of kidney from a Finnish-Landrace lamb with immune complex–mediated glomerulonephritis. The labeled antisheep globulin reveals the presence of granular deposits characteristic of membranoproliferative glomerulonephritis in many glomeruli. (Angus KW, Gardiner AC, Morgan KT, et al. Mesangiocapillary glomerulonephritis in lambs. II. Pathological findings and electron microscopy of the renal lesions. *J Comp Pathol.* 1974;84:319–330 [Tizard IR, Veterinary Immunology. 2016; 10 edition. Elsevier.])

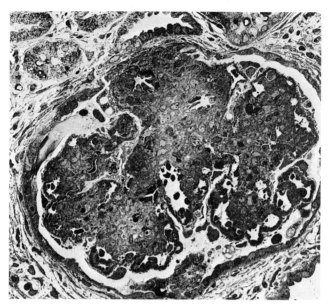

Fig. 13.7 A thin section of glomerulus from a Finnish-Landrace lamb with membranoproliferative glomerulo-nephritis. The primary lesion in this case is mesangial proliferation with some basement membrane thickening. (Angus KW, Gardiner AC, Morgan KT, et al. Mesangiocapillary glomerulonephritis in lambs. II. Pathological findings and electron microscopy of the renal lesions. *J Comp Pathol.* 1974;84:319–330 [*Tizard IR, Veterinary Immunology. 2016; 10 edition. Elsevier.*])

CANINE GLOMERULOPATHY

A familial glomerulopathy has been reported to occur in English and American Cocker Spaniels as a result of the presence of abnormal collagen IV in renal basement membranes. Dalmatians and Bull Terriers are also reported to suffer from autosomal dominant glomerulopathies. A familial glomerulopathy also has been reported to occur in Bernese Mountain Dogs. It is associated with the development of MPGN and interstitial nephritis.

C3 deficiency inherited as an autosomal recessive condition has been described in Brittany Spaniels. Many of these dogs develop MPGN, leading to renal failure. The lesions show mesangial proliferation, thickening of the glomerular capillary wall, and deposition of electron-dense deposits in the mesangium and subendothelial space. The deposits contain both IgG and IgM.

Sources of Additional Information

Chronic Active Hepatitis

Bexfield N. Canine idiopathic chronic hepatitis. *Vet Clin Small Anim.* 2017;47:645–663.

Dyggve H, Kennedy LJ, Meri S, et al. Association of Doberman hepatitis to canine major histocompatibility complex II. *Tissue Antigens.* 2010;77:30–35.

Dyggve H, Meri S, Spillmann T, et al. Antihistone autoantibodies in Dobermans with hepatitis. *J Vet Intern Med.* 2017;31:1717–1723.

Liaskos C, Mavropoulos A, Orfanidou T, et al. The immunopathogenic role of antibodies in canine autoimmune hepatitis: lessons to learn from human autoimmune hepatitis. *Autoimmune Highlights.* 2012;3:87–93.

Webster CRL, Center SA, Cullen JM, et al. ACVIM consensus statement on the diagnosis and treatment of chronic hepatitis in dogs. *J Vet Int Med.* 2019;33:1173–1200.

Weiss DJ, Armstrong PJ, Mruthyunjaya A. Anti-liver membrane protein antibodies in dogs with chronic hepatitis. *J Vet Intern Med.* 1995;9:267–271.

Autoimmune and Immune Complex Nephritis

Aresu L, Pregel P, Bollo P, et al. Immunofluorescence staining for the detection of immunoglobulins and complement (C3) in dogs with renal disease. *Vet Rec.* 2008;163:679–683.

Banks KL. Animal model: anti-glomerular basement membrane antibody in horses. *Am J Pathol.* 1979;94:443–446.

Cianciolo RE, Mohr FC, Aresu L, et al. World Small Animal Veterinary Association Renal Pathology Initiative: classification of glomerular diseases in dogs. *Vet Pathol.* 2016;53:113–135.

Harris CH, Krawiec DR, Gelberg HB, et al. Canine IgA glomerulopathy. *Vet Immunol Immunopathol.* 1993;36:1–16.

Kurts C, Panzer U, Anders H-J, et al. The immune system and kidney disease: basic concepts and clinical implications. *Nature Revs Immunol.* 2013;13:738–753.

Mansfield CS, Mooney CT. Lymphocytic-plasmacytic thyroiditis and glomerulonephritis in a boxer. *J Small Anim Pract.* 2006;47:396–399.

McSloy A, Poulsen K, Fisher PJ, et al. Diagnosis and treatment of a selective immunoglobulin M glomerulopathy in a Quarter Horse gelding. *J Vet Intern Med.* 2007;21:874–877.

Rossi F, Aresu L, Martini V, et al. Immune-complex glomerulonephritis in cats: a retrospective study based on clinicopathological data, histopathology, and ultrastructural features. *BMC Vet Res.* 2019. doi:10.1186/s12917-019-2046-y.

Yabuki A, Shimokawa Miyama T, Kohyama M, et al. Canine IgA nephropathy: a case report. *J Vet Med Sci.* 2016;78:513–515.

Autoinflammatory Diseases

As described in Chapter 3, immune-mediated diseases usually involve a mixture of both dysfunctional innate and adaptive responses. The importance of each type of response varies among diseases. Thus there is a continuum from purely autoinflammatory disease at one extreme to purely autoimmune disease at the other. In this chapter are discussed those immune-mediated diseases that involve predominantly dysfunctional innate immune responses.

Innate autoimmunity, otherwise called autoinflammation, when first conceived, encompassed a set of monogenic human diseases marked by recurrent episodes of systemic and organ-specific inflammation caused by dysregulation of the innate immune system. Since this initial definition, our concept of autoinflammatory diseases has been greatly expanded. While initially encompassing only innate immunity, it is apparent that many such systemic diseases play an important role in both autoimmune and even immunosuppressive disorders. Many have very complex genotypes and phenotypes involving uncontrolled NF-κB activation. Among these complex, multifactorial inflammatory diseases are mixed pattern disorders such as reactive arthritis (described in Chapter 17) and polygenic disorders such as systemic lupus erythematosus, rheumatoid arthritis, and antineutrophil cytoplasmic antibody (ANCA)–associated vasculitis (described in Chapters 15, 16, and 18, respectively).

A consistent feature of all these is the overproduction of proinflammatory cytokines. For example, type 1 interferons are overproduced in systemic lupus erythematosus, tumor necrosis factor-alpha (TNFα) and IL6 are overproduced in rheumatoid arthritis, interleukin-23(IL23) is overproduced in human inflammatory bowel disease, and IL17 is overproduced in reactive arthritis. As a result, affected animals suffer from recurrent fevers, hyperinflammation, and eventual systemic amyloidosis. These diseases, if left untreated, may be relentless and cause severe tissue damage and eventual death.

Even under normal circumstances, acute inflammation, the quintessential reaction of innate immunity, may be painful and uncomfortable. This is usually, however, a temporary state and subsides once the invading organisms are eliminated and the damaged tissues heal. Under some circumstances, however, inflammation may become uncontrollable. Chronic, unresolved inflammation is often a result of inherited defects in immune regulatory processes. Many such diseases have been identified in humans as well as a few in domestic animals. In the latter case, these are often associated with specific dog breeds. On the other hand, there are also many auto-inflammatory diseases of unknown etiology with no obvious genetic or breed links. These too may be considered to result from a failure to control innate immune responses. These diseases or syndromes are often interrelated and may have many overlapping clinical features. Their common feature is extensive and uncontrolled inflammation.

Examples of autoinflammatory diseases include systemic lupus erythematosus, rheumatoid arthritis, reactive arthritis, vasculitis, and Sjögren syndrome. Although these diseases all have some form of autoimmune component, they do not simply result from autoantibodies causing tissue destruction. In humans, many are also associated with the presence of immune complexes and complement in tissues resulting in chronic inflammation. Many result from uncontrolled inflammatory cytokine production, different forms of programed cell death driven by specialized inflammasomes, or abnormalities in the complement system. (Inflammasomes are multimeric immune signaling complexes that drive innate immunity). Their initiating factors are often unknown, but all exhibit a significant genetic predisposition, commonly with linkage to the major histocompatibility complex. It is also important to point out that a loss of control of inflammation is a key component of the aging process (Box 14.1).

BOX 14.1 ■ Inflammaging

As animals age, their immune system changes. These changes affect many immune parameters when compared to the young and healthy. For example, aging of the immune system, immunosenescence, is associated with a decline in cell-mediated immunity and an increase in innate immunity. Beginning with thymic involution, T-cell numbers drop over time, while memory cells accumulate. There is also a shift in the helper T (Th) cell balance from Th1 to Th2 responses, associated with a decline in interleukin-2 (IL2) production.

Aging is also associated with the progressive development of a chronic low-grade inflammation, a process called inflammaging. This is probably a result of the gradual accumulation of damaged or dying cells and organelles over time. These dying cells generate senescence-associated DAMPs that act through TLR2 and IL1β to activate the NF-κB pathway. This in turn causes chronic activation of the innate immune system. Over time, this chronic activation results in a change in the phenotype of cells such as macrophages. These cells release a mixture of proinflammatory molecules in a condition known as the senescence-associated secretory phenotype (SASP). The SASP macrophages produce increased quantities of tumor necrosis factor-alpha (TNFα), IL6, matrix metalloproteases, and monocyte chemoattractant protein. Proinflammatory cytokines such as TNFα, IL6, and C-reactive protein levels in the bloodstream gradually increase over time.

Generation of SASP is the main driver of age-related inflammation. At low levels, SASP macrophages may be protective, but as the levels of proinflammatory cytokines increase, they eventually provoke the development of many of the chronic diseases of aging such as heart disease, neurodegeneration, and arthritis. Therefore in some respects inflammaging can be considered a manifestation of innate autoimmunity.

As noted elsewhere, Th17 cells play an important role in the pathogenesis of many immune-mediated inflammatory diseases in animals. The numbers of Th17 cells have been assessed over time in dogs, and it has been found that these numbers are positively correlated with age, a finding compatible with the concept of inflammaging. Thus in dogs under 1 year of age, the proportion of CD3+ CD4+ IL17+ T cells averaged 1.52%; in dogs 1 to 5 years, the average was 3.81%; while in dogs 6 years of age or older, they averaged 7.49%.

DAMPs, Damage-associated molecular patterns

Akiyama S, Asahina R, Ohta H, et al. Th17 cells increase during maturation in peripheral blood of healthy dogs. *Vet Immunol Immunopathol.* 2019;209:17–21.
Franceschi C, Garagnani P, Vitale G, et al. Inflammaging and garb-aging. *Trends Endocrinol Metabol.* 2017. doi.org/10.1016/j.tem.2016.09.005.

Autoinflammatory Diseases

SHAR-PEI FEVER SYNDROME

Shar-Peis are an ancient Chinese breed that came close to extinction in the 1950s when the Communist authorities taxed them heavily. However, a few were exported to the United States in the 1970s. Their offspring have been heavily selected for a wrinkled skin phenotype. This wrinkled skin results from excessive deposition of hyaluronic acid (HA) in the extracellular tissue of the upper dermis (Fig. 14.1). Blood levels of HA are also elevated in these dogs, a condition called hyaluronanosis. The HA synthase gene *HAS2* is overexpressed in dermal fibroblasts from Shar-Peis. As a result, HA is deposited throughout the skin, often in microscopic "lakes" and macroscopic vesicles. These deposits result in extensive and thick skin folding around the head and the hocks. Selection for folds around the mouth ("meatmouth") has been especially extensive. It is these meatmouth dogs that appear to be most susceptible to developing the fever syndrome.

Unfortunately, HA acts as an alarmin so that if it escapes into tissues, it serves as a danger signal that activates the innate immune system. HA interacts with cells such as macrophages to induce production of excessive IL1β and IL6. These cytokines act on the hypothalamus to cause a fever. The development of wrinkled skin and the development of a fever are therefore related. Both are associated with a mutation in a regulatory region located about 350 kB upstream of the gene for *HAS2*. This mutation is a 16.1-kB duplication whose copy number is related to *HAS2* expression and disease. (Unaffected dogs of other breeds have only one copy.) The proportion of Shar-Peis within the US population with this mutation is now estimated to be as high as 23%. A second, modifier gene locus affects the subsequent development of amyloidosis.

Clinical Disease

Shar-Peis present with recurrent unprovoked episodes of fever and inflammation. They have 12- to 48-hour episodes of high fever accompanied by localized arthritis, especially in one or both tibiotarsal joints. These attacks may occur every few weeks. However, acute phase reactants such

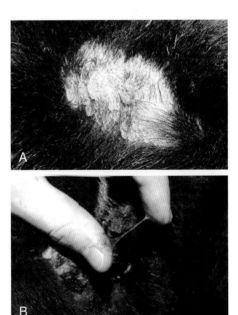

Fig. 14.1 Shar-Pei fever. (A) Multiple mucin-filled vesicles on the back of an adult Shar Pei. (B) The same dog where the vesicle has ruptured and viscous hyaluronic acid is released. (Congenital Diseases from Small Animal Dermatology. 2017; Edited by: Keith A. Hnilica and Adam P. Patterson. Elsevier.)

as serum amyloid A remain high between episodes so that the dogs eventually develop reactive amyloidosis. Amyloid is deposited in multiple organs, including the kidney, liver, spleen, gastrointestinal tract, and myocardium. Renal amyloidosis and kidney or liver failure lead to early death.

Diagnosis and Treatment

There is no specific diagnostic test for this syndrome prior to amyloid deposition, and a presumptive diagnosis is based solely on clinical signs. While IL6 levels are increased during fever episodes, they are inconsistently elevated between episodes and cannot be used to screen for the disorder. Renal biopsy and staining with Congo red are necessary for the definitive diagnosis of renal amyloidosis.

Colchicine treatment has been recommended for the treatment of Shar-Pei fever syndrome in an effort to prevent amyloid deposition and its progression into renal failure.

CANINE HYPERTROPHIC OSTEODYSTROPHY

Canine hypertrophic osteodystrophy (HOD) is an uncommon inflammatory bone disease, also known as metaphyseal osteopathy. It occurs in young, rapidly growing, large-breed dogs such as Irish Setters, Great Danes, Irish Wolfhounds, and especially Weimaraners. Occasional cases have been reported in other canine breeds. The Weimaraner breed is prone to a multiorgan inflammatory form of the disease with severe gastrointestinal, respiratory, and neurologic signs.

HOD is characterized by metaphyseal necrosis, hemorrhage, and inflammation. It affects young dogs during periods of rapid growth and diminishes once their bone plates have closed; thus it causes an acute-onset bilateral lameness. Both fore- and hind limbs are equally affected so that it affects the radius, ulna, and tibia. The vertebral bodies may also be affected. Affected dogs have significantly elevated levels of multiple inflammatory cytokines, including IL1β, IL18, IL6, GM-CSF, CXCL10, TNFα, and IL10. These cytokines may remain elevated, even in recovered dogs. Systemic signs include anorexia, depression, fever, and gastrointestinal, nervous, and respiratory issues, in addition to symmetric bone lesions with painful, swollen metaphyses. Radiologic examination shows radiolucent zones in the distal metaphyses, flared diaphyses, and the formation of new periosteal bone (Fig. 14.2).

These dogs may also have a preexisting immune dysfunction with low concentrations of one or more immunoglobulin classes, recurrent infections, and inflammatory disease. (Low levels of IgG, IgM, or IgA in blood are documented inconsistently in HOD-affected dogs.) The cause of HOD remains unknown, with earlier speculations of vitamin C deficiency or overnutrition now discounted. A heritability for HOD of 0.68 suggests a significant genetic effect.

HOD is a vaccination-proximate disease. Approximately 70% of the Weimaraners diagnosed with HOD have been reported to have received a multivalent vaccine within 1 to 2 weeks of disease onset. The disease is reported to develop within 10 days after administration of modified-live canine distemper vaccine. It is possible that the condition is triggered in genetically susceptible animals by prior vaccination, although it is equally likely that the onset of disease simply coincides with the recommended age of dog vaccination. It is important to note that there have been reports of Weimaraners with HOD that had not received any vaccines within the previous 3 weeks, confirming that proximity to vaccination is not a mandatory trigger for its development.

HOD is not the only problem suffered by young Weimaraners. Recurrent febrile episodes associated with systemic inflammatory signs have also been recognized in this breed. The term *hyperinflammatory syndrome* has been used to describe collectively not only HOD but also aseptic meningitis, postvaccinal reactions with high fever and/or nodular skin disease, and an immunodeficiency syndrome. There is likely to be a common underlying cause for all these inflammatory diseases that has yet to be identified.

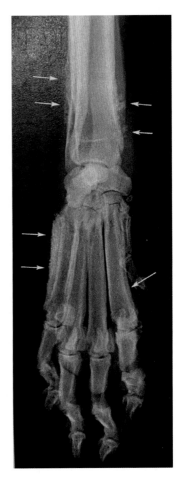

Fig. 14.2 Radiograph of the manus of a dog with hypertrophic osteodystrophy. There is an irregular periosteal reaction *(arrows)* that is most pronounced on the lateral aspect of the fifth metacarpal bone and on the medial aspect of the distal radius. There is a less pronounced periosteal reaction on the medial aspect of the manus. (G Allan and S Davies. Orthopedic diseases of Young and Growing dogs and cats from In Thrall DE. Textbook of Veterinary Radiology, 7ed 2018. Elsevier.)

Clinical Disease

Males and females are equally affected, and the age of onset is typically 8 to 16 weeks of age. Dogs with HOD present with anorexia, depression, fever, vomiting, lymphadenopathy, and swollen, painful metaphyses. The dogs may also suffer from an ocular and nasal discharge, skin pustules, rectal bleeding, vulvovaginitis, and respiratory tract inflammation. Many dogs have self-limiting small bowel diarrhea coincident with the onset of fever and joint pain. They also show pain and soft tissue swelling over the affected bones. Lameness is associated with swelling of the growth plates in the long bones.

Diagnosis and Treatment

Diagnosis of HOD relies on history, clinical signs, and the presence of characteristic radiographic findings at the growth plate of long bones. It is essential to rule out infectious causes for the fever and bone pain. Hematologic findings include a neutrophilic leukocytosis and a monocytosis. Alkaline phosphatase is elevated reflecting bone necrosis. Some animals may also be hypogammaglobulinemic. Biopsies show severe neutrophilic inflammation, subperiosteal hemorrhage, and trabecular necrosis. Prompt recognition of the disease and appropriate treatment are the keys to a good outcome.

Treatment of HOD has traditionally relied on rest, carefully calibrated use of nonsteroidal antiinflammatory drugs (NSAIDs), and opiate analgesics as necessary. NSAIDs and rest are appropriate for self-limiting disease, but corticosteroids should be used for severe, progressive disease when radiographic changes in the growth plates are consistent with HOD. In most cases, the disease is self-limiting, and most dogs recover in several weeks subsequent to physeal closure. Dogs that recover may have residual skeletal deformities.

SWEET SYNDROME

Sweet syndrome in humans is an acute febrile neutrophilic dermatosis. Affected individuals develop pyrexia and a neutrophilia in addition to the dermatosis. They develop painful papules or nodules containing a diffuse mature neutrophilic infiltrate within the superficial dermis. The syndrome results from the overexpression of proinflammatory cytokines, especially granulocyte colony-stimulating factor (G-CSF). This causes excessive neutrophil production and eventually results in a massive sterile inflammatory response. The localization in the skin is believed to be Th17-cell mediated. Classic Sweet syndrome is idiopathic, but other forms may be drug induced or paraneoplastic.

A similar syndrome has been described in dogs. Affected animals develop fever, lymphadenopathy, and a severe leukocytosis. Extracutaneous lesions include a vasculitis, immune-mediated hemolytic anemia, hepatopathy, and thrombocytopenia. Skin lesions, including a sterile neutrophilic dermatitis with ulcerations, erythema, and crusting, develop after 3 to 4 weeks. Similar canine cases may result from adverse reactions to the drug carprofen. Treatment with dexamethasone supplemented with mycophenolate mofetil has been reported to be effective.

STERILE NODULAR PANNICULITIS

Panniculitis refers to inflammation of subcutaneous fat. While often of unknown etiology, some forms have also been associated with pancreatic disease, systemic lupus erythematosus, rheumatoid arthritis, colitis, and hepatitis. Miniature Dachshunds, Poodles, Australian Shepherds, Brittany Spaniels, and neutered and young dogs appear to be most susceptible. Affected dogs develop multiple skin nodules that ulcerate, fistulate, and drain a yellowish oily exudate, but other deeper subcutaneous nodules may persist (Fig. 14.3). At the same time, affected dogs show evidence of systemic disease, including lethargy, anorexia, depression, and fever. The disease appears to come in waves. Some dogs may develop a concurrent arthritis.

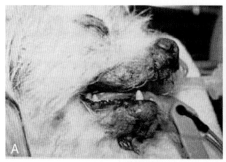 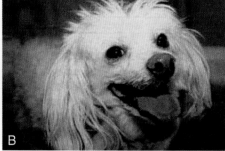

Fig. 14.3 Sterile nodular panniculitis in a Poodle mix with the plaque form of sterile nodular dermatitis (A) and after treatment (B). (Schissler J., Sterile Pyogranulomatous Dermatitis and Panniculitis Sterile Pyogranulomatous Dermatitis and Panniculitis Vet Clin Small Anim 2019; 49:27–36.)

The cutaneous or subcutaneous nodules may show a septal or diffuse pattern with a neutrophil and macrophage infiltration. Lymphocytes and plasma cells may also be present in the infiltrate. Clinical pathology generally shows a neutrophilia that may include a left shift, increased alkaline phosphatase, hypoalbuminemia, and proteinuria. Diagnosis requires exclusion of infectious causes. Immunosuppressive therapy with oral glucocorticoids appears to be effective. This may be supplemented, if necessary, with cyclosporine, azathioprine, or tetracycline plus niacinamide.

CANINE CHRONIC ULCERATIVE STOMATITIS

As its name suggests, canine chronic ulcerative stomatitis is a progressive and painful inflammatory disease of the oral mucosa. Maltese Terriers, Cavalier King Charles Spaniels, Labrador Retrievers, and Greyhounds appear to be the most susceptible breeds. Dogs develop painful mucosal ulcers that vary in size and distribution. As a result, affected animals refuse to eat and lose weight due to chronic oral pain.

The lesions are characteristically lichenoid with a dense inflammatory cell infiltrate developing between the superficial mucosal epithelium and the subepithelial connective tissue. These lesions contain large numbers of B and T cells, including FoxP3$^+$ cells, in other words Treg cells, and large numbers of IL17-producing cells. They also contain plasma cells, neutrophils, and mast cells. Interestingly, the IL17$^+$ cells are CD3$^-$, suggesting that they are not T cells. They appeared to be primarily mononuclear cells, but their role is unclear. Their numbers correlate negatively with lesion severity scores. While originally believed to be associated with the presence of periodontal disease, this does not now appear to be the case. The lesions are very different. There is no evidence that autoantibodies are involved in their pathogenesis, but it appears likely that this disease may reflect the results of a local imbalance between Th17 and Treg cells, resulting in excessive mucosal IL17 production.

Canine IgG4-Related Diseases

IgG4-related diseases are a group of autoinflammatory disorders characterized by excessive IgG4 production. While antibodies of the IgG4 subclass have been considered biologically inert, they play a prominent role in diverse autoimmune and immunologically mediated diseases in both humans and dogs. These antibodies can react with many autoantigens and as a result cause diverse diseases. IgG4 antibodies have a unique ability to exchange their Fab arms between molecules. This is a process that makes them functionally monovalent and amplifies their pathogenicity. In addition, IgG4 antibodies can activate macrophages that then cause extensive tissue fibrosis. IgG4-related abnormalities have also been reported in many other lymphocyte populations such as Th2 cells, Treg cells, and CD8$^+$ cytotoxic T cells. Likewise, affected individuals develop abnormalities in innate immunity, including activation of macrophages, mast cells, basophils, and dendritic cells.

IgG4-related disease in humans is an insidiously progressive fibroinflammatory disease. It is characterized by the development of tumorlike masses in many different organs. It presents as a multiorgan disease and can cause significant organ dysfunction, failure, and death. The tumorlike lesions are characterized by a dense infiltration of oligoclonal IgG4-positive plasma cells (Fig. 14.4). Affected organs include the lacrimal glands, the major salivary glands, pancreas, bile ducts, retroperitoneum, lungs, kidney, aorta, meninges, and thyroid. Paradoxically, serum IgG4 levels are normal in many patients. In progressive cases, death may result from periaortitis, retroperitoneal fibrosis, or pachymeningitis.

The IgG4$^+$ B cell and plasma cell infiltration of the lesions is accompanied by infiltration of the fibrotic stroma with CD4$^+$ T cells and M2 macrophages. The T cells contribute to the development of fibrosis by inducing local apoptosis, while the macrophages produce profibrotic cytokines

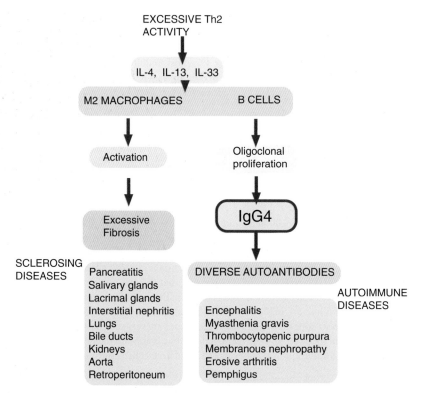

Fig. 14.4 The major features of immunoglobulin G4 *(IgG4)* disease. It probably originates as a result of excessive helper T type 2 *(Th2)* cell function. This in turn activates the wound healing process and so generates a severe sclerosing disease as a result of uncontrolled fibroblast activation. The generation of excessive amounts of IgG4 from B cells results in the production of diverse autoantibodies and autoimmune diseases. *IL,* Interleukin.

such as IL10, IL33, and CCL18. BAFF (a B-cell–stimulating cytokine) is also overproduced. In the human disease, the newly produced IgG4 is directed against diverse autoantigens such as carbonic anhydrase, plasminogen binding protein, lactoferrin, pancreatic secretory trypsin inhibitor, amylase, galectin-3, the acetylcholine receptor, and laminin-511. Thus these IgG4 autoantibodies may also cause diseases such as myasthenia gravis, pemphigus vulgaris, thrombocytopenic purpura, and pancreatitis. As might be expected, the more diverse autoantibodies are produced, the more severe the disease.

TYPE 1 AUTOIMMUNE PANCREATITIS

IgG4-related disease also occurs in dogs. Like the human disease, it is a systemic fibroinflammatory disease characterized by the infiltration of affected tissues with massive numbers of IgG4-positive plasma cells. The pancreas appears to be the preferred target organ so that dogs typically develop a lymphoplasmacytic sclerosing pancreatitis. The pancreas is infiltrated with a dense polyclonal infiltrate of plasma cells, layers of fibrosis, and obliterative phlebitis. IgG4+ plasma cells may account for more than 40% of all the lymphocytes and plasma cells in the infiltrate. The infiltration eventually results in tissue damage and organ fibrosis. Lesions are not, however, restricted to the pancreas. IgG4-positive B cells may also infiltrate other organs such as the salivary glands, periorbital tissues, retroperitoneum, kidney, biliary tract, lungs, and thyroid (Fig. 14.5).

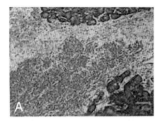 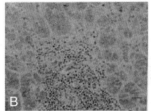 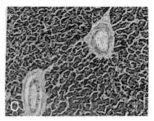

Fig. 14.5 Hematoxylin and eosin–stained sections of pancreas from (A) an English Cocker Spaniel, (B) a Great Dane crossbreed, and (C) a normal pancreas, showing the characteristic mononuclear cell infiltrates of IgG4–mediated pancreatitis. (Coddou MN, Constantino-Casas F, Scase T, et al. Chronic inflammatory disease of the pancreas, kidney, and salivary glands of English Cocker Spaniels and dogs of other breeds shows similar histological features to human IgG4-related disease. *J Comp Pathol.* 2020;177:18–33.)

Chronic IgG4-mediated type 1 pancreatitis occurs in English Cocker Spaniels and other breeds such as Huskies. The developing inflammation results in abdominal discomfort and eventual loss of both endocrine and exocrine functions. On histopathology, the lesions are characterized by interlobular fibrosis and a dense perivascular B-cell accumulation. Infiltration with IgG4+ B cells is also observed in the kidneys, salivary glands, tear ducts, and lacrimal glands of affected dogs. Tumorlike swellings may develop in the salivary glands.

Clinical Disease

Chronic type 1 autoimmune pancreatitis occurs in many dog breeds, but English Springer and Cocker Spaniels tend to be overrepresented. Affected dogs develop an exocrine pancreatic insufficiency with a combination of signs such as steatorrhea, weight loss, and a positive response to pancreatic enzyme supplementation. They may also develop diabetes mellitus with polydipsia and polyuria and persistent hyperglycemia, proteinuria, and possibly ketonuria. Some animals may also develop keratoconjunctivitis sicca (see Chapter 8).

Diagnosis and Treatment

IgG4 disease resembles the plasma cell tumor, multiple myeloma. Increased concentrations of oligoclonal IgG4 in the bloodstream are highly suggestive but not pathognomic. It is often associated with an enlarged hypoechoic pancreas on ultrasound. The lacrimal glands may be grossly normal even when infiltrated with plasma cells. Diagnosis depends on finding the characteristic histopathology and increased numbers of IgG4+ cells in affected tissues.

Animals and humans respond positively to glucocorticoid treatment, supplemented by cyclophosphamide if necessary.

TYPE 2 AUTOIMMUNE PANCREATITIS

The most common cause of an exocrine pancreatic deficiency in dogs is atrophy associated with lymphocyte and plasma cell infiltration (i.e., type 2 autoimmune disease). The disease has a high heritability as shown by its prevalence in German Shepherd Dogs and Rough-Coated Collies. It has also been reported in juvenile Greyhounds, Beagles, and English Setters. Genetic studies have suggested that certain MHC genes are associated with the disease. One haplotype containing a novel class I DLA-88 allele is highly associated with the disease, while other haplotypes may confer protection. There are no apparent gender differences.

The autoimmune attack results in selective destruction of the acinar cells that produce digestive enzymes. At the end stage, no acinar tissue remains. The acini are replaced by atypical parenchyma, ductal structures, and adipose tissue. Large clusters of lymphocytes may be present and form follicles. Biopsies from subclinical cases indicate that the lymphocyte infiltration is most marked in the border zone between affected and nonaffected parenchyma. It then spreads into the acinar tissues. It is clear that the lymphocytic infiltration precedes the atrophy of the acini. The infiltrating lymphocytes are primarily CD4$^+$ and CD8$^+$ T cells, but plasma cells are present as well. The CD8$^+$ T cells are associated with areas of pancreatic necrosis. Some of these dogs have low levels of antibodies against pancreatic acinar cells, so type 2 disease also has an autoimmune component. A possible autoantigen has been identified as acinar cell lactoferrin.

Unlike type 1 IgG4 disease, the predominant infiltrating cells in type 2 pancreatitis are almost all T cells with equal numbers of CD4$^+$ and CD8$^+$ cells. The cytotoxic T cells predominate in areas of acinar cell destruction. Type 2 pancreatitis is not associated with any abnormalities in IgG4 levels, nor does it affect organs other than the pancreas.

Clinical Disease

Signs of type 2 disease usually appear between 1 and 5 years of age. Dogs present with signs of abdominal discomfort and maldigestion. They lose weight despite a good appetite. They may have diarrhea, steatorrhea, or loose stools. Their feces are a pale color, either yellowish or gray, and are soft and loose. The diarrhea is accompanied by flatulence. Many cases remain subclinical as long as sufficient acinar tissue remains.

Diagnosis and Treatment

The diagnosis of exocrine pancreatic function is best achieved using pancreatic function tests. Two such tests are recommended. The TLI (trypsin-like immunoreactivity) test uses a radioimmunoassay to measure the amount of trypsinogen that has entered the bloodstream from the pancreas. Low values indicate pancreatic insufficiency. This may be detected before the appearance of clinical disease. While TLI is the best test for exocrine pancreatic insufficiency, it may be falsely elevated as a result of inflammation. Conversely, PLI (pancreatic lipase immunoreactivity) in blood is considered the best test to measure the severity of the pancreatic inflammation. The lipase leaks from damaged acinar cells into the bloodstream where it can be measured by enzyme-linked immunosorbent assays (see Chapter 20).

BOX 14.2 ■ Is Equine Laminitis an Autoinflammatory Disease?

Laminitis, a crippling inflammatory disease syndrome of horses, is a consequence of several different systemic diseases. These include endocrine disease, malnutrition, sepsis, and altered weight bearing. Studies on horses with chronic laminitis have demonstrated that their leukocytes produce more IFNγ than leukocytes from normal horses; however, they showed no differences in immunoglobulin levels or detectable rheumatoid factor. Unlike other autoimmune and autoinflammatory diseases, there is no apparent linkage between laminitis susceptibility and the MHC complex. Thus there is no evidence to support the concept that laminitis is autoimmune in nature.

Studies on lamellar tissue from horses with supporting limb laminitis have, however, demonstrated upregulation of the genes for IL17A as well as those encoding the IL17 inflammatory pathway. This is probably a secondary consequence of cell stress and tissue damage rather than primary causation. It can be argued therefore that while the initiating factors of laminitis are not immunologic, chronic cell stress acting through the NF-κB pathway can result in the development of autoinflammatory processes.

IFNγ, Interferon-gamma; *IL,* interleukin; *MHC,* major histocompatibility complex.

Steelman SM, Johnson D, Wagner B, et al. Cellular and humoral immunity in chronic equine laminitis. *Vet Immunol Immunopathol.* 2013;153:217–226.

Cassimeria L, Engiles JB, Galantino-Homer H. Interleukin 17A pathway target genes are upregulated in *Equus caballus* supporting limb laminitis. *PLOSOne.* 2020. doi.org/10.1371/journal.pone.0232920.

Treatment of exocrine pancreatic insufficiency is by oral pancreatic enzyme replacement. Uncoated tablets, raw chopped pancreas, and powdered formulations appear to be most effective.

Sources of Additional Information

Abeles V, Harrus S, Angles JM, et al. Hypertrophic osteodystrophy in six Weimaraner puppies associated with systemic signs. *Vet Rec.* 1999;145:130–134.

Anderson JG, Kol A, Bizikova P, et al. Immunopathogenesis of canine ulcerative stomatitis. *PLOSOne.* 2020. doi:10.1371/journal.pone.0227386.

Anderson JG, Peralta S, Kass PH, et al. Clinical and histopathologic characterization of canine ulcerative stomatitis. *Vet Pathol.* 2017;54:511–519.

Coddou MN, Constantino-Casas F, Scase T, et al. Chronic inflammatory disease of the pancreas, kidney, and salivary glands of English Cocker Spaniels and dogs of other breeds shows similar histological features to human IgG4-related disease. *J Comp Pathol.* 2020;177:18–33.

Colopy LJ, Shiu K-B, Snyder LA, et al. Immunoglobulin G4-related disease in a dog. *J Vet Int Med.* 2019;33:2732–2738.

Contreary CL, Outerbridge CA, Affolter VK, et al. Canine sterile nodular panniculitis: a retrospective study of 39 dogs. *Vet Dermatol.* 2015;26:451 -e105.

Foale RD, Herrtage ME, Day MJ. Retrospective study of 25 young Weimaraners with low serum immunoglobulin concentrations and inflammatory disease. *Vet Rec.* 2003;153:553–558.

Kastner DL, Aksentijevich I, Goldbach-Mansky R. Autoinflammatory disease reloaded: a clinical perspective. *Cell.* 2010;140:784–790.

Koneczny I. Update on IgG4-mediated autoimmune diseases: new insights and new family members. *Autoimm Rev.* 2020. doi:10.1016/j. autrev.2020.102646.

Liu C, Zhang PM, Zhang W. Immunological mechanisms of IgG4-related disease. *J Transl Autoimmun.* 2020. doi:10.1016/j.jtauto.2020.100047.

O'Kell AL, Inteeworn N, Diaz SF, et al. Canine sterile nodular panniculitis: a retrospective study of 14 cases. *J Vet Intern Med.* 2010;24:278–284.

Ollson M, Meadows JRS, Truvé K, et al. A novel unstable duplication upstream of *HAS2* predisposes to a breed-defining skin phenotype and a periodic fever syndrome in Chinese Shar-Pei dogs. *PLOS Genet.* 2011. doi:10.1371/journal.pgen.1001332.

Perugino CA, Stone JH. IgG4-related disease: an update on pathophysiology and implications for clinical care. *Nature Rev Rheumatol.* 2020. doi:10.1038/s41584-020-0500-7.

Safra N, Hitchens PL, Maverakis E, et al. Serum levels of innate immunity cytokines are elevated in dogs with metaphyseal osteopathy (hypertrophic osteodystrophy) during active disease and remission. *Vet Immunol Immunopathol.* 20126;179:32-35.

Watson PJ, Roulois A, Scase T, et al. Characterization of chronic pancreatitis in English Cocker Spaniels. *J Vet Intern Med.* 2011;25:797–804.

Woodard JC. Canine hypertrophic osteodystrophy: a study of the spontaneous disease in littermates. *Vet Pathol.* 1982;19:337–354.

Zen Y, Bogdanos DP, Kawa S. Type 1 autoimmune pancreatitis. *Orphanet J Rare Dis.* 2011;6:82–92.

Systemic Lupus Erythematosus

In the previous chapters, we reviewed many different autoimmune diseases that were, for the most part, mediated by autoantibodies targeted against a single organ or cell type. In many cases these reflected a breakdown in tolerance to a specific autoantigen and the emergence of a small number of self-reactive B- or T-cell clones. However, there are other autoimmune and inflammatory diseases where control is lost over much of the immune system. In effect, these animals suffer a generalized breakdown of peripheral tolerance. These diseases or syndromes are interrelated and have many overlapping clinical features. One common feature is extensive and uncontrolled inflammation in multiple tissues or organs. Thus the dysfunction encompasses both the innate and adaptive immune systems. These diseases may be considered to be located in the middle of the spectrum between purely autoimmune and purely autoinflammatory diseases.

Examples of these systemic immune-mediated diseases include systemic lupus erythematosus (SLE), rheumatoid arthritis, nonerosive forms of arthritis, systemic vasculitis, and Sjögren syndrome. Although each of these diseases is associated with some degree of autoimmunity, they do not simply result from tissue damage caused by antibodies and T cells. Many of their lesions are associated with the presence of immune complexes and activated complement components in tissues. Many result from uncontrolled inflammatory cytokine production or from defects in the regulation of the complement system. Their initiating factors are largely unknown, although they all exhibit a significant genetic predisposition, commonly with linkage to the major histocompatibility complex (MHC). As with other autoimmune diseases, microbial dysbiosis is also consistently associated with their development. As a result, affected animals develop multiple autoantibodies, T-cell dysfunction, impaired apoptosis, and multiorgan inflammation. The most significant of these diseases is SLE.

Predisposing Factors

SLE is a complex syndrome that occurs in humans, other primates, mice, dogs, cats, and horses. It is characterized by diverse clinical signs and a wide variety of disease courses that fluctuate over time, and as a result both diagnosis and treatment are challenging. The factors that trigger the development of SLE are multiple and poorly defined, but as with other autoimmune diseases the three major groups of predisposing factors are environmental, hormonal, and genetic.

ENVIRONMENTAL FACTORS

One important predisposing factor for many forms of lupus is exposure to ultraviolet (UV) light. Both UV-A and UV-B light can penetrate the skin and damage epithelial basal cells. The short-wave UV-B (290–320 nm) can penetrate the epidermis, whereas the longer wave UV-A (320–400 nm) can penetrate as far as the dermis. UV-A contributes to the generation of reactive oxygen species, whereas UV-B can cause DNA breakage. Cells damaged by UV light undergo apoptosis and release nucleic acids into the tissues. In cases of lupus, the damaged cells are consequently attacked by antibodies and cytotoxic T cells. UV light elicits a neutrophil-dependent injury response. Not only are neutrophils attracted to UV light-exposed skin in lupus patients, but the activated cells also disseminate systemically and trigger inflammation in the kidney in an interleukin-17 (IL17)–dependent manner, thus there is a direct link between exposure to UV light and kidney damage in lupus patients.

Drugs are important triggers of systemic lupus. At least 90 drugs are known to cause a lupuslike disease in humans, and they account for about 10% of cases; 90% of these patients experience arthritis, and about half develop myositis. Lupus symptoms do not usually develop immediately on taking a drug but may take from months to years to fully develop. Offending drugs include hydralazine, procainamide, sulfadiazine, isoniazid, methyldopa, quinidine, minocycline, and chlorpromazine. Hydralazine and procainamide carry the highest risk. Both inhibit DNA methylation and can induce lupuslike lesions in healthy humans. Monoclonal antibodies that block tumor necrosis factor-alpha (TNFα) and interferon (IFN) signaling may also induce a lupuslike syndrome. These include infliximab, etanercept, and adalimumab. A lupuslike disease may develop in cats treated with the antithyroid drug propylthiouracil.

Aged individuals and lupus patients share features of immunosenescence. This appears to result from dysbiosis in the gut microbiota. Thus both show alterations in their Firmicutes/Bacteroidetes ratio (increased Bacteroidetes and Proteobacteria are associated with enhanced inflammation), a decrease in microbial diversity, and decreased production of antiinflammatory short-chain fatty acids.

Some infectious agents may trigger lupus in susceptible individuals. While no obvious viral trigger has been identified in humans, Epstein-Barr virus nuclear antigen cross-reacts with the lupus autoantigen Ro, suggesting possible molecular mimicry. As discussed in Box 15.1, some evidence exists for a role of an infectious trigger for lupus in dogs.

BOX 15.1 ■ A Viral Cause of Systemic Lupus Erythematosus?

It has been suggested by many investigators that endogenous retroviruses may serve as the link between the genome, the environment, and the development of systemic lupus erythematosus (SLE). Endogenous retroviruses are retroviral gene sequences integrated into the animal genome. For example, concordance rates for developing SLE are as low as 30% between monozygotic twins. This clearly indicates that genetic factors are by no means the major driving causes of this disease. It has been suggested that endogenous and exogenous retroviruses may epigenetically control the many immune system genes dysregulated in lupus. Likewise, the retroviral nucleic acids, it is suggested, may serve as activators of TLR7. Some retroviruses such as human immunodeficiency virus may cause disease syndromes that resemble SLE, and there is limited evidence that human endogenous retroviruses may play a pathogenic role in SLE.

New Zealand Black (NZB) mice spontaneously develop a disease that closely resembles human lupus. The retroviral envelope glycoprotein gp70 is found in the sera of both normal and NZB mice; however, only NZB mice spontaneously develop gp70–anti-gp70 immune complexes. These immune complexes are deposited in the mouse glomeruli and cause glomerulonephritis.

There is some evidence that a similar endogenous retrovirus may play a role in SLE in dogs. When dogs with lupus are bred, the number of affected offspring is higher than can be accounted for genetically, suggesting that the disease may be vertically transmitted. A type C retrovirus has been suggested as a potential trigger of canine lupus. Epidemiologic evidence also tends to support an environmental or possibly infectious cause for lupus, since it has been reported that pet dogs living in contact with human SLE patients are themselves at a higher risk of developing antinuclear antibodies and clinical SLE.

Chiou S-H, Lan J-L, Lin S-L, et al. Pet dogs owned by lupus patients are at a higher risk of developing lupus. *Lupus.* 2004;13:442–449.

Quimby FW, Gebert R, Datta S, et al. Characterization of a retrovirus that cross-reacts serologically with canine and human systemic lupus erythematosus (SLE). *Clin Immunol Immunopathol.* 1978;9:194–210.

HORMONAL FACTORS

Lupus in humans is predominantly a disease of young adult women, suggesting that hormonal factors play a key role. The female:male gender ratio may be as great as 15:1, depending on the age and ethnic group affected. One reason for this relates to the two X chromosomes in females. It is no coincidence that some toll-like receptors with genes on the X chromosomes such as TLR7 and TLR8 are more active in females than males, and these play a key role in the body's response to free nucleic acids. The gene encoding CD40 is also located on the X chromosome and may play a role in promoting excessive immune function (Box 15.2). Hormones also play an important role; thus pregnancy aggravates the disease. In lupus-prone NZB/MZW mice, estrogens accelerate the development of disease, whereas androgens have an opposite effect. Curiously, unlike humans and mice, there does not appear to be a gender bias in dogs with SLE.

GENETIC FACTORS

A predisposition to develop SLE in humans is associated with many different genes (Fig. 15.1). As a result, its worldwide prevalence varies from 3 to 517 cases per 100,000 individuals. Some cases can be caused by inherited deficiencies of the complement components C1q or C4. Lack of C4 results in a failure to eliminate self-reactive B cells, whereas lack of C1q results in decreased removal of necrotic cell debris. Likewise, loss-of-function mutations in the Fas or Fas-ligand genes that mediate T-cell killing of unneeded lymphocytes cause a lupuslike disease in humans, mice, and cats (see Chapter 22). Recent evidence suggests that a gain of function mutation in the TLR7 gene can also cause human lupus. Much more commonly, however, lupus is caused by the cumulative effects of many different genes. Most of the single nucleotide polymorphisms (SNPs) associated with lupus susceptibility are found in the noncoding regions of genes linked to the immune response. Some increase sensitivity to autoimmune diseases in general, while others specifically affect SLE. Genes

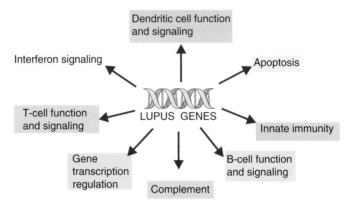

Fig. 15.1 Some of the many different genes and their targets that determine susceptibility to systemic lupus.

associated with dendritic cell functions, immune complex processing, T-cell functions and signaling, apoptosis, and B-cell functions have all been implicated. Epigenetic changes in keratinocytes caused by environmental factors such as UV light have also been linked to lupus.

Pathogenesis

Lupus is a complicated disease syndrome resulting from the interaction of multiple factors, both genetic and environmental, and diverse pathogenic processes (Fig. 15.2). The most important of these are linked to defects in the way dead and dying cells are handled by the immune system.

ABNORMAL APOPTOSIS

Apoptosis is a physiologic form of cell death that ensures that dying cells retain their contents as they break up into small apoptotic bodies. In healthy tissues, these apoptotic bodies display signals that ensure they are rapidly and completely phagocytosed by phagocytes, thus preventing cell membrane rupture and the release of proinflammatory damage-associated molecular patterns (DAMPs). This effectively prevents the accumulation of dead cells in normal tissues, and as a result, billions of cells are removed by apoptosis daily without triggering inflammation.

Two problems with apoptosis develop in lupus patients. First, their macrophages are unable to effectively remove apoptotic cell debris promptly. As a result of this "waste disposal defect," the debris accumulates in tissues. Second, rather than undergoing normal apoptosis, many cells die through other programmed death pathways, namely pyroptosis and NETosis. As a result, cellular DNA is released into tissues in large amounts. The effects of these apoptosis defects are most obvious in the skin of affected animals, where UV radiation damages and kills keratinocytes. Evidence suggests that normal lymphocytes can protect keratinocytes from apoptosis. In lupus patients, however, the lymphocytes fail to do so, perhaps as a result of a local epidermal transforming growth factor-beta (TGFβ) deficiency that permits excessive inflammation to develop. In humans, lupus skin lesions are commonly restricted to the bridge of the nose and the area around the eyes subjected to UV radiation from sunlight. A similar situation is seen in dogs.

SOURCES OF DNA

A defining feature of SLE is the production of antinuclear antibodies (ANA). The nucleic acids that trigger ANA production come from four major sources: (1 and 2) cells dying as a result of pyroptosis and NETosis, (3) platelet mitochondria, and (4) bacterial infections (Fig. 15.3). The defective clearance of cell debris together with cell death by other mechanisms generates an abundance of immunostimulatory and potentially antigenic DNA, RNA, and chromatin.

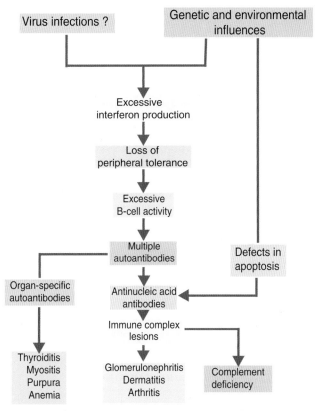

Fig. 15.2   A simplified overview of the pathogenesis of systemic lupus.

Pyroptosis

Pyroptosis is a form of programed cell death characterized by the formation of pores in the cell membrane, the release of IL1 and IL18, and DNA fragmentation. Cell swelling is followed by a breakdown in membrane integrity and the escape of cell contents. This is normally a defensive process that prevents replication of intracellular microbial invaders. Pyroptosis is triggered by the formation of a specialized protein complex, a pyroptosome, that activates multiple caspases. The caspases in turn activate IL1 and IL18 as well as a pore-forming effector protein called gasdermin D. The activated gasdermin D binds to cell membrane lipids and forms oligomeric pores in the plasma membrane. These pores permit the escape of IL1 and IL18 into the tissues. The dying cells eventually rupture as a result of increased osmotic pressure, thus releasing the rest of their contents into the tissues. These contents include both nuclear and mitochondrial DNA. When first released, the cellular DNA is largely intact and consists of very long strands. However, it is rapidly fragmented into much smaller pieces of about 166 base pairs—about the length of a strand of DNA wrapped around a single nucleosome. Mitochondrial DNA is released at the same time. It is a potent proinflammatory DAMP since its nucleotide composition reflects its microbial origins. Thus gasdermins also promote NETosis.

NETosis

Neutrophils exposed to pathogen-associated molecular patterns (PAMPs), DAMPs, and inflammatory mediators acting through pattern-recognition receptors (PRRs), especially their toll-like receptors, can expel their chromosomal DNA in the form of neutrophil extracellular traps (NETs).

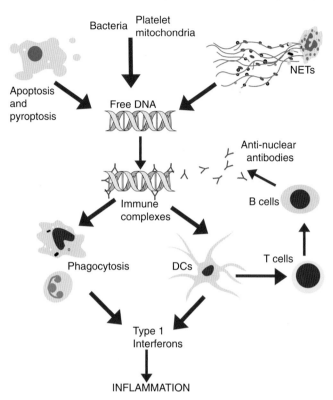

Fig. 15.3 The sources of DNA that can trigger the production of antinuclear antibodies in systemic lupus erythematosus and the consequences of immune complex formation. *NETs,* Neutrophil extracellular traps.

These traps normally capture and neutralize invading pathogens. This form of cell death is called NETosis. NETosis is related to pyroptosis since both caspases and gasdermin D are needed to rupture the neutrophil membrane. The cells then release decondensed chromatin, RNA and DNA, together with neutrophil granule proteins such as myeloperoxidase and elastase. The components of these NETs can be endocytosed by antigen-processing cells while the escaped DNA binds to TLR9. NETosis therefore provides a source of potential autoantigens in SLE as well as triggering inflammation.

In lupus cases, ANA may bind to NETs and protect them against digestion by nucleases. As a result, intact NETs are trapped in the glomerular capillaries and so cause lupus nephritis. In addition, when this DNA is opsonized by ANA and taken up by macrophages, the cells are triggered to produce large amounts of type I IFN via intracellular DNA sensors and the NF-κB pathway. This IFN plays a critically important role in lupus by suppressing regulatory T (Treg) functions.

Platelet Activation

Platelets possess toll-like receptors and Fc receptors and can therefore be activated by immune complexes. While blood platelets have no nuclei, they each contain, on average, about three mitochondria (about 27% of the mitochondrial DNA in blood). Once activated, the platelets release these mitochondria either as extracellular vesicles or simply as free mitochondria. These mitochondria can be ingested by phagocytic cells and activate intracellular DNA receptors. Given their numbers in peripheral blood and the fact that they are chronically activated in lupus cases, it appears that platelets are a significant source of the DNA that forms immune complexes.

Bacterial Sources

Animals predisposed to lupus may respond to bacterial infections by producing antibodies against bacterial DNA. These antibodies may cross-react with their own DNA. For example, the NZB/NZW mouse strain develops a lupuslike syndrome when immunized with bacterial DNA. It is possible that this bacterial DNA may be the initial trigger that starts the anti-DNA antibody cascade in lupus patients.

INNATE IMMUNE RESPONSES TO DNA

DNA Receptors

Cells of the innate immune system, especially plasmacytic dendritic cells, express diverse pattern-recognition receptors that can bind both foreign and self-nucleic acids. These include endosomal receptors such as TLR3 that binds double-stranded RNA, TLR7 and TLR8 that bind single-stranded RNA, and TLR9 that binds microbial DNA. Cytosolic nucleic acid receptors include retinoic acid-inducible gene 1 (RIG-1) that binds 5′-triphosphate RNA and melanoma differentiation associated gene-3 (MDA3) that binds long double-stranded RNAs. While their normal function is to recognize nucleic acids from invading bacteria and viruses, they can also bind related nucleic acids such as those from mitochondria. The DNA will bind to TLR7 and TLR9 and activate the NF-κB pathway. This results in the production of large quantities of the type I IFNs, especially IFNα, as well as proinflammatory cytokines such as IL1, IL6, IL12, and TNFα. In a normal situation, this would act to block viral and bacterial invasion. In lupus, this mechanism overreacts possibly because of exposure to excessive amounts of cellular DNA.

Interferons

The development of symptomatic lesions in lupus patients is closely associated with overproduction of type 1 IFNs by plasmacytoid dendritic cells (pDCs) to such an extent that systemic lupus has been classified by some investigators as an "interferonopathy." The level of IFNα correlates with disease activity, especially in cutaneous disease; 60% to 80% of human patients have increased expression of IFN-stimulated genes in peripheral blood. IFNs normally block viral infections by triggering innate immunity. IFN promotes inflammation by promoting macrophage differentiation and activating both Th1 and Th17 cells. The excessive production of IFNα in lupus in effect is a grossly exaggerated antiviral response. Fc receptor– and toll-like receptor–mediated uptake of immune complexes and nucleic acids further activates pDCs and triggers more IFNα production. The IFN effectively suppresses Treg activities and causes a generalized loss of peripheral tolerance. Type III IFNs are also increased in lupus patients and may contribute to the immune dysregulation and tissue damage.

B-CELL RESPONSES TO DNA

Antibody-DNA complexes bind to the pattern-recognition receptor TLR9 and activate B cells by triggering both their toll-like receptors and Fc receptors. Overactive B cells and long-lived plasma cells are central to the pathogenesis of lupus since they are the source of the autoantibodies responsible for its characteristic lesions. These activated B cells show enhanced toll-like receptor, antigen, and B-cell activating factor (BAFF) receptor signaling, in addition to responding to many different autoantigens. BAFF is a cytokine produced by myeloid cells. It supports the survival of autoreactive B cells and prevents their apoptosis. BAFF is commonly overexpressed in SLE and Sjögren syndrome.

ANTINUCLEAR ANTIBODIES

The hallmark of all forms of lupus is the development of autoantibodies against nuclear components, including DNA, histones, ribonucleoproteins, and chromatin. Anti-DNA antibodies generally bind to conserved epitopes on DNA molecules. They can bind to both single- and double-stranded DNA, although they require large fragments of DNA to form stable immune complexes.

ANA are found in 97% to 100% of dogs with lupus compared to only 16% to 20% of normal animals. About 16 different nuclear antigens have been identified in humans. There are two different types of ANA. The first type includes autoantibodies to DNA and closely linked nucleosomal contents such as histones and DNA-histone complexes. The second type consists of antibodies directed against RNA-binding proteins. These binding proteins, such as SSA/Ro, SSB/La, and Sm, are normally attached to specific RNA molecules in the cytoplasm (see Box 8.1). Dogs mainly develop autoantibodies against histones and ribonucleoproteins. In humans, antibodies to DNA are generally specific for SLE, whereas antibodies to the RNA-binding proteins are also produced in other inflammatory diseases such as Sjögren syndrome and rheumatoid arthritis. ANA levels can fluctuate greatly over time, spiking, for example, during disease flares, whereas the levels of antibodies to the RNA-binding proteins tend to be stable irrespective of the disease status.

OTHER B-CELL RESPONSES

Although the production of ANA is characteristic of SLE, many other autoantibodies are also produced by these animals, confirming a loss of peripheral tolerance and grossly abnormal B-cell function (Fig. 15.4). The B cells of affected animals show abnormalities in signaling and migration, overexpression of CD40L, and enhanced production of IL6 and IL10. Their loss of tolerance is also due in part to upregulation of B-cell transcription factors such as AP-1 as a result of elevated IFN levels. It is therefore probable that the production of multiple autoantibodies in lupus is a combined result of defective apoptosis, excessive IFN production, overstimulation of B cells, and a consequent failure of peripheral tolerance. (Box 15.2)

As a result, lupus B cells target a diverse array of nuclear, cytoplasmic, and membrane antigens. Autoantibodies to red cells induce a hemolytic anemia. Antibodies to platelets induce a thrombocytopenia. Antilymphocyte antibodies may interfere with immune regulation. About 20% of dogs with lupus produce antibodies to IgG (rheumatoid factors). Antibodies to phospholipids interfere with platelet functions and may cause immunothrombosis and vasculitis. Antibodies to

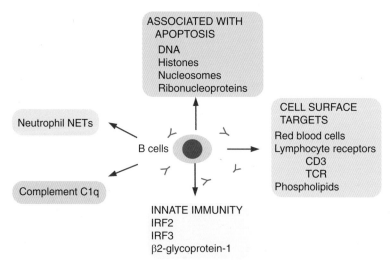

Fig. 15.4 Some of the targets of the multiple autoantibodies generated in systemic lupus.

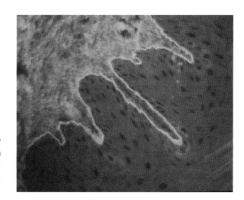

Fig. 15.5 An indirect immunofluorescence assay shows deposition of immunoglobulin G on the skin basement membrane (a lupus band). (Courtesy Dr. FC Heck [Tizard IR. *Veterinary Immunology*. 10th ed. Elsevier; 2016].)

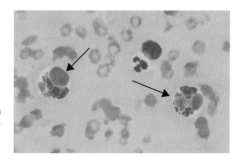

Fig. 15.6 Two lupus erythematosus cells *(arrows)* from a dog with systemic lupus erythematosus. Original magnification × 1300. (From Tizard IR. *Veterinary Immunology*. 10th ed. Elsevier; 2016.)

complement C1q are associated with renal disease. Antimuscle antibodies may cause myositis, and antimyocardial antibodies may provoke myocarditis or endocarditis.

Autoantibodies to skin basement membrane cause the characteristic lupus dermatitis characterized by changes in epidermal thickness, focal mononuclear cell infiltration, collagen degeneration, and immunoglobulin deposits at the dermoepidermal junction. These deposits form a lupus band that is seen in many other autoimmune skin diseases in addition to lupus (Fig. 15.5). The results of all this excessive immune reactivity are also reflected in a polyclonal gammopathy, enlargement of lymph nodes and spleen, and thymic enlargement with germinal center formation. ANA can also bind to the nuclei of degenerating cells to produce round or oval structures called hematoxylin bodies in the skin, kidney, lung, lymph nodes, spleen, and heart. Within the bone marrow, opsonized cell nuclei may be phagocytosed, giving rise to lupus erythematosus (LE) cells (Fig. 15.6).

The diversity of autoantibodies produced in lupus can cause an equally great variety of clinical symptoms. Polyarthritis, fever, proteinuria, anemia, and skin diseases are the most common abnormalities, but pericarditis, myocarditis, myositis, lymphadenopathy, and pneumonia have all been reported.

IMMUNE COMPLEX FORMATION

Renal failure is the cause of death in up to 60% of human lupus patients. It results from the deposition of immune complexes in the glomeruli. Immune complexes, especially those containing nuclear material such as DNA and chromatin from NETs, are produced in large amounts within the bloodstream. Normally, circulating antigen-antibody complexes are captured by Fc receptors and removed by macrophages in the liver and spleen. In lupus patients, as a result of defects in Fc and complement receptors, they are not completely removed, and the surplus complexes are filtered out in the renal glomeruli. There the NETs bind to basement membrane laminin, and the immune complexes accumulate in the basement membrane and subendothelial areas. Their presence results in local inflammation and cell proliferation that eventually causes a membranoproliferative glomerulonephritis. Extracellular vesicles derived from activated and dying cells can also deliver DNA-containing immune complexes and complement components to the glomeruli.

Immune complexes, NETs, and extracellular vesicles may also be deposited in arteriolar walls, where they cause an inflammatory arteritis and provoke immunothrombosis, or in synovia, where they provoke polyarthritis. Antibodies to blood cells may activate complement and so result in cytopenias. Some autoantibodies may cross the blood-brain barrier and so cause neurocognitive defects. Other B cells produce antiphospholipid antibodies and so induce an antiphospholipid syndrome (see Chapter 11).

Complement

In humans and other primates, complement components normally mediate the efficient clearance of apoptotic cells and immune complexes. Complement deficiencies, especially C1q or C4 deficiency, are therefore associated with the development of lupuslike syndromes. Some lupus patients may have a deficiency of the complement receptor CD35. As a result, complement-containing immune complexes are not bound to red cells or platelets and therefore are not removed from the circulation. In about one-third of lupus patients, autoantibodies are directed against C1q. Their presence is also associated with the development of renal disease.

T-CELL ABNORMALITIES

Lymphopenia is a marked feature of systemic lupus, and it correlates with disease activity. This is a result of a reduction in circulating CD8$^+$ cell numbers, whereas CD4$^+$ cell numbers are relatively unaffected. T-cell antigen receptor functions are also altered in lupus. The TCR-CD3 complex, instead of signaling through the CD3ζ chain as in normal T cells, signals through the common gamma chain of the Fc receptor. As a result, effector T-cell signaling is reduced. Reduced production and signaling by IL2 together with increased IL17 production occur in some lupus patients. As a result, cell-mediated cytotoxicity, whether mediated by CD8$^+$ T cells or by natural killer (NK) cells, is significantly reduced. In addition, the numbers of CD4$^+$ FoxP3$^+$ Treg cells are reduced in lupus patients.

Canine Systemic Lupus

SLE is a rare disease that affects dogs between 2 and 12 years of age. Any gender predisposition in this species is debatable. The disease occurs in Rough Collies, German Shepherd Dogs, Nova Scotia Duck Tolling Retrievers, and Shetland Sheepdogs, but Beagles, Irish Setters, Old English Sheepdogs, Poodles, and Afghan Hounds are also susceptible. Lupus (or positive lupus serology) may occur in healthy related animals, confirming the significance of genetic factors. A study of Nova Scotia Duck Tolling Retrievers has identified five gene loci associated with the SLE disease complex in this breed. The products of four of these loci are involved in T-cell activation through the NF-κB pathway (see Fig. 2.4). Likewise, dogs possessing the MHC class I antigen DLA-A7 are at increased risk, while those possessing DLA-A1 and -B5 are at decreased risk of developing the disease (see Box 15.1).

Several attempts have been made to establish breeding colonies of lupus dogs by selective mating of affected animals. This has been relatively successful as the animals become more inbred. Likewise, the prevalence of lupus dropped in colonies where there was extensive outbreeding.

CLINICAL DISEASE

Lupus is insidious and progressive, so the severity of the lesions and the number of organ systems involved gradually increases if left untreated. The most characteristic presentation in dogs is a fever accompanied by a symmetric, nonerosive polyarthritis. As many as 90% of dogs with lupus develop joint disease. These animals have obviously painful muscles and a shifting lameness. Fournel and colleagues in Lyon reported on 75 cases in dogs and showed that other common presenting signs included glomerulonephritis resulting in renal failure and proteinuria (65%), skin disease, especially skin ulcers and vesicles (60%), lymphadenopathy or splenomegaly (50%), leukopenia (20%), immune-mediated hemolytic anemia (13%), and thrombocytopenia (4%). Dogs may also develop myositis (8%) or pericarditis (8%) and neurologic abnormalities such as seizures (1.6%).

In addition to a severe lymphopenia, affected dogs have an increased CD4/CD8 T-cell ratio as a result of a major loss of $CD8^+$ cells with a much smaller loss of $CD4^+$ cells. The CD4/CD8 ratio may climb as high as 6, compared with a normal value of about 1.7. This lymphopenia results from damage to the bone marrow, and myelonecrosis has been recorded in canine lupus.

Lupus skin lesions are highly variable but are commonly restricted to areas exposed to sunlight (Fig. 15.7). Mucocutaneous or mucosal ulcers and erosions develop most commonly. Skin lesions also include scaling, erythema, alopecia, crusting, and scarring. They primarily affect the face, pinnae, and distal limbs. Skin biopsies show a lichenoid interface dermatitis with an obvious loss of basal or suprabasal cells. There may be subepidermal vacuolation and basement membrane thickening as well.

A different lupus-related disease has been described in Gordon Setters. These dogs develop a symmetric onychodystrophy with malformations and loss of the claws (Fig. 15.11). As a result, affected animals show lameness, severe discomfort, and acute foot pain. Some also develop ANA. A related disease of Gordon Setters may be black hair follicular dysplasia. In this disease, dogs begin to shed their black hair without normal regrowth. The remaining black hair is either short and stiff or thin and easily removed. Many affected Setters have positive ANA titers. These two diseases, occurring in the same breed and often in the same individual, are almost certainly closely related.

DIAGNOSIS

With this great variety of clinical presentations to choose from, it is not surprising that lupus is difficult to diagnose in dogs. A simple diagnostic rule for lupus is therefore the following: Suspect lupus in an animal with multiple inflammatory disorders such as those described previously and a positive ANA test. A positive ANA test is a mandatory diagnostic criterion, despite its limitations.

ANA are normally detected by immunofluorescence assays (Fig. 15.8). Cultured cells or frozen sections of mouse or rat liver on a microscope slide are used as the source of antigen.

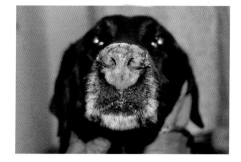

Fig. 15.7 Erythematous, depigmented, ulcerated, and crusted nasal lesions of facial discoid lupus erythematosus in a German Shepherd Dog.
(Banovic F. *Vet Clin Small Anim* 2019; 37–45.)

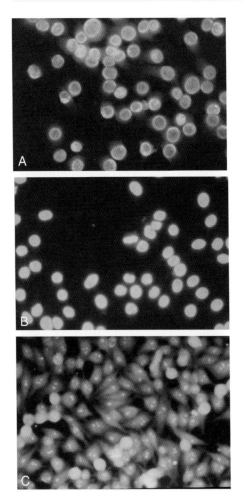

Fig. 15.8 Three positive antinuclear antibody reactions. These are indirect fluorescent antibody reactions in which dog serum under test is layered onto a cell culture. After washing, the bound antibody is detected using a fluorescent antiglobulin. Although "rim" fluorescence (A) has traditionally been considered a positive reaction, the staining pattern obtained appears to depend in large part on the way the cells are fixed. These can therefore show diffuse staining (B) or nucleolar fluorescence (C). Positive nucleolar fluorescence suggests the presence of antiribonucleoprotein antibodies rather than anti-DNA antibodies. (Courtesy Dr. FC Heck [Tizard IR. *Veterinary Immunology*. 10th ed. Elsevier; 2016].)

The patient's serum is applied, and the slide is incubated. Any unbound antibodies are then washed off. Bound antibodies are revealed by incubating the tissue sections in a fluorescein-labeled antiglobulin and then rewashing. On examination, if positive, the cell nuclei will fluoresce. Several different nuclear staining patterns have been described in humans and their clinical correlations identified. In animals, staining patterns have been less thoroughly investigated, and their significance is less clear. Homogeneous staining of the complete nucleus or staining of the nuclear rim is considered of greatest diagnostic significance and generally confirms lupus. Nucleolar fluorescence or a speckled fluorescence pattern suggests that the autoantibodies are directed against ribonucleoproteins, as in cases of Sjögren syndrome or dermatomyositis. Some normal dogs, dogs undergoing treatment with certain drugs (griseofulvin, penicillin, sulfonamides, tetracyclines, phenytoin, procainamide), and some dogs with liver disease or a lymphosarcoma may also have detectable ANA. Dogs infected with *Bartonella vinsonii, Ehrlichia canis,* and *Leishmania infantum* also have ANA. Dogs infected with multiple vectorborne organisms are especially likely to be ANA positive, thus nonspecific ANA positivity may be a result of many different neoplastic, inflammatory, and autoimmune diseases. ANA test results must therefore be used with caution.

Lupus dogs can also develop autoantibodies against interleukin enhancer-binding factors 2 and 3 (ILF2 and ILF3). These are found exclusively in dogs that show a speckled nuclear staining pattern on immunofluorescence. They are also found with a low frequency in dogs with Sjögren syndrome. ILF2 and ILF3 are transcription factors required for the expression of IL2 and IL13. Suppression by these autoantibodies may account in part for the lack of IL2 in lupus patients.

A relatively simple test that may assist in the diagnosis of SLE is the LE cell test. LE cells, as previously mentioned, are neutrophils that have phagocytosed nuclear material from other apoptotic cells. Their presence may be detected in the bone marrow and occasionally in buffy coat preparations from animals with lupus. It is usually necessary, however, to produce them in vitro. This can be accomplished by allowing the blood of an affected animal to clot and then incubating it at 37°C for 2 hours. During this time, normal neutrophils will phagocytose the nuclei of any nearby apoptotic cells. The clot is then disrupted by pressing it through a fine mesh. The resulting cell suspension is centrifuged, and the buffy coat is smeared, stained, and examined. If positive, the smear will show some neutrophils containing a round pink inclusion. These are LE cells. The inclusion is often very large and displaces the nucleus of the ingesting cell (see Fig. 15.6). Unfortunately, LE cells are not a totally reliable diagnostic feature of systemic lupus in domestic animals since there is a high prevalence of both false-positive and false-negative results. For clinical purposes, the LE cell assay has been largely replaced by the simpler and more sensitive indirect immunofluorescence assays. These in turn are being replaced by other sensitive and specific assays such as solid phase immunoassays and laser addressable bead-based multiplex assays (see Chapter 20).

TREATMENT

Lupus usually responds well to immunosuppressive doses of corticosteroids (prednisolone or prednisone), accompanied, if necessary, by cyclophosphamide, azathioprine, or chlorambucil. However, more drastic measures, such as plasmapheresis, may be needed in refractory cases. In general, SLE can be managed but rarely cured. Specific problems such as liver or kidney failure may also need to be addressed.

FELINE SYSTEMIC LUPUS

SLE is uncommon in cats, in which it usually presents as an antiglobulin-positive anemia. About half of feline lupus cases also develop skin disease. Other clinical manifestations include fever, hemolytic anemia, thrombocytopenia, polyarthritis, and glomerulonephritis. The skin lesions may include alopecia with an erythematous scaling and crusting dermatosis that can occur anywhere on the body. Administration of propylthiouracil to cats may result in the development of an antiglobulin-positive anemia as well as positive ANA reactions. The ANA test must be interpreted with care in cats since many normal cats are ANA positive.

EQUINE SYSTEMIC LUPUS

SLE is a very rare disease of horses. In these cases, the disease has presented as a generalized skin disease. Animals develop an exfoliative dermatitis with alopecia, mucocutaneous ulceration, scaling, and crusting. Some affected horses may be almost totally hairless. Leukoderma develops on the face and trunk. Systemic manifestations include fever, anorexia, and weight loss. Affected horses may also have uveitis, glomerulonephritis, synovitis, and lymphadenopathy with lymphedema in the lower limbs. An antiglobulin-positive anemia and thrombocytopenia with purpura may develop. Affected horses are ANA positive, although LE cell tests are equivocal in this species. Skin biopsies show an interface dermatitis containing lymphocytes, plasma cells, and histiocytes with basal cell degeneration and IgG deposition on the skin basement membrane (a lupus band) (see Fig. 15.5).

If SLE is suspected, an LE test should be conducted and at least two other autoimmune conditions identified. These may include hemolytic anemia, thrombocytopenia, or glomerulonephritis in addition to the skin lesions. Treatment requires immunosuppressive doses of glucocorticoids, perhaps supplemented with other immunosuppressants such as azathioprine or cyclosporine. However, treatment of the reported equine cases has been unsuccessful.

Lupus-Related Skin Diseases

CUTANEOUS (DISCOID) LUPUS ERYTHEMATOSUS

Despite its name, cutaneous lupus erythematosus (CLE) is a skin disease that is distinctly different from SLE. It can present clinically in many diverse ways (Fig. 15.9). The term *discoid* derives from the circular coin-sized lesions that develop in humans.

The initial steps in the development of CLE are probably triggered by skin damage due to UV radiation. The UV radiation causes susceptible keratinocytes to produce cytokines and other proinflammatory molecules. The cytokines activate local innate immune responses. DNA released from apoptotic cells and NETs activates some toll-like receptors. Type 1 IFNs are generated and activate adaptive immune responses, first DCs and then Th1 responses and cytotoxic T cells. Nearby NK cells are also activated. These in turn activate local Th17 responses, and this results in yet more inflammation. The mixture of T cells, NK cells, and cytokines contributes to the local tissue damage by attacking and killing keratinocytes. The release of cell debris, especially nuclear antigens, reactivates the innate immune pathways, causes the pDCs to produce yet more IFNs, and thus generates a self-amplifying inflammatory cycle. Nuclear autoantigens such as SSA/Ro are also induced by the IFNs and promote further ANA production. Local accumulation of immune complexes may also contribute to the inflammatory process.

Clinical Disease

CLE occurs in dogs, cats, horses, and humans. It is not a systemic disease. Its lesions are restricted to the skin. ANA and LE tests are negative or weakly positive. Facial discoid lupus has been described in Collies and Collie crosses, German Shepherd Dogs, Siberian Huskies, and Shetland Sheepdogs. The age of onset is between 1 and 7 years. Nasal lesions predominate with erythema, erosions, scaling, and crusting ulcers. Scaling and loss of pigment involves the

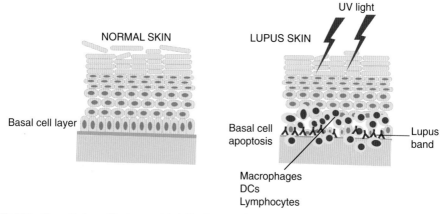

Fig. 15.9   The pathology of the lupus-related skin diseases. Thus a linear lichenoid infiltrate develops along the interface between the epidermis and dermis. This is associated with basal cell apoptosis and deposition of immunoglobulins, a lupus band, along the basement membrane. *DC*, Dendritic cell; *UV*, ultraviolet.

nasal planum and the bridge of the nose. The lesions may spread to the lips, periocular skin, and genitals (see Fig. 15.7). Occasionally, the feet may be affected, and some dogs may develop oral ulcers.

Diagnosis and Treatment

A skin biopsy is required for diagnosis. Histopathology of CLE cases shows characteristic lesions at the dermoepidermal junction and basal cell degeneration (Fig. 15.10). There is an interface inflammation, with vacuolar degeneration, apoptosis, loss of basal cells, and basement membrane thickening accompanied by a lymphoplasmacytic infiltration. The basement membrane thickening may be patchy and multifocal. This is the classical bandlike pattern of an interface dermatitis (also called a lichenoid infiltrate). C3, IgA, IgG, or IgM may be detected in the skin basement membrane in a typical lupus band.

CLE is usually treated with corticosteroids, and the prognosis is good. Retinoids and tetracycline antibiotics have also been used for their steroid-sparing effect. Since the lesions are exacerbated by sunlight, it is appropriate to use sunscreens and encourage the owner to keep the animal out of intense sunlight.

FELINE CUTANEOUS LUPUS

Cutaneous lupus in cats is characterized by a nonpruritic scaling and crusting dermatitis almost totally confined to the pinnae of the ear. There may be some ulceration and papule or pustule formation. Skin biopsies show a mononuclear infiltration of the basal cell layer with degeneration of basal cells. Direct immunofluorescence of skin sections shows a lupus band. Affected cats have negative or low ANA titers and negative LE cell tests. Treatment with corticosteroids is effective.

GENERALIZED CLE

A generalized form of cutaneous lupus has been reported to occur in Chinese Crested dogs, Labrador Retrievers, and some other breeds. The median age of onset is 9 years. Animals develop classical discoid plaques. Lesions show adherent scales, follicular plugs, peripheral hyperpigmentation, erythema, erosions, ulcers, scaling, and crusting. These develop below the neck and on the trunk, abdomen, and legs. The lesions eventually result in scarring, depigmentation, or hyperpigmentation. Animals sometimes show evidence of pruritus and pain.

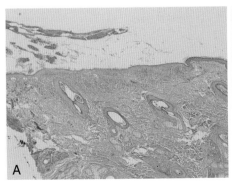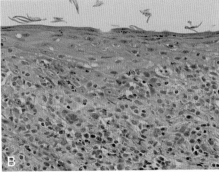

Fig. 15.10 The histopathology of cutaneous lupus. (A) A low-power view (4×) showing the interface dermatitis, bandlike infiltration of lymphocytes, histiocytes, and plasma cells. (B) A high-power view (40×) showing apoptotic cells at the level of the basal cell layer and interface dermatitis. (Courtesy of Dr. Dominique Wiener.)

Immunofluorescence shows the presence of IgG, IgM, and C3 in the dermoepidermal basement membrane zone. Although these dogs have low positive ANA titers, they do not progress to systemic lupus. Affected animals respond well to steroid treatment but often relapse when doses are reduced.

MUCOCUTANEOUS CLE

This form of cutaneous lupus primarily occurs in middle-aged German Shepherd Dogs and their crosses. Females are overrepresented. Affected dogs develop perimucosal skin lesions. Erosions and ulcers develop mainly on the anus as well as in the perigenital and periocular regions. Lesions occasionally develop on the lips. The lesions show crusting and hyperpigmentation. The ulcers may become secondarily infected. Scarring is not usually seen. While some dogs may show evidence of discomfort when urinating and defecating, there may be no other systemic signs. The lesions show a typical lupus histology with a lymphoplasmacytic interface dermatitis and basal keratinocyte apoptosis and loss. Animals have a positive IgG lupus band on skin biopsy, but ANA tests are negative. Treated dogs respond well to glucocorticoids, with remission occurring within a few weeks. Dogs may, however, relapse when the drug dose is tapered.

VESICULAR CLE

A unique form of CLE is restricted to Collies (Rough and Border), Shetland Sheepdogs, and their crosses. The dogs present with erythema and multiple flaccid skin vesicles that slough, leaving erosions. The lesions are found on the glabrous skin of the abdomen, axillae, and groins, as well as within in the concave pinnae and perimucosal areas. Secondary bacterial infections are common. The lesions show typical lupus histopathology (i.e., a lymphocytic interface dermatitis with prominent basal cell vacuolation resulting in apoptosis). The amount of cell death is sufficient to cause skin separation and vesicle formation. Up to half the infiltrating lymphocytes are CD8$^+$ cytotoxic T cells, whereas CD4$^+$ cells are less common. Langerhans cells are also present in the infiltrate. Direct immunofluorescence staining shows an IgG lupus band. IgG may also be deposited around blood vessels and within basal cells. The serum of most affected dogs contains autoantibodies directed against a diversity of nuclear antigens, including soluble SSA/Ro, SSB/La, and Sm. Anti-Ro and -La are most common. Affected animals make antibodies against type VII collagen as well as ANA. Animals respond to treatment with glucocorticoids and cyclosporine, together with UV avoidance and the use of sunscreens.

EXFOLIATIVE CLE

This scaly, generalized dermatosis occurs mainly in young adult German Short-Haired Pointers and Vizslas. It is an inherited disease transmitted as an autosomal recessive trait associated with a SNP located on chromosome 18. Skin lesions include erythema, scaling, follicular casts, and some scarring. Dyspigmented plaques appear. The lesions first appear on the muzzle, pinnae, and trunk but spread to the limbs, sternum, and ventral abdomen. Affected dogs may also show systemic signs such as a generalized lymphadenopathy, as well as arthralgia and a stiff gait. Others may develop anemia and thrombocytopenia. Histology shows a dermal T-cell lymphocyte infiltrate with some hyperkeratosis. The T cells affect the sebaceous glands. Immunofluorescence shows the presence of IgG deposits, but some dogs may have IgM, IgA, or C3 deposits on their epidermal basement membrane as well. Affected animals respond poorly to immunosuppressive therapy.

Nailbed Diseases

SYMMETRIC LUPOID ONYCHOMADESIS (ONYCHODYSTROPHY)

Symmetric lupoid onychomadesis (SLO) is an acute disease in which dogs lose multiple claws on all four paws over a period of 3 to 4 months. The disease occurs in Gordon Setters, German Shepherd Dogs, Bearded Collies, Rhodesian Ridgebacks, Giant Schnauzers, and some other breeds. This breed prevalence suggests a genetic predisposition. The haplotype DLA-DRB1*01801/DQA1*00101/DQB1*00802 appears to be significantly linked to SLO in Gordon Setters. Males are overrepresented in Norwegian Gordon Setters.

Affected dogs show sudden nail loss but no other disease (Fig. 15.11). Histologic features include an interface dermatitis with formation of subepidermal clefts, basal cell vacuolization and apoptosis, lymphoplasmacytic subepidermal infiltration, and fibroplasia. A few macrophages may also be present. Thus the inflammatory infiltrate forms a parallel band to the basement membrane (a lichenoid pattern) similar to that observed in discoid lupus erythematosus. There is also local pigmentary incontinence. There may be secondary bacterial infection of the nailbed. ANA have been detected in 3 of 10 Gordon Setters with clinical SLO as well as in 5 of 13 with black hair follicular dysplasia. This suggests the two diseases may be autoimmune in origin and related.

Clinical Disease, Diagnosis, and Treatment

The age of onset of SLO in dogs is between 2 and 7 years, with a mean of 3.9 years. Affected dogs show sudden discomfort, pain, and lameness, as well as toe licking. Their nails fall off, and there is subsequent sloughing of one or more claw plates. Within a few weeks, the condition may generalize. Multiple claws soon become affected. The regrowing claws are short, dry, deformed, and brittle. Survivors may have chronically misshapen claws (see Fig. 15.11).

It is of course important to rule out bacterial and fungal infections and demodex by cytology. An affected dewclaw is ideal for histology. Similar histology is seen in cutaneous LE, but in SLO, ANA are not consistently present.

In addition to treating secondary infections, the nails should be trimmed and any loose nails removed under anesthesia. Immunosuppressive therapy is appropriate using prednisolone and cyclosporine, azathioprine, or pentoxifylline. Nicotinamide plus doxycycline therapy has been used with success. Essential fatty acid supplementation has also been recommended.

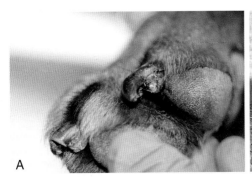 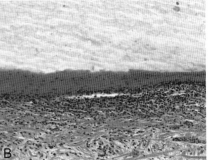

Fig. 15.11 Symmetric lupoid onychomadesis (onychodystrophy). (A) The nail distortion typical of symmetric lupoid onychomadesis. (Courtesy of Dr. Robert Kennis.) (B) Nailbed epithelium with a lymphocytic interface dermatitis. Note artificial cleft formation due to weakening of the dermoepidermal junction. 20× magnification, H&E stain. (Courtesy of Dr. Dominique Wiener.)

BOX 15.2 ■ The CD40-CD40L Pathway

CD40 is expressed on antigen-presenting cells, including dendritic cells and B cells. Its ligand CD40L is found on activated CD4+ helper T cells. Their interaction is essential for a successful antibody response, cytokine production, the formation of germinal centers, and immunoglobulin class switching (see Fig. 2.5). CD40L expression on B cells, T cells, and monocytes is significantly upregulated in systemic autoimmune diseases such as systemic lupus erythematosus, Sjögren syndrome, polymyositis, pemphigus, immunoglobulin G4 disease, and rheumatoid arthritis. This overexpression of CD40L is correlated with the development of inflammation in nonlymphoid tissues as well as a poor clinical outcome. Collectively, this suggests that aberrant signaling between CD40 and its ligand may play a role in the pathogenesis of these autoimmune diseases. Blockade of the CD40 pathway with humanized monoclonal antibodies against CD40L has shown encouraging results in the treatment of some of these diseases.

Karnell JL, Rieder SA, Ettinger R, et al. Targeting the CD40-CD40L pathway in autoimmune diseases: humoral immunity and beyond. *Adv Drug Deliv Rev.* 2019;141:92–103.

Sources of Additional Information

Banovic F. Canine cutaneous lupus erythematosus: newly discovered variants. *Vet Clin Small Anim.* 2018;49:37–45.

Bonnhorst JØ, Hanssen I, Moen T. Antinuclear antibodies (ANA) in Gordon Setters with symmetrical lupoid onychodystrophy and black hair follicle follicular dysplasia. *Acta Vet Scand.* 2001;42:323–329.

Bremer HD, Landegren N, Sjöberg R, et al. ILF2 and ILF3 are autoantigens in canine systemic autoimmune disease. *Nature.* 2018. doi:10.1038/s41598-018-23034-w.

Chabanne L, Fournel C, Caux C, et al. Abnormalities of lymphocyte subsets in canine systemic lupus erythematosus. *Autoimmunity.* 1995;22:1–8.

Chiou S-H, Lan J-L, Lin S-L, et al. Pet dogs owned by lupus patients are at higher risk of developing lupus. *Lupus.* 2004;13:442–449.

Fournel C, Chabanne L, Caux C, et al. Canine systemic lupus erythematosus. I. A study of 75 cases. *Lupus.* 1992;1:133–139.

Gestermann N, Di Domizio J, Lande R, et al. Netting neutrophils activate autoreactive B cells in lupus. *J Immunol.* 2018;200:3364–3371.

Karnell JL, Rieder SA, Ettinger R, et al. Targeting the CD40-CD40L pathway in autoimmune diseases: humoral immunity and beyond. *Adv Drug Deliv Revs.* 2019;141:92–103.

Olivry T, Linder KE, Banovic F. Cutaneous lupus erythematosus in dogs, a comprehensive review. *BMC Vet Res.* 2018. doi:10.1186/s12917-018-1446-8.

Olivry T, Savary KCM, Murphy KM, et al. Bullous systemic lupus erythematosus (type 1) in a dog. *Vet Rec.* 1999;145:165–169.

Pisetsky DS. Evolving story of autoantibodies in systemic lupus erythematosus. *J Autoimmun.* 2019. doi:10.1016/j.jaut.2019.102356.

Rossi MA, Messinger LM, Linder KE, et al. Generalized canine discoid lupus erythematosus responsive to tetracycline and niacinamide therapy. *J Am Anim Hosp Assoc.* 2015;51:171–175.

Steimer T, Bauer A, Kienzle E, et al. Canine symmetrical lupoid onychomadesis in bearded collies. *Vet Dermatol.* 2018;30:411 -e124.

Tsokos GC. Autoimmunity and organ damage in systemic lupus erythematosus. *Nature Immunol.* 2020;21:605–614.

Wilbe M, Jokinen P, Truvé K, et al. Genome-wide association mapping identifies multiple loci for a canine SLE-related disease complex. *Nat Genet.* 2010;42:250–254.

Zhou X, Yan J, Lu Q, et al. The pathogenesis of cutaneous lupus erythematosus: the aberrant distribution and function of different cell types in skin lesions. *Scand J Immunol.* 2020. doi:10.1111/sji.12933.

Rheumatoid Arthritis

As described in Chapter 1, the innate immune system in the form of inflammation serves as an important stimulus for adaptive immune responses. Triggers of inflammation such as infections, environmental insults, and signals from the body's commensals can also serve to initiate many autoimmune diseases. Innate immune responses also play a key role in mediating the consequences of autoimmunity. The organ damage resulting from an autoimmune attack is also a result of innate mechanisms. The activation of cells by proinflammatory cytokines, the generation of tissue-degrading enzymes, and the production of potent oxidants that destroy tissues can all result from uncontrolled innate immunity. This progression from innate immunity to adaptive immunity to innate immunity again is well seen in the erosive inflammatory joint diseases typified by rheumatoid arthritis (RA).

Rheumatoid Arthritis

The most important immune-mediated erosive polyarthritis in humans is RA. This is a common, crippling syndrome that affects about 1% of humans—mainly women, smokers, and people with a family history of the disease. A very similar disease is seen in domestic animals, especially dogs. It is characterized by dysfunctional innate immunity, including immune complex formation and complement dysregulation; by adaptive autoimmune responses against posttranslationally modified proteins; by T-cell dysregulation; and by macrophage activation in joints resulting in cartilage and bone destruction.

RA is a chronic immune-mediated systemic inflammatory disease. Clinical RA develops after many years of asymptomatic autoimmunity. Eventually self-tolerance erodes sufficiently for effector T cells to invade joints, for regulatory mechanisms to fail, and for uncontrolled inflammation to cause severe tissue damage. The loss of T-cell tolerance derives from accumulated defects in their DNA repair mechanisms.

Clinically, RA commences as a lymphocytic synovitis with neutrophils in the joint fluid. Cytokines such as interleukin-6 (IL6) and tumor necrosis factor-alpha (TNFα) are released, and inflammation develops progressively. As the inflammation continues and becomes more severe, the synovia swell and proliferate. The synovial lining becomes thickened and hyperplastic. Outgrowths of this hyperplastic synovia eventually invade the joint cavities in the form of pannus. Pannus consists of fibrous vascular tissue that spreads over a joint surface and releases proteases that erode and destroy the articular cartilage and, ultimately, neighboring bony structures. Systemic lesions, including amyloidosis, arteritis, glomerulonephritis, and lymphatic hyperplasia, are occasional complications of RA. Because of the involvement of so many different inflammatory and autoimmune pathways it has been suggested that RA should be considered a common syndrome resulting from the generation of joint inflammation by many different routes.

PREDISPOSING FACTORS

Environmental Factors

Many stimuli may trigger RA in animals with a high-risk genetic background. Infectious agents implicated in the human disease include Epstein-Barr virus (a herpesvirus), parvoviruses, and mycobacteria. Infections may also trigger the development of erosive arthritis in domestic mammals. *Mycoplasma hyorhinis, Erysipelothrix rhusiopathiae,* and *Borrelia burgdorferi* can each cause a chronic arthritis that resembles RA. Dogs with RA have antibodies to canine distemper in their synovial fluids. Immune complexes can be precipitated out of rheumatoid synovial fluid of dogs, and analysis of these complexes by Western blotting has detected the presence of distemper virus antigens. Thus distemper virus may be present in some canine rheumatoid joints and may play a role in its pathogenesis. These antibodies are not present in dogs with osteoarthritis, a nonimmune-mediated disease.

As pointed out elsewhere, the intestinal microbiota appear to play an important role in predisposing to diseases such as RA. RA patients have significant and consistent changes in their microbiota (and in their intestinal bacteriophage communities!) when compared to healthy patients. Thus certain intestinal bacteria, the segmented filamentous bacteria, promote helper T type 17 (Th17) cell responses. These same bacteria appear to fine-tune regulatory T-cell responses and so influence the severity of autoimmune arthritis. Intestinal bacteria also influence the ability of an animal to generate neutrophil extracellular traps (NETs). Increased NET formation in RA has been postulated to be the stimulus for production of rheumatoid factors (RF) and anticitrullinated protein antibodies (ACPA) since these intracellular molecules are exposed when NETs are released into the extracellular environment. Many RA patients as well as those with systemic lupus and Sjögren syndrome make autoantibodies specifically directed against NET antigens. In humans, inflammation of the oral mucosa in the form of periodontitis caused by *Porphyromonas gingivalis* is also associated with increased susceptibility to RA. It has been suggested that *Porphyromonas* is highly effective in citrullinating proteins and hence stimulates the production of ACPA.

Genetic Factors

In humans, about 12% to 15% of monozygotic twins both develop RA. This compares to 1% of dizygotic twins. More than 100 gene loci have been associated with RA susceptibility, and these account for ~15% of the phenotypic variation in the disease. Variants located within the major histocompatibility complex (MHC) class II region (HLA-DR) account for more than 40% of its known heritability. This susceptibility is associated in part with the presence of a conserved 5-amino acid sequence (residues 71–74) located in the third hypervariable region of the antigen-binding groove of the beta chain of certain HLA-DRB1 alleles. This is known as the RA shared epitope. This sequence together with variant amino acids at positions 11 and 13 form part of the antigen-binding pocket on the MHC molecule. These variants bind citrullinated proteins especially strongly and as a result determine RA susceptibility. It is important to note that this same RA shared epitope is found on canine DLA-DRB1 and is associated with susceptibility to RA in some dog breeds.

Genetic studies on dogs with RA have also identified three other DLA-DRB1 alleles that are associated with disease risk: DLA-DRB1*002, DRB1*009, and DRB1*018. Some MHC class III genes also affect susceptibility to canine RA. For example, possession of the C4 allotype C4-4 is associated with the development of autoimmune polyarthritis. The remaining non–HLA-associated susceptibility genes are located in noncoding gene regions often associated with histone markers or enhancers of CD4+ T-cell functions. Other RA-associated genes are associated with B-cell pathways, cytokine pathways, cell proliferation, and hematopoiesis.

Pathogenesis

The development of RA is progressive and takes many years. It develops in three distinct phases (Fig. 16.1). In the first phase, genetically predisposed individuals begin to produce autoantibodies. These autoantibodies are neither obviously pathogenic nor directed against joint tissues, so patients may live for many years showing no symptoms. In the second phase, they begin to develop a symptomatic acute T-cell–mediated synovitis. This in turn transitions into the third phase, a chronic destructive arthritis leading to irreversible bone loss and tissue injury. Although RA was once considered to be purely an autoimmune disease, it is now best considered as a chronic immune-mediated syndrome that may be triggered by autoimmunity but eventually involves the malfunction of many different immune cell types, especially T cells.

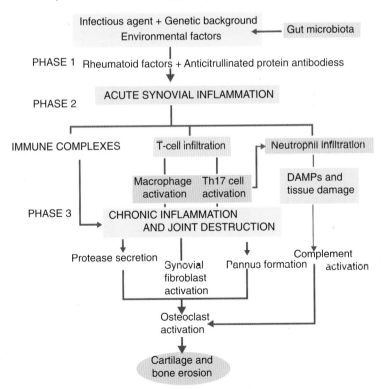

Fig. 16.1 A schematic diagram showing the stages by which rheumatoid arthritis develops. *DAMPs,* Damage-associated molecular pattern molecules; *Th17,* helper T cell type 17.

PHASE 1: THE PRODUCTION OF AUTOANTIBODIES

The autoantibodies that are characteristic of RA are directed against two major groups of autoantigens: immunoglobulin G (IgG) and citrullinated proteins.

Rheumatoid Factors

The presence of autoantibodies directed against IgG in RA patients was first described in 1940 by the Norwegian investigator Erik Waaler. He called these antibodies rheumatoid factors (Fig. 16.2). RF are directed against epitopes on the C_H2 domains of the heavy chains of antigen-bound IgG. They can belong to any immunoglobulin class, including IgE, although IgG RF are by far the most common. RF can bind to each other and as a result may generate very large, stable immune complexes. They cannot bind to immunoglobulins in solution but only to the new heavy chain epitopes exposed when immunoglobulins change their shape on binding to antigen. The IgG produced by RA patients is also less glycosylated than normal IgG, and it may be that this abnormal IgG can act as an immunogen in a susceptible animal. RF are also produced in systemic lupus erythematosus (SLE) and other diseases where extensive immune complex formation occurs. It is of interest to note also that RF can be detected in the synovia of pigs suffering from *Erysipelothrix* polyarthritis.

RF are detected by serologic assays (see Chapter 20). For example, RF can agglutinate antibody-coated particles. In humans, latex beads coated with IgG are used for this purpose. In dogs, it may be easier to make a canine anti–sheep-erythrocyte serum and coat sheep erythrocytes with

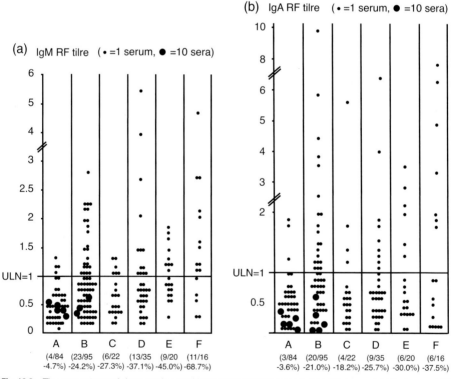

Fig. 16.2 The percentage of dogs testing positive for rheumatoid factors. (a) IgM rheumatoid factor, and (b) IgA rheumatoid factor in *(A)* normal sera, *(B)* sera from dogs with unclassified polyarthritis, *(C)* rheumatoid arthritis sera, *(D)* systemic lupus erythematosus sera, *(E)* dogs with leishmaniasis or heartworm disease, and *(F)* pyometra sera. (Chabanne L, Fournel C, Faure JR, et al. IgM and IgA rheumatoid factors in canine polyarthritis. *Vet Immunol Immunopathol.* 1993;39:365–379.)

BOX 16.1 ■ Natural Anti-IgG Antibodies in Dogs

Healthy normal dogs possess circulating autoantibodies against immunoglobulin G (IgG). They have several different specificities. Some are rheumatoid factors directed against the heavy chain of the IgG molecule. Others are directed against the antigen-binding arm of IgG, the Fab region. A third type is directed toward cryptic epitopes located in the immunoglobulin hinge region. These autoantibodies will only react with paired Fab regions (Fab'2). They persist for at least 2 years. The significance and functions of the Fab-binding antibodies remain unclear. They have, however, the potential to interfere with monoclonal antibody therapy in dogs and interfere with some diagnostic immunoassays.

Bergman D, Backstrom C, Hansson-Hamlin H, et al. Pre-existing canine anti-IgG antibodies: implications for immunotherapy, immunogenicity testing and immunoassay analysis. *Nature Sci Rep.* 2020. doi. org/10.1038/s41598-020-69618-3.

this in a subagglutinating dose. After washing, these antibody-coated red cells will agglutinate when mixed with RF-positive dog serum.

Although RF are of diagnostic importance, their clinical significance is less clear. Thus in humans they can be detected many years before the onset of clinical disease. RF are found in joint fluid, where their titer tends to correlate with the severity of the lesions. The lesions themselves may be exacerbated by intraarticular inoculation of autologous immunoglobulins. Nevertheless some individuals with erosive arthritis may have no detectable RF, and it is not uncommon to find others who have no arthritis despite the presence of RF in their serum serum (Box 16.1).

Citrullinated Proteins

The selective process that establishes central tolerance eliminates developing T cells that can respond to AIRE-induced self-peptides. Thymic selection cannot, however, induce tolerance to proteins that are chemically modified after translation. As a result, posttranslational modifications such as citrullination and carbamylation may make proteins antigenic unless suppressed by peripheral tolerance mechanisms. Of human RA patients, 80% to 90% make autoantibodies against citrullinated proteins. (Citrulline is derived from the amino acid arginine by conversion of its amino group [=NH] to a ketone [=O] in a process called citrullination or deimination [Fig. 16.3].) This chemical change, mediated by enzymes called deiminases, occurs in proteins after they have been translated from RNA and fundamentally alters their tertiary structure and behavior. Thus arginine is positively charged, and citrulline is neutral. As a result, citrullinated proteins are more hydrophobic and fold differently resulting in alterations in both shape and function. It is these changes that also make citrullinated proteins antigenic.

The binding specificity of these autoantibodies (i.e., ACPA) is highly variable but includes citrullinated epitopes on multiple self-proteins, including fibrinogen, vimentin, fibronectin, collagen, and histones, among others. Citrullinated proteins are expressed in stressed or inflamed tissues. They are also generated in large amounts in neutrophil NETs. (Cigarette smokers and

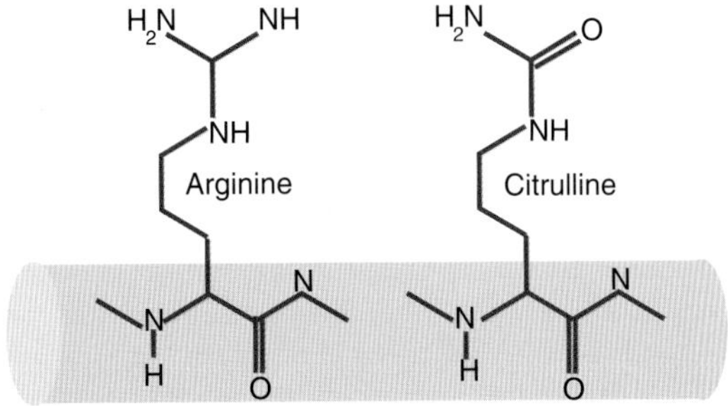

Fig. 16.3 Citrulline is generated from arginine by deimination. This occurs after a protein is translated by RNA. As a result, tolerance to citrullinated proteins can only be maintained by peripheral tolerance mechanisms.

those with periodontitis generate citrullinated proteins in the lungs and mouth, respectively, probably by inducing NET formation.) As with RF, patients may develop high levels of autoantibodies to ACPA long before they develop clinically significant arthritis. They may form immune complexes in joints and can activate macrophages promoting their differentiation into osteoclasts. The key initial lesion in RA may therefore involve autoimmunity directed against ACPA.

As indicated earlier, both RF and ACPA may appear many years before the development of clinical arthritis, but they gradually increase to peak around the time of disease onset. ACPA are specific for this disease (88%–96%), whereas RF are found in many other autoimmune diseases. ACPA are considered risk factors for erosive joint destruction. A subset of human patients may also develop autoantibodies against other posttranslationally modified proteins as a result of carbamylation or acetylation.

Drug-induced suppression of B cells in RA patients results in significant clinical improvement suggesting that these cells play a key role in its pathogenesis. More than 30% of ACPA-positive B cells have been shown to be activated. They produce large quantities of proinflammatory cytokines and are resistant to the effects of inhibitory signals. ACPA-positive B cells in blood and the synovial membranes produce large quantities of IL8 (CXCL8). IL8 is a potent chemoattractant for neutrophils, and neutrophils are the most abundant inflammatory cells in rheumatoid synovial fluid. Thus persistent signaling by ACPA-positive B cells contributes to this persistent neutrophil activation and inflammation.

PHASE 2: THE DEVELOPMENT OF SYNOVIAL INFLAMMATION

Eventually RA proceeds from the systemic production of apparently nonpathogenic autoantibodies to focusing on joints and the development of acute synovial inflammation. It is unclear just what triggers this switch, but it may reflect the unique structure of synovial blood vessels.

Synovial capillaries are fenestrated so that relatively large gaps exist between their endothelial cells. As a result, these vessels are up to 50 times more permeable than conventional capillaries. Water and small solutes (<12 kDa) can readily pass into the tissues, although proteins such as albumin and clotting factors are retained. In addition, the synovial lining cells do not form tight junctions with their neighbors, and there is no underlying basement membrane. Solutes and small proteins from the bloodstream can therefore readily gain access to synovial tissues as well as the synovial fluid.

The healthy synovium consists of a lining layer composed of two types of synoviocytes, macrophage-like cells called type A synoviocytes and fibroblast-like cells called type B synoviocytes. This layer is normally about two to three cells deep. Beneath this is a sublining layer of connective tissue that contains small blood and lymphatic vessels as well as fibroblasts and clusters of macrophages. The thin lining layer responds to inflammation by thickening to 10 to 12 cells as a result of fibroblast and macrophage growth, the production of extracellular matrix by the fibroblasts, and the production of inflammatory cytokines by the macrophages. As a result of these structural features, joints are uniquely capable of developing and sustaining localized inflammation.

The deposition of RF and ACPA-containing immune complexes within the synovia and articular cartilage activates complement and generates anaphylatoxins. The anaphylatoxins C5a and C3a attract neutrophils that then swarm into the joint and release their proteases and oxidants. Dendritic cells are also attracted and produce proinflammatory cytokines, including IL1, TNFα, IL6, IL12, and the interferons.

It is clear, however, that immune complexes alone cannot explain the severity of the subsequent inflammatory response. Pathogen-associated molecular patterns (PAMPs) and damage-associated molecular patterns (DAMPs) also act through pattern-recognition receptors (PRRs) to activate T cells and fibroblasts. Once it becomes inflamed, the synovium increases in vascularity, thickens as a result of synovial cell hyperplasia, and is invaded by T cells, neutrophils, and macrophages. CD4+ T cells accumulate in the synovia where they are activated by exposure to the inflammatory environment. In the presence of reactive oxygen species released during inflammation, the T cells differentiate and proliferate. They also undergo premature aging and a loss of

DNA repair mechanisms (see Chapter 3), and as a result they undergo a behavioral shift. Instead of differentiating into long-lived memory cells they develop into short-lived tissue invasive, proinflammatory effector cells. These short-lived T cells soon die as a result of pyroptosis; however, in the process they generate large amounts of proinflammatory cytokines.

Unregulated activation of Th17 cells also occurs in RA patients. Th17 numbers in blood are elevated as are levels of IL6, IL17, and IL21. Activated Th17 cells are found within affected joints. The IL17 upregulates numerous inflammation-related genes in synovial fibroblasts. Activated synovial fibroblasts activate intracellular complement (C3), which reprograms their bioenergetics. This results in the accumulation of yet more neutrophils in the synovial fluid. These cells in turn sustain the inflammatory environment and promote local T- and B-cell activation.

At this stage neutrophils are the dominant cell type in the joint fluid followed by T cells, B cells, and macrophages in the synovia. While T cells predominate in and are distributed throughout the synovia, B cells and plasma cells tend to occur in focal aggregates. Defects in the programed death process result in a failure to remove dead and dying neutrophils, enhancing the inflammation still further. Immune complexes from RA sera activate monocytes so that they become proinflammatory M1 cells. Macrophage-derived cytokines also promote synovial angiogenesis.

PHASE 3: PROGRESSION TO CHRONIC TISSUE DESTRUCTION

The switch from acute to chronic inflammation in joints is associated with activation of type B synoviocytes, also called fibroblast-like synoviocytes (FLS) caused by the multiple proinflammatory molecules generated by T cells, especially Th17 cells and neutrophils. FLS are normally found in the intimal lining layer of the synovium. When activated by IL-17, they proliferate, upregulate genes encoding MHC proteins and complement C3, and act as antigen-presenting cells. They also activate their inflammasomes and so turn on the genes for the three proinflammatory cytokines, IL-1β, TNF-α and IL-6. The C3 causes them to increase glycolysis so they can thrive under hypoxic conditions. They suppress autophagy, making them apoptosis- resistant. Their mitochondria also generate increased amounts of reactive oxygen species.

As the disease progresses, synovial lining cells, small blood vessels, and fibroblasts proliferate. The synovial lining thickens enormously as a result of the proliferation of resident synovial fibroblasts and invasion by macrophages. This inflamed synovia eventually forms a layer of invasive granulation tissue (called pannus) that grows into the joint space where it infiltrates and destroys the articular cartilage, ligaments, and bone (Fig. 16.4). The pannus contains proliferating activated synovial fibroblasts together with lymphocytes, plasma cells, and neutrophils. Large numbers of activated macrophages (type Λ synoviocytes) are also found in the pannus. Fibroblast and macrophage activation is accompanied by phagocytosis of tissue debris leading to protease escape and the release of more DAMPs. Activated platelets enter the joint space and aggravate the process by producing yet more IL1.

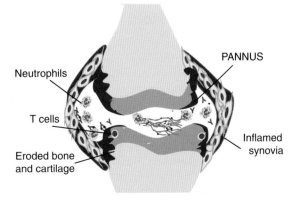

Fig. 16.4 The features of a joint affected by rheumatoid arthritis. It becomes swollen and painful because of inflamed synovia. A layer of pannus grows over and erodes the cartilage and bone. The predominant cell within the synovial fluid is the neutrophil, but T cells are abundant in the pannus and synovia.

PANNUS

Neutrophils

T cells

Inflamed synovia

Eroded bone and cartilage

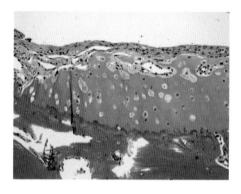

Fig. 16.5 A layer of pannus growing over the surface of articular cartilage. Notice how the underside is invading and eroding the cartilage surface. (Courtesy of Dr Roy Pool.)

Erosive joint destruction by invasive pannus is a defining feature of RA (Fig. 16.5). The growing pannus is able to invade and destroy joint cartilage through its production of proteases such as collagenase, stromelysin, and gelatinase. The flood of cytokines stimulates cartilage degradation by the activated FLS and by stimulating their release of these proteases. Metalloproteases-2 and -9 from chondrocytes and macrophages degrade both articular cartilage and nearby ligaments.

The growth of pannus and its accompanying cytokine release eventually leads to bone erosion and the characteristic joint pathology of RA. Macrophage-derived osteoclasts are responsible for this erosive bone destruction. The differentiation of macrophages into bone-destroying osteoclasts is driven by a member of the TNF receptor superfamily called RANKL (receptor activator for NF-κB ligand). RANKL is produced by B cells, Th1, and Th17 cells, and most importantly by activated FLS. Thus it and other macrophage-activating mediators are produced in large quantities by the growing pannus. RANKL binds and activates osteoclasts and is the direct cause of the bone destruction so characteristic of this form of arthritis.

Collagen Autoantibodies

Late in the disease progression, autoantibodies to collagen may develop. Type II collagen is the predominant protein in articular cartilage. Autoantibodies to type II collagen can be detected in the serum and synovial fluid of dogs with RA, infective arthritis, and osteoarthritis. They appear to circulate in the form of immune complexes. These antibodies may result from epitope spreading following citrullination of collagen. Affected humans also develop a T-cell–mediated response to denatured collagen II and III. While the collagen-anticollagen immune complexes may play a role in RA pathogenesis, they appear to be secondary to the disease process. Arthritic horses can also develop antibodies to collagens I and II. An autoimmune disease that closely resembles RA can be induced in experimental rats or sheep immunized with type II collagen (see Chapter 22).

Canine Rheumatoid Arthritis

Erosive polyarthritis is not common in dogs. It is most often encountered in middle-aged toy breeds and Shetland Sheepdogs. There is no sex predilection. Dogs with RA may present with chronic depression, lethargy, anorexia, and fever, in addition to lameness, stiffness, and a reluctance to move, which tends to be most severe after rest (e.g., immediately after waking in the morning). The animals may be very unwilling to walk or stand. The arthritis is symmetric with synovial swelling as a result of the effusions into the joints. The joints become warm as the blood flow increases, but because the inflammation is restricted to the synovia the skin rarely becomes red. The animal may show depression and fatigue as a result of the systemic effects of IL1 and TNFα. Muscle atrophy may also be obvious. Some animals may simply show lameness without systemic signs. The disease mainly affects peripheral joints, especially the carpometacarpal and tarsometatarsal joints, that develop symmetric swelling and stiffness. Crepitus, laxity, and subluxation gradually develop. RA tends to be progressive and eventually leads to severe joint erosion and deformities. In advanced cases affected joints may fuse as a result of the formation of bony ankyloses. Radiologic findings are variable, but the swelling usually involves soft tissues only, and there may be subchondral bone lysis, cartilage erosion, and narrowing of the joint space. Soft tissue lesions include periarticular fibrosis, hyperplasia, and villous hypertrophy of the synovium.

DIAGNOSIS

The diagnosis of RA in animals is based on 10 criteria established for human RA:

1. Stiffness
2. Pain on manipulation of at least one joint
3. Arthritis persisting for at least 3 months
4. Periarticular soft tissue swelling
5. Typical radiographic changes showing irregular joint surfaces, subchondral bone destruction resulting in punched-out lesions along the joint surface; loss of mineralization at the epiphysis; periarticular calcification in the soft tissue; increases or decreases in the joint space; and extensive bone destruction resulting in gross joint deformity (Fig. 16.6)

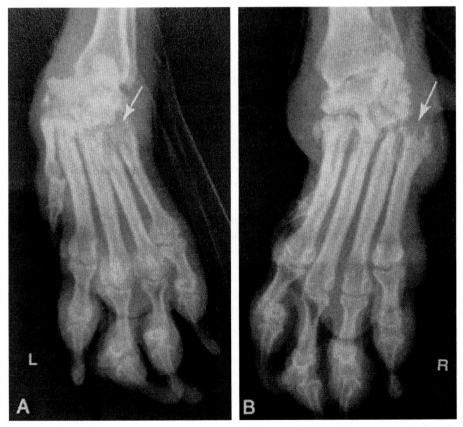

Fig. 16.6 Dorsopalmar radiographs of the left (A) and right (B) manus of a dog with immune-mediated erosive arthropathy. There is subluxation of the left antebrachiocarpal joint and the right carpometacarpal joint. There is also subluxation of distal interphalangeal joint in each manus. Numerous subchondral lytic erosive lesions are present *(white arrows)*. (G Allan and S Davies. Radiographic signs of Joint Disease in Dogs and Cats from In Thrall DE. Textbook of Veterinary Radiology, 7ed 2018. Elsevier.)

6. Inflammatory but sterile synovial fluid
7. Symmetric deformations of the distal joints
8. Presence of RF in serum
9. Characteristic histopathology in the synovia such as pannus formation
10. Extraarticular lesions such as a lymphadenopathy

Most of these signs should have been present for at least 6 weeks. If five are positive, then this is suggestive of RA; if seven or more are positive, then this is considered diagnostic.

RF may also be present in the serum and synovial fluid of some dogs with osteoarthritis, including cruciate ligament disease and septic arthritis, thus the measurement of RF in dogs is of doubtful specificity. In addition, steps should be taken to exclude SLE (by testing for antinuclear antibodies) and to exclude any infectious causes such as Lyme disease. In practice, arthrocentesis should be performed on several joints and the synovial fluid cultured and examined. Cytologic evaluation of sterile synovial fluid with a protein concentration of greater than 3.0 g/dL and a nucleated cell count of greater than 3000 cells/mL consisting of more than 12% neutrophils identifies an inflammatory arthritis, especially when supported by radiographic evidence of bone erosion. The synovial lymphocyte count in dogs with erosive polyarthritis is much greater than in dogs with nonerosive polyarthritis.

There appears to be no published data reporting on the presence of ACPA in dogs with RA. This is an area worth studying given their importance in the human disease (Box 16.2).

TREATMENT

Treatment of canine RA tends to be unsatisfactory. In general, mild cases may be treated conservatively with nonsteroidal antiinflammatory drugs (NSAIDs). These include carprofen, deracoxib, etodolac, firocoxib, meloxicam, and tepoxalin. NSAIDs are generally the first choice in treating early, mild cases of RA. Corticosteroids such as prednisolone should be reserved for late, severe cases in which NSAIDs have proved inadequate. Steroid injections into affected joints will usually produce rapid relief and clinical remission; however, rheumatoid joints are still subjected to stress, bone erosion may not be slowed, and the corticosteroids can delay healing and permit further articular degeneration. Their use may therefore permit joint damage to proceed unabated.

Short-term (2-week) systemic glucocorticosteroid therapy followed by tapering of the dose may be effective. If the response is unsatisfactory then the prednisolone may be combined with

---

BOX 16.2 ■ Autoantibodies to CTLA-4 in Dogs With Rheumatoid Arthritis and Other Autoimmune Diseases

As described in Chapter 2, cytotoxic T-lymphocyte–associated antigen 4 (CTLA-4) is a T-cell surface molecule that suppresses immune responses. In some cancer patients, for example, it prevents T-cell–mediated destruction of cancer cells. Monoclonal antibodies designated checkpoint inhibitors can block this CTLA-4–mediated suppression and so act as potent T-cell stimulators. In a survey of dogs with assorted autoimmune diseases, Khatlani et al. found that many of these animals possessed auto-antibodies directed against CTLA-4. They found these antibodies in 31.8% of dogs with rheumatoid arthritis, 20% of dogs with systemic lupus, and 12.5% of dogs with pemphigus. They were not detected in dogs with immune-mediated hemolytic anemia or in normal dogs. While unproven, it is entirely probable that these autoantibodies contribute to the excessive T-cell activity observed in these diseases. Exacerbation of rheumatoid arthritis has been reported in cancer patients receiving anti–CTLA-4 immune checkpoint therapy.

Khatlani TS, Ma Z, Okuda M, et al. Autoantibodies against T-cell costimulatory molecules are produced in canine autoimmune diseases. *J Immunother.* 2003;26:12-20.

other immunosuppressants such as azathioprine or cyclophosphamide. Newer immunosuppressants such as leflunomide or methotrexate may also be effective, although data on their effectiveness are limited. Monoclonal antibodies to TNFα (infliximab), CD4, thymocytes, or IL2R have helped to prevent bone erosions in humans, as has administration of recombinant TNFα receptors bound to IgG (etanercept). Slow-acting immunosuppressive agents, such as the gold salts, sodium aurothiomalate, and aurothioglucose, and antimalarials, such as chloroquine, are also used in humans, but they are expensive, results have been erratic, and experience with these in animals is limited. Appropriate surgery may improve joint stability and reduce pain. The prognosis for RA is generally poor as a result of the progressive joint destruction, and lifelong treatment may be required.

POLYARTHRITIS OF GREYHOUNDS

An erosive polyarthritis has been reported in young greyhounds (3–30 months of age). On necropsy this appears to be distinctly different from RA. The animals develop a subacute nonsuppurative synovitis accompanied by ulcerated erosions and extensive necrosis of the deep articular cartilage but relative sparing of the superficial cartilage in the limb joints. There is minimal bone damage but only moderate pannus formation. There are no extraarticular lesions and no evidence of an infectious cause. Its etiology is unknown.

Feline Erosive Polyarthritis

Two forms of erosive polyarthritis have been identified in cats: rheumatoid-like arthritis and feline periosteal proliferative polyarthritis.

RHEUMATOID-LIKE ARTHRITIS

This is a slowly developing polyarthritis with lameness gradually worsening over a period of months. Middle-aged and older cats may develop erosive polyarthritis in multiple joints. This is clinically similar to canine RA in that there is synovial inflammation leading to synovial villous hypertrophy, pannus formation, and detectable RF. Siamese cats may be predisposed. Treatment is as in dogs, thus NSAIDs such as meloxicam and carprofen may be used for mild cases. Glucocorticoids such as prednisolone may be used in severe cases. This may be supplemented by methotrexate, azathioprine, or leflunomide in refractory cases, otherwise the prognosis is poor.

PERIOSTEAL PROLIFERATIVE POLYARTHRITIS

This form of idiopathic arthritis occurs mainly in male cats. It is commonest in young adults under 5 years of age. Affected animals show an acute onset of typical arthritic signs, namely lethargy and a stiff gait. There may be pain and swelling of the carpal and tarsal-metatarsal joints. There may be generalized muscle atrophy and local lymphadenopathy as well, but systemic illness and fever do not develop. Synovial fluid shows a moderate to severe sterile neutrophil pleocytosis. After about 10 to 12 weeks, radiologically apparent lesions develop. They show periarticular soft tissue swelling and significant periosteal proliferation. The proliferating periosteal new bone formation increases around the hocks and tarsi until it results in osteophyte bridging and joint ankylosis. Lytic lesions develop, and periarticular erosions occur around the joint. This is a predominantly neutrophilic synovitis (90%) and tenosynovitis, but the proportion of lymphocytes and plasma cells in the lesions increases over time. Synovial biopsy eventually shows chronic synovitis, with villous hypertrophy and dense lymphocyte and plasma cell infiltrates. Radiology shows severe subchondral and marginal erosions eventually resulting in extensive bone destruction and joint deformity. There may be calcification in the soft tissue surrounding the joints. Feline RF assays are not commercially available, but experimental studies have shown their presence in some but not all cases. (These RF-positive cases should perhaps be classified as RA.) This form of arthritis has also been associated with feline leukemia virus, immunodeficiency virus, and syncytium-forming virus infections.

Treatment with glucocorticoids and analgesics may reduce pain and discomfort but does not reverse bone changes. Aggressive treatment with immunosuppressives such as prednisolone, cyclophosphamide, methotrexate, or leflunomide may be effective; however, relapses are common.

Sources of Additional Information

Rheumatoid Arthritis

Cheng Z, Meade J, Mankia K, et al. Periodontal disease and periodontal bacteria as triggers for rheumatoid arthritis. *Best Pract Res Clin Rheumatol*. 2017;31:19–30.

Firestein GS, McInnes IB. Immunopathogenesis of rheumatoid arthritis. *Immunity*. 2017;46:183–196.

Hoikhman R, Kudlackova H, Babak V, et al. Detection of IgM-rheumatoid factor and anti-citrullinated protein antibodies in healthy horses and their comparison. *Vet Immunol Immunopathol*. 2018;202:141–146.

Kim K, Bang S-Y, Lee H-S, et al. Update on the genetic architecture of rheumatoid arthritis. *Nat Rev Rheumatol*. 2017. doi:10.1038/nrrheum.2016.176.

Kristyanto H, Blomberg NJ, Slot LM, et al. Persistently activated, proliferative memory autoreactive B cells promote inflammation in rheumatoid arthritis. *Sci Transl Med*. 2020. doi:10.1126/scitranslmed.aaz5327.

Nygaard G, Firestein GS. Restoring synovial homeostasis by targeting fibroblast-like synoviocytes. *Nat Rev Rheumatol*. 2020;16:316–333.

Scherer HU, Häupl T, Burmester GR. The etiology of rheumatoid arthritis. *J Autoimmunity*. 2020. doi:10.1016/j.jaut.2019.102400.

Timoney J. Antibody and rheumatoid factor in synovia of pigs with *Erysipelothrix* polyarthritis. *J Comp Pathol*. 1971;81:243–248.

Weyand CM, Goronzy JJ. The immunology of rheumatoid arthritis. *Nat Immunol*. 2021;22:10–18.

Canine Rheumatoid Arthritis

Carter SD, Bell SC, Bari ASM, et al. Immune-complexes and rheumatoid factors in canine rheumatoid arthritides. *Ann Rheum Dis*. 1989;48:986–991.

Chabanne L, Fournel C, Faure JR, et al. IgM and IgA rheumatoid factors in canine polyarthritis. *Vet Immunol Immunopathol*. 1993;39:365–379.

Huxtable CR, Davis PE. The pathology of polyarthritis in young greyhounds. *J Comp Pathol*. 1976;86:11–21.

Lewis RM. Rheumatoid arthritis.. *Vet Clin Small Anim Pract*. 1994;24:697–701.

May C, Hughes DE, Sd Carter, et al. Lymphocyte populations in the synovial membranes of dogs with rheumatoid arthritis. *Vet Immunol Immunopathol*. 1992;31:289–300.

Ollier WER, Kennedy LJ, Thomson W, et al. Dog MHC alleles containing the human RA shared epitope confer susceptibility to canine rheumatoid arthritis. *Immunogenetics*. 2001;53:669–673.

Shaughnessy ML, Sample SJ, Abicht C, et al. Clinical features and pathological joint changes in dogs with erosive immune-mediated polyarthritis: 13 cases (2004-2012). *J Amer Vet Med Assoc*. 2016;249:1156–1164.

Feline Polyarthritis

Hannah FY. Disease modifying treatment for feline rheumatoid arthritis. *Vet Comp Orthop Traumatol*. 2005;18:94–99.

Seronegative Nonerosive Arthropathies

In this and the remaining disease chapters, we focus on predominantly inflammatory diseases in which tissue damage and destruction are not associated with direct autoimmune attack on cellular targets. Many are, however, mediated by the inflammation resulting from the deposition of immune complexes and activated complement in tissues, as well as by aberrant behavior of the interleukin-23 (IL23)/IL17 axis. These diseases can be subdivided into primary diseases, in which the trigger may be an autoantigen or remains unknown, and secondary diseases, where the triggering immune stimulus is derived from infectious agents, neoplasia, or drugs. The major targets of these inflammatory diseases are the joints, blood vessels, and walls of the large and small intestines.

The nonerosive seronegative arthropathies, unlike rheumatoid arthritis, are characterized by inflammation that is largely confined to the joint capsule and synovia and in which the joint cartilage or bone is not destroyed. Many of these cases resemble rheumatoid arthritis clinically but may be differentiated by their nonerosive character and the absence of autoantibodies such as rheumatoid factors (RF) and anticitrullinated protein antibodies (ACPA). Inflammation (enthesitis) at the sites of tendon attachments to bones is often a defining characteristic of these arthropathies. In many cases, they probably result from type III immune complex–mediated hypersensitivity reactions developing within the synovia and joint capsule (Fig. 17.1). In other cases, they appear to be mediated by inappropriate helper T type 17 (Th17) cell responses resulting in a neutrophil-dominated inflammation. In still other cases, they may result from chronic overproduction of tumor necrosis factor (TNF). It is also fair to say that in many cases their pathogenesis is unknown or speculative. Thus rather than the autoantibodies and aberrant T-cell responses of rheumatoid arthritis, these arthritides are driven primarily by innate immune mechanisms and not by autoimmune processes. In humans, they are classified as reactive arthritis/undifferentiated spondyloarthropathy. These arthropathies are then divided into two subtypes: axial and peripheral. In humans, a common presentation is the development of ankylosing spondylitis (fusion of

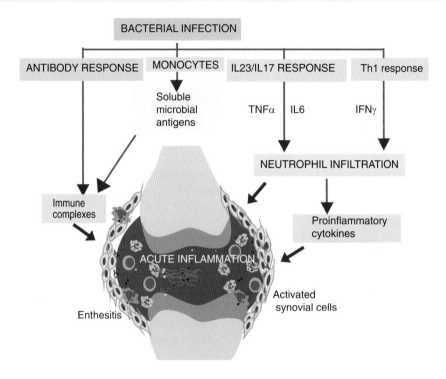

Fig. 17.1 The pathogenesis of nonerosive polyarthritis. Unlike rheumatoid arthritis in which the destructive lesion is largely mediated by activated T cells and synovial fibroblasts, the nonerosive immune-mediated arthritides probably result from both a type III hypersensitivity reaction occurring as a result of immune complexes forming within synovial vessels and helper T type 17 cell activation likely initiated at inflammatory sites elsewhere in the body. *IFNγ,* Interferon-gamma; *IL,* interleukin; *Th1,* helper T type 1, *TNFα,* tumor necrosis factor-alpha.

the spinal joints). However, ankylosing spondylitis is rare in the major domestic species. It has been described in the dog but appears to be uncommon and sporadic. Another animal disease that resembles human spondyloarthropathies is *Erysipelothrix*-mediated spinal disease in swine. Primates such as the great apes can also develop these spondyloarthropathies. Thus axial disease is rarely reported in domestic species. Peripheral reactive polyarthritis is much more common.

Reactive Polyarthritis

One form of nonerosive arthritis in humans and dogs is the acute inflammatory joint disease that develops 1 to 4 weeks after a gastrointestinal, respiratory, or urogenital infection. This so-called reactive arthritis commonly presents as a mono- or polyarthritis affecting the lower limbs in humans. Organisms associated with these reactive arthritides include *Chlamydia, Yersinia, Shigella, Salmonella, Campylobacter,* and some *Clostridia.* These are all gram-negative aerobic or microaerophilic bacteria with lipopolysaccharides in their outer membrane. However, viable organisms cannot be isolated from the inflamed joints. The joint inflammatory fluids remain sterile. As described later, these reactive arthropathies share similar manifestations of sterile joint inflammation and enthesis.

The pathophysiology of reactive polyarthritis is not fully understood, and two theories have been proposed to explain it. One theory, the arthritogenic peptide hypothesis, suggests that circulating peptides derived from intestinal bacteria can penetrate the intestinal epithelium, circulate, and enter synovial vessels, where they either trigger a local type III hypersensitivity response or cross-react with structurally similar self-peptides to trigger a local autoimmune response. A second theory, the aberrant cellular trafficking hypothesis, suggests that signals emanating from the gastrointestinal microbiota result in circulating Th17 cells and/or antigen-bearing macrophages homing in specifically on the joints. While the pathogenesis of reactive arthropathies remains unclear, it is apparent that many are triggered by intestinal dysbiosis or enteric disease. For example, 50% to 70% of human reactive arthritis patients have coexisting intestinal inflammation. Thus changes in the gut microbiota can increase the production of an epithelial cell protein called zonulin. Zonulin causes the disassembly of the tight junctions between intestinal epithelial cells. This opens gaps between the cells that permit the entry of many pathogen-associated molecular pattern molecules such as endotoxins and so stimulate inflammasome activation and proinflammatory cytokine release. Under experimental conditions in mice, chronic overstimulation by exposure to TNF results in activation of synovial fibroblasts and intestinal fibroblasts, and this can result in the simultaneous development of both arthritis and colitis.

In humans, the development of these forms of arthritis is also associated with the major histocompatibility complex–human leukocyte antigen (MHC-HLA) class I allele B27, but no comparable susceptibility allele has been identified in domestic animals (Box 17.1). A single nucleotide polymorphism of the IL23 receptor gene is also a known risk factor in humans.

PATHOGENESIS

Once immune cells and antigens reach the joints, there are two leading theories as to how reactive arthritis develops. One suggests that it is due to immune complex deposition in synovial blood vessels. The other suggests that it is due to uncontrolled Th17 cell activation. They are not mutually incompatible.

Immune Complex Arthropathies

Typically, animals with reactive arthritis suffer from neutrophil-mediated inflammation in multiple joints. As pointed out in Chapter 16, synovial capillaries are fenestrated. As a result, soluble macromolecules smaller than 12 kDa can pass from the bloodstream into the synovial tissues and joint fluid. However, large molecular aggregates such as immune complexes will be retained. Thus as in the glomeruli of the kidneys, it is possible that circulating antigens produced by microbial invaders or commensals may be bound by antibodies, form immune complexes, lodge in synovial capillary walls, activate complement, and trigger acute inflammation. The inducing antigens may circulate in the form

---

BOX 17.1 ■ The Role of HLA-B27

It has long been known that in humans and other primates, there is a close association between possession of the major histocompatibility complex (MHC) antigen HLA-B27 and the development of many arthropathies. It is present in 50% to 80% of patients with these diseases. B27-positive patients develop more severe and more persistent arthritis than B27-negative patients. It has long been theorized that HLA-B27 presents certain bacterial antigens to T cells in way that triggers T-cell responses, resulting in autoimmune disease, especially directed against autoantigens in spinal joints and triggering ankylosing spondylitis. However, B27-expressing monocytes have a reduced ability to prevent the intracellular replication of *Salmonella*. B27 might also enhance endotoxin-induced tumor necrosis factor-alpha production in macrophages. Thus the effects of HLA-B27 may result from a combination of alterations in antigen presentation coupled with changes in macrophage behavior.

Zhang L, Zhang Y-J, Chen J, et al. The association of HLA-B27 and *Klebsiella pneumoniae* in ankylosing spondylitis: a systematic review. *Microb Pathogen*. 2018;117:49-54.

of intracellular organisms, fragments of organisms, or soluble microbial antigens. This immune complex hypothesis is supported by the observation that affected animals may also develop similar lesions elsewhere, such as uveitis, dermatitis, glomerulonephritis, and possibly inflammatory bowel disease.

Activation of the Th17 Pathway

The joint fluids of affected individuals contain a complex mixture of proinflammatory cytokines. These include transforming growth factor-beta (TGFβ), IL6, IL10, IL12, IL17, and interferon-gamma (IFNγ). When the levels of these cytokines in reactive arthritis are compared with their levels in rheumatoid arthritis joint fluids, differences stand out. Levels are approximately equal for TGFβ, IL10, and IL12. However, reactive synovial fluid contains about twice as much IL6, three times more IFNγ, and six to seven times more IL17 than rheumatoid arthritis joint fluid. This is clearly a Th17-predominant profile. It has been suggested therefore that reactive arthropathies may also result from a generalized Th1 and Th17 cell response triggered by bacterial infections or gut dysbiosis. *Chlamydia, Salmonella,* and *Yersinia* have all been shown to induce Th1 and Th17 responses. The cytokine IL23 produced by antigen-presenting cells is required for the production of Th17 cells (Fig. 17.2). Studies have suggested that much of this IL23 originates in the Paneth cells of the inflamed intestine. IL23-producing cells have also been found within arthritic joints. IL17 production is further stimulated by the simultaneous presence of TGFβ and IL6. Th17 cells originating in the intestine or in another localized infection site may enter the circulation and subsequently converge on joints. Once within the synovia, IL17 is produced and binds to cell surface receptors (IL17RA thru RE) that signal through NF-κB. IL17 stimulates the production of granulocyte macrophage (GM) colony-stimulating factor (CSF) leading to a neutrophilia. Locally, it also promotes the recruitment and survival of macrophages. IL17 triggers production of many other cytokines, such as IL1 and TNFα from macrophages, and IL6, GM-CSF, and IL8 from synovial fibroblasts, in addition to multiple chemokines and inflammatory mediators such as prostaglandins. IL17 attracts neutrophils and macrophages to inflammatory sites as a result of stimulating IL6 production.

CANINE POLYARTHRITIS

Dogs may develop several distinct forms of nonerosive polyarthritis. These can be divided into three major categories: primary idiopathic arthritis, arthritis secondary to systemic lupus, and arthritis associated with a concurrent polymyositis. Breeds predisposed to developing polyarthritis include German Shepherd Dogs, Irish Setters, Shetland Sheepdogs, Cocker Spaniels, and Springer Spaniels. The main clinical features of all these are stiffness, pyrexia, anorexia, and lethargy.

The vast majority of canine polyarthritis cases are nonerosive and predominantly neutrophil mediated. It is believed therefore that the triggering antigen must first diffuse into the synovia, where it encounters circulating antibodies within local blood vessels. Immune complexes form and are deposited between and beneath vascular endothelial cells. Complement components activated by the classical pathway will be deposited here as well.

Immune complexes formed in the synovia must be removed. They first bind to Fc and complement receptors on cells. The most widespread of these Fc receptors is FcγRII expressed on neutrophils. Immune complexes binding to these receptors activate the neutrophils and stimulate their production of oxidants, leukotrienes, prostaglandins, cytokines, and chemokines. Immune complexes also bind to synovial mast cells through FcγRIII and trigger the release of their granule contents, most notably TNFα. All these mediators promote a synovitis by acting on vascular endothelium and stimulating neutrophil adherence and emigration.

Neutrophil proteases also act on C5 to generate the small but highly active complement peptide C5a. C5a promotes further neutrophil accumulation and degranulation. Neutrophils, attracted by C5a and mast cell–derived TNFα, bind the complexes and promptly phagocytose

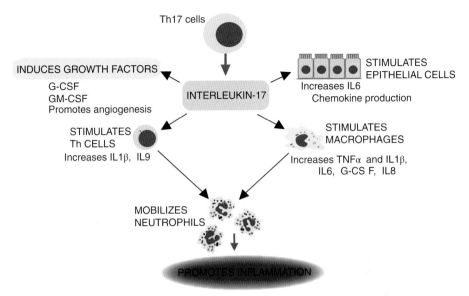

Fig. 17.2 The role of interleukin *(IL)*–17 in promoting acute inflammation. *G-CSF,* Granulocyte colony-stimulating factor; *GM-CSF,* granulocyte macrophage colony-stimulating factor; *Th17,* helper T type 17.

them. Eventually the immune complexes are digested and destroyed. During this process, however, proteases and oxidants are released into the tissues. Neutrophil proteases disrupt collagen fibers and destroy cartilage and ground substances, basement membranes, and elastic tissue. As a result of all this, inflammation and destruction of blood vessel walls cause edema and synovial vasculitis. The identity of the initiating antigen(s) is in most cases unknown.

Canine idiopathic polyarthritis has been classified into four types (Fig. 17.3). Type I disease is polyarthritis alone with no obvious underlying disease. Type II disease is a reactive arthritis associated with infections in the respiratory or urinary tract, tooth infections, or cellulitis. Type III disease is associated with the presence of enteric diseases such as gastroenteritis, diarrhea, or ulcerative colitis. It is not clear whether this type of disease is truly distinguishable from type II disease. Type IV disease is a paraneoplastic arthritis associated with the presence of tumors, including seminomas and carcinomas. In general, the histopathology and clinical presentation of each of these types is identical. The differences lie in the underlying conditions and presumably the nature of the triggering antigens.

Type I Idiopathic Immune-Mediated Polyarthritis

A stand-alone idiopathic polyarthritis is the most common of the nonerosive arthropathies, accounting for 50% to 80% of canine cases. Idiopathic polyarthritis does not have a sex predilection, and about half of the cases are seen in young to middle-aged dogs between 1 and 10 years of age. Sporting dogs and large breeds such as Rottweilers, Retrievers (both Labrador and Golden), German Shepherd Dogs, and Cocker Spaniels are overrepresented. The clinical signs are highly variable, but most of these animals develop fever, anorexia, weight loss, and lethargy. Affected animals may have effusions in multiple joints and are reluctant to walk. Many but not all may be lame and have a history of stiffness after rest. The most commonly affected joints are the stifle, elbow, and carpus. The lesions are usually bilateral. The onset of lameness tends to be sudden but may be associated with obvious muscle atrophy. There is no significant joint erosion, only periarticular soft tissue swelling and synovial effusions. Some cases may develop proliferative periosteal changes. Some but not all cases may have joint pain detectable by physical examination. Some cases may also

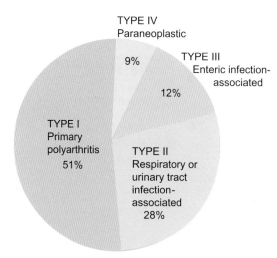

Fig. 17.3 The relative prevalence of the different types of nonerosive reactive polyarthritis in dogs. (Data from Bennett D. Immune-based non-erosive inflammatory joint disease of the dog. 3. Canine idiopathic polyarthritis. *J Small Anim Pract.* 1987;28:909-928.)

show evidence of spinal pain. These cases are negative for RF and antinuclear antibody (ANA), and importantly, the joint fluid is sterile.

Synovial biopsies show hypertrophy with a neutrophil or a mononuclear cell infiltration, or both. There are large numbers of cells in the synovial fluid, with neutrophils predominating (Fig. 17.4). Fibrin deposits are seen in most cases, as is fibrosis. Most lesions contain immunoglobulin M (IgM), IgG, and complement, and some contain IgA-producing plasma cells. Some affected dogs may also develop a glomerulopathy, while about a quarter may also develop a steroid-responsive meningitis. Serum levels of C-reactive protein and IL6 are elevated. Animals respond well to corticosteroids. Leflunomide appears to be an effective alternative to oral corticosteroids for the treatment of this disease. This disease has a good prognosis, but recurrence rates are high.

An inherited form of type I polyarthritis is the juvenile polyarthritis syndrome that develops in Akitas between the ages of 9 weeks and 8 months. These dogs develop a cyclic high fever lasting 24 to 48 hours before resolving and severe, incapacitating joint pain with soft tissue swelling. Radiology shows hepatosplenomegaly and lymphadenopathy. Some animals may also develop meningitis or meningoencephalitis. Their erythrocytes may be immunoglobulin positive. Synovial fluid shows no evidence of infection, although large numbers of neutrophils are present. Proteomic analysis of the fluid may show increased protein content due to elevated immunoglobulins. Some dogs respond positively to corticosteroid treatment. In refractory cases, azathioprine may also be required.

Type II (Reactive) Polyarthritis

These cases are associated with the presence of an inflammatory or infected focus in tissues elsewhere in the body. Thus they have been associated with urinary or respiratory tract bacterial, fungal, and viral infections, heartworm, leishmaniasis, ehrlichiosis, and Lyme borreliosis, as well as periodontal disease. They account for 15% to 25% of polyarthritis cases. The underlying causal infection may be located anywhere in the body. Noninfectious inflammation such as acute pancreatitis may also trigger type II polyarthritis.

A drug-induced polyarthritis can develop 5 to 20 days after drug treatment, and clinical signs are similar to the other canine polyarthropathies. Implicated drugs include sulfonamides such as sulfadiazine-trimethoprim, phenobarbital, penicillins, and cephalexin. Animals may also show other signs of drug hypersensitivities such as skin lesions. Clinical improvement should be seen within 24 hours of stopping the drug.

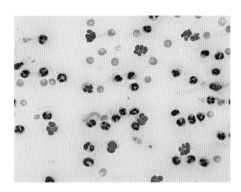

Fig. 17.4 Synovial fluid from an adult Labrador Retriever with immune-mediated polyarthritis with an extremely high nucleated cell count that was predominantly neutrophilic. Note the absence of bacteria. Original magnification × 20. (Courtesy Dr. Mark Johnson.)

One specific form of reactive polyarthritis is vaccine induced. This develops within about 3 to 15 days after vaccination. The polyarthritis is transient and usually resolves within a few days. Distemper vaccine appears to be one source of the inciting antigen. Thus antidistemper virus antibodies have been detected in synovial fluid in some cases, and these may therefore result in the development of immune complexes within joints. Vaccine-induced disease tends to be a sudden-onset acute inflammatory arthritis. There are high leukocyte counts in the joint fluid. Affected animals respond rapidly to nonsteroidal antiinflammatory drugs (NSAIDs). Akitas appear to be especially predisposed to developing these vaccine-related reactions.

Type III (Enteropathic) Polyarthritis

Type III disease is a reactive polyarthritis associated with hepatic or gastrointestinal diseases, including inflammatory bowel disease. It is not very common, accounting for only about 5% of canine polyarthritis cases. It has been reported as occurring in dogs infected with *Salmonella* or *Campylobacter*. It has been suggested that increases in intestinal permeability during such infections may permit microbial antigens to enter the body and trigger both Th17- and immune-complex–mediated disease. In humans and other primates, a form of reactive polyarthritis has been associated with intestinal *Klebsiella* infections. These human diseases primarily affect intervertebral joints, causing ankylosing spondylitis.

Type IV (Paraneoplastic) Polyarthritis

This form of polyarthritis is associated with the presence of a neoplasm elsewhere in the body. It is the least common form of polyarthritis, accounting for about 2% of cases. It has occurred in association with diverse carcinomas such as squamous cell or mammary carcinomas, sarcomas, and lymphomas. It is believed to result from soluble antigen released from cancer cells forming immune complexes that are then filtered out in synovial vessels.

Diagnosis and Treatment

It is first necessary to rule out infectious causes of the polyarthritis and identify any associated diseases. Animals may have evidence of systemic inflammation such as a leukocytosis, nonregenerative anemia, and hypoalbuminemia. Examination of synovial fluid from affected joints should include cytologic analysis and culturing for the presence of bacteria. The quantity and state of the synovial fluid may vary between joints so multiple joints should be sampled, especially the carpal, tarsal, and stifle joints. An ANA test may be performed to exclude lupus. Radiology should be used to determine if bone and joint structures are significantly damaged.

Treatment will depend on the underlying cause. Analgesia using NSAIDs may be used initially until any infectious cause is definitively excluded. NSAIDs should not be administered concurrently with corticosteroids, and a washout period of about 7 days is recommended before commencing steroid therapy. In the case of idiopathic disease where infection has been definitely excluded, glucocorticosteroids may be used until remission is achieved. If corticosteroids prove insufficient, then they may be supplemented by cytotoxic drugs such as azathioprine, cyclophosphamide, or leflunomide.

FELINE POLYARTHRITIS

Infectious polyarthritis is very much more common than primary immune-mediated arthritis in cats. Immune-mediated joint diseases are very uncommon. Affected cats may be in obvious pain, show a reluctance to walk, or have a stiff gait. Chronic progressive disease of male (rarely female) cats is characterized by a polyarthritis with either osteopenia or periosteal new bone formation. Periarticular erosions and eventual collapse or subchondral erosions, joint instabilities, and deformities closely resembling those of rheumatoid arthritis are also seen. Affected cats may be infected with feline syncytia-forming virus (FeSFV), feline leukemia virus (FeLV), or both. (The prevalence of FeSFV in these cats is 2 to 4 times higher, and the incidence of FeLV is 6 to 10 times higher than in nonarthritic cats.) It is described here because of suggestions that it is of immune origin, and cyclosporine has been used successfully to treat some cases. These suggestions are also based on the massive lymphocyte and plasma cell infiltration of affected joints and the simultaneous presence of an immune complex–mediated glomerulonephritis.

Primary immune-mediated polyarthritis in cats must be diagnosed by exclusion. All infectious causes must have been eliminated and the cat shown not to be suffering from systemic lupus erythematosus (SLE) or reactive polyarthritis. Diagnosis is thus based largely on a positive response to glucocorticosteroid therapy.

Reactive polyarthritis occurs in response to infections, neoplasia, or certain drugs. These infections include toxoplasmosis, FeLV, feline infectious peritonitis, pyelonephritis, or respiratory disease.

Cats should not be treated with immunosuppressive agents until all infectious causes of arthritis have been definitely excluded. Corticosteroids lessen the severity of clinical signs. Combination therapy with corticosteroids and azathioprine or cyclophosphamide can induce remissions.

EQUINE POLYARTHRITIS-POLYSYNOVITIS

Polyarthritis has been reported in foals in association with a lupuslike syndrome. Affected foals (up to 3 months of age) develop multiple swollen joints involving all four limbs and a persistent fever. In some cases, synovial sheaths, including tendon sheaths and bursae, are also affected. The synovial effusions are sterile, but synovial biopsies show lymphocyte and plasma cell infiltration with some immunoglobulin deposits. The cells in the joint fluid are mainly neutrophils. These animals are negative for RF, ANA, and LE cells. Many of these foals have a lesion within the thorax, especially *Prescottella (Rhodococcus) equi* pneumonia. It is possible that immune complexes originating in the lung lesions may lodge in the synovial vessels and trigger the synovitis. The polyarthritis usually resolves once the primary lesion heals.

A primary immune-mediated polyarthritis has also been recorded in horses. In these cases, animals lose weight and develop an intermittent fever and effusions in multiple joints, leading to stiffness. They have systemic signs of inflammation, including anemia, leukocytosis, hyperfibrinogenemia, and hyperglobulinemia. The synovial fluid is sterile, and immunoglobulins are present in the synovial membrane. The condition usually resolves with steroid and immunosuppressive therapy.

Other Inflammatory Arthritides

LUPUS POLYARTHRITIS

Among the most frequent signs of SLE in dogs is a nonerosive polyarthritis. It is estimated that up to 90% of canine lupus patients develop arthritis. Thus affected dogs develop stiffness and persistent lameness, especially after rest. The joints are obviously painful on palpation.

Some dogs may also suffer from a simultaneous polymyositis with megaesophagus. Some Nova Scotia Duck Tolling Retrievers may develop concomitant steroid-resistant meningitis-arteritis. In that breed, susceptibility is associated with homozygosity of the MHC haplotype DLA-DRB1*00601/DQA1*005011/DQB1*02001. Most affected dogs also possess ANA. Diagnosis is contingent on making a firm diagnosis of systemic lupus. Thus it is necessary to show multisystem involvement, a significant titer of serum ANA, and immunopathologic features consistent with lupus (see Chapter 15). Its clinical presentation of an acute synovitis is similar to other nonerosive polyarthritides. Treatment is as for lupus, but dogs may require lifelong immunosuppressive and antiinflammatory medication.

SLE-associated polyarthritis in cats is very uncommon. In this species, it is most commonly associated with dermatitis, fever, and glomerulonephritis. Synovial fluid must be collected and analyzed when evaluating feline arthritis. Cats should also be tested for feline immunodeficiency virus and FeLV. However, affected cats are usually RF and ANA negative, and their serum immunoglobulin levels tend to be close to normal (Box 17.2).

POLYARTHRITIS-POLYMYOSITIS SYNDROME

A disease characterized by both nonerosive polyarthritis and polymyositis is recognized in young dogs. Most recorded cases have been seen in Spaniels. The animals develop painful joints, fever, lethargy, weakness, muscle atrophy, and muscle pain. The arthritis is usually symmetric and involves multiple joints. The animals may also have a symmetric inflammatory myopathy with myalgia that eventually results in atrophy and muscle contracture. Muscle biopsies show a neutrophil or mononuclear cell infiltrate, or both, with muscle fiber atrophy and degeneration. Synovial biopsies show a neutrophil and mononuclear cell infiltration with a fibrinous exudate. The synovial fluid contains high numbers of white cells, especially neutrophils. IgG, IgM, and complement are deposited in the walls of the synovial blood vessels. These dogs test negative for both ANA and RF. Animals may be treated with corticosteroids and immunosuppressive agents such as cyclophosphamide.

CRUCIATE LIGAMENT RUPTURE

Cranial cruciate ligament disease is the commonest cause of hindlimb lameness in adult dogs. It is usually a result of a progressive degeneration that results in eventual rupture of the ligament. The

---

BOX 17.2 ■ Canine Psoriatic Arthritis

About 20% of arthritis cases in humans are classified as psoriatic arthritis, so named because the arthritis is associated with the simultaneous presence of the skin disease psoriasis and the absence of rheumatoid factor. It also commonly involves enthesitis, dactylitis, and axial involvement and it has significant cardiovascular comorbidities. Its pathogenesis is unclear, but it appears to involve activation of the interleukin-23/helper T type 17 pathway and dysregulated tumor necrosis factor (TNF) production. Patients respond well to anti-TNF monoclonal antibody therapy.

A single case of psoriatic arthritis has been reported in a 4-year-old spayed female Pug mix that presented with skin lesions and a deforming arthritis. Biopsy of the skin lesions showed severe hyperplastic parakeratotic hyperkeratosis with an infiltration of lymphocytes and plasma cells, corresponding to the characteristic features described in human psoriasis. The animal was given nonsteroidal antiinflammatory drugs to treat the pain and inflammation, while the skin lesions were treated with topical steroids, topical vitamin D, and a topical keratinolytic. The dog showed a rapid and complete recovery.

Regan SA, Marsella R, Ozmen I. First report of a psoriatic-like dermatitis and arthritis in a 4-year-old female spayed pug mix. *Case Reps Vet Med.* 2015. doi.org/10.1155/2015/912509.

reasons for this progressive degeneration are complex and unclear. Possible causes include genetic, conformational, inflammatory, and immune-mediated mechanisms. They are not mutually exclusive. The degeneration is associated with a progressive loss of ligament fibroblasts, which results in collagen fibril disruption. While genetic and conformational causes predominate, environmental factors such as obesity and neutering status play a role. Interestingly, immunologic abnormalities have also been associated with its spontaneous rupture.

Studies on dogs with osteoarthritis as well as with spontaneous cruciate ligament rupture have shown that up to 90% may possess antibodies against type I and type II collagens in their sera and synovia (Box 17.3). Collagen I is the predominant structural protein in cruciate ligaments, whereas collagen II predominates in joint cartilage. In addition, the synovia of dogs with ruptured ligaments contains B cells, IgG-positive plasma cells, and numerous MHC class II$^+$ dendritic cells. Thus it resembles the infiltrates encountered in rheumatoid arthritis. Canine joints in which the anterior cruciate ligament has ruptured contain increased numbers of CD4$^+$, CD8$^+$, and double-negative (CD4$^-$CD8$^-$) T cells. Likewise, the macrophages within these joints have a predominantly M1 activated phenotype, whereas healthy dog joints contain primarily M2 macrophages.

However, ligament rupture is an end-stage disease, and these observations raise the question, are these autoantibodies, lymphocytes, and macrophages the cause or the consequence of ligament rupture? Autoantibodies to both type I and type II collagen are found in synovial fluid following cruciate ligament rupture (secondary to osteoarthritis), usually bound in the form of immune complexes. Their presence is probably secondary to tissue damage, since in a prospective study, there was no evidence that the development of antibodies to type I collagen preceded cruciate ligament rupture. There is also no evidence to suggest that anticollagen antibodies alone can cause ligament damage. Thus synovial titers of these antibodies were measured in dogs with a unilateral rupture. Some of these dogs eventually developed a contralateral rupture, but this was not correlated with the presence of anticollagen I antibodies. IL8 levels rise in joints prior to cruciate ligament rupture, implying that inflammation precedes rupture. It is therefore believed that early deterioration of the cruciate ligament results in the release of collagen I into the joint. This collagen is antigenic and so triggers a B-cell response and the production of anticollagen antibodies. These in turn form immune complexes, resulting in a local inflammation. These immune complexes may contribute to further ligament deterioration.

BOX 17.3 ■ Osteoarthritis

Osteoarthritis, a common form of degenerative arthritis in aged dogs and humans, has generally been considered to result from "wear and tear" on joints and is not considered an autoimmune disease. However, over time, prolonged stress acts on joint cells, such as chondrocytes and osteocytes, through mechanoreceptors. This stress on the cells, together with the insidious process of inflammaging, eventually results in activation of the innate immune pathways and the development of a low-grade inflammation involving all joint tissues. Kinases are activated, resulting in increased expression of proinflammatory cytokines, metalloproteases, and reactive oxygen species. The metalloproteases may cause the release of fibronectin into the synovium so triggering a synovitis. Macrophages, T cells, and mast cells are commonly found in the synovia of affected joints. Chondrocytes can produce proinflammatory cytokines, including both tumor necrosis factor-alpha and interleukin-1β. It has been reported that about 50% of dogs with osteoarthritis have antibodies to type II collagen in their serum and synovial fluid. This is believed to be a secondary response to chronic joint damage. Thus although mechanically initiated, osteoarthritis also has an autoinflammatory component.

Bari ASM, Carter SD, Bell SC, et al. Anti-type II collagen antibody in naturally occurring canine joint diseases. *Brit Jour Rheumatol.* 1989;28:480-486.
Konttinen Y, et al. Osteoarthritis as an autoinflammatory disease caused by chondrocyte-mediated inflammatory responses. *Arthritis Rheum.* 2012;64:613-616.

RELAPSING POLYCHONDRITIS

Recurrent inflammation of cartilaginous tissue (i.e., relapsing polychondritis) has been reported in humans, dogs, and cats. This disease is characterized by recurrent inflammatory episodes involving cartilage and other proteoglycan-rich tissues such as the eye, heart tissues, joints, and the inner ear. This results in progressive deformation of structures such as the pinnae, the nasal cartilage, and polyarthritis. The cartilage is infiltrated with plasma cells and lymphocytes. Circulating antibodies against collagens II, IX, and XI are found in affected humans, suggesting that these may serve as target antigens. Collagen II predominates in cartilage and may be the major target. The cartilage matrix protein matrilin-1 is also an important autoantigen.

This rare disease has been reported in young to middle-aged cats. Animals present with bilateral swelling of the pinnae accompanied by curling, wrinkling, erythema, and pain. Some affected cats may be febrile, with lethargy and anorexia. Biopsy of the lesions shows inflammation, degeneration, and necrosis accompanied by a dense lymphocytic infiltrate with some multinuclear giant cells and local fibrosis. In cats, it has also been associated with mild ocular disease (keratitis) and cardiomegaly (left ventricular dilatation). A similar lesion in kittens has been associated with CD3[+] T cells found in close approximation to degenerating chondrocytes, suggesting that T-cell–mediated cytotoxicity may be occurring. Application of topical tacrolimus cream has led to resolution of the lesions within a few weeks. Relapsing polychondritis may also respond to glucocorticoid therapy, but results are inconsistent. Dapsone has been used successfully, and spontaneous remissions have been reported.

Sources of Additional Information

Canine Polyarthritis

Clements DN, Gear RN, Tattersall J, et al. Type I immune-mediated polyarthritis of dogs: 39 cases (1997-2002). *J Amer Vet Med Assn.* 2004;224:1323–1327.

Foster JD, Sample S, Kohler R, et al. Serum biomarkers of clinical and cytological response in dogs with idiopathic immune-mediated polyarthropathy. *J Vet Intern Med.* 2014;28:905–911.

Grapes NJ, Packer RMA, De Decker S. Clinical reasoning in canine cervical hyperesthesia: which presenting features are important?. *Vet Rec.* 2020. doi:10.1136/vr.105818.

Idowu OA, Heading KL. Type I immune-mediated polyarthritis in dogs and lack of a temporal relationship to vaccination. *J Small Anim Pract.* 2018;59:183–187.

Johnson K, Mackin A. Canine immune-mediated arthritis: part 1: pathophysiology. *J Amer Anim Hosp Assn.* 2012;48:71–82.

Johnson K, Mackin A. Canine immune-mediated arthritis: part 2: diagnosis and treatment. *J Amer Anim Hosp Assn.* 2012;48:12–17.

Qaiyum Z, Lim M, Inman RD. The gut-joint axis in spondylarthritis: immunological, microbial, and clinical insights. *Semin Immunopathol.* 2021;43:173–192.

Sikes D, Hayes FA, Prestwood AK, et al. Ankylosing spondylitis and polyarthritis of the dog: physiopathologic changes of tissues. *Am J Vet Res.* 1970;31:703–712.

Stull JW, Evason M, Carr AP, et al. Canine immune-mediated polyarthritis: clinical and laboratory findings in 83 cases in western Canada (1991-2001). *Can Vet J.* 2008;49:1195–1203.

Webb AA, Taylor SM, Muir GD. Steroid-responsive meningitis-arteritis in dogs with noninfectious, nonerosive, idiopathic, immune-mediated polyarthritis. *J Vet Intern Med.* 2002;16:269–273.

Whitworth F, Adamantos S, Frowde P, et al. Ligament laxity in nonerosive immune-mediated polyarthritis in dogs: five cases (2009-2017). *J Amer Anim Hosp Assn.* 2019;55:210–214.

Feline Polyarthritis

Pedersen NC, Pool RR, O'Brien T. Feline chronic progressive polyarthritis. *Am J Vet Res.* 1980;41:522–535.

Cruciate Ligament RuptureDoom M, de Bruin T, de Rooster H, et al. Immunopathological mechanisms in dogs with rupture of the cranial cruciate ligament. *Vet Immunol Immunopathol.* 2008;125:143–161.

Niebauer GW, Wolf B, Bashey RI, et al. Antibodies to collagen types I and II in dogs with spontaneous cruciate ligament rupture and osteoarthritis. *Arthr Rheum.* 1987;30:319–327.

Immune-Mediated Vascular Disease

Vasculitis, as its name implies, is inflammation of the blood vessel walls. Several forms of immune-mediated vasculitis have been described in domestic animals. They can be classified according to the types and sizes of blood vessels affected or according to the nature and location of the inflammatory infiltrate within vessel walls. Their precise relationships are often unclear. They can, however, be readily subdivided into those that affect large blood vessels such as arteries and those that occur within small blood vessels and cause microangiopathies (Fig. 18.1).

Arteritis

CANINE JUVENILE POLYARTERITIS

Canine juvenile polyarteritis syndrome is another name for steroid-responsive meningitis-arteritis described in Chapter 7. The disease has also been called canine pain syndrome or Beagle pain syndrome because animals may suffer from severe generalized pain during the acute stages of the disease. It is a necrotizing arteritis that primarily affects Beagles between 3 and 18 months of age. However, it can also affect dogs of other and mixed breeds. Affected animals show episodes of distress with a persistent fever greater than 40°C. They adopt a characteristic hunched stance with lowered head and a stiff gait, indicating severe neck pain. They may show evidence of abdominal pain as well. Their pharyngeal mucosa may also be inflamed. These episodes generally last 3 to 7 days. The animals are anorexic during their febrile period. The disease may become remitting and relapsing with regular cycling at 15- to 45-day intervals.

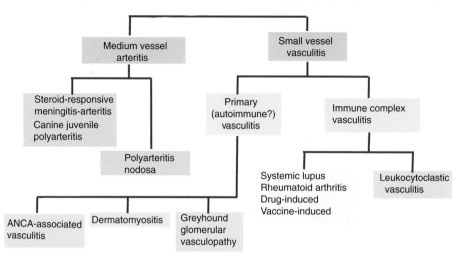

Fig. 18.1   A simplified scheme classifying the major forms of immune-mediated vasculitis occurring in the dog. *ANCA,* Antineutrophil cytoplasmic antibodies.

Animals usually have a marked leukocytosis (>25,000 white blood cells/mL) with a mature neutrophilia (>15,000/mL) and elevated acute phase proteins. Dogs also have consistently elevated serum immunoglobulin A (IgA), less consistent increases in IgM, and usually normal IgG levels. They are hypoalbuminemic. Blood B-cell numbers are increased, but T cells are decreased, as is their response to mitogens (perhaps resulting in a loss of regulatory T cells). Antineutrophil cytoplasmic autoantibodies (ANCA) are present in some affected dogs, but animals are usually negative for anti-nuclear antibodies (ANA) or rheumatoid factors. Macrophage activation is obvious when the blood mononuclear cells are cultured. Multinucleated giant cells may also develop in these cultures. Dogs have elevated platelet counts. Cerebrospinal fluid analysis shows a moderate to severe neutrophil pleocytosis.

On necropsy, affected animals show few gross lesions, although there may be some hemorrhage within lymph nodes. Histologically, the dogs have a systemic vasculitis and perivasculitis. In acute cases, there is necrotizing vasculitis with fibrinoid necrosis and a massive inflammatory cell infiltration involving small and medium-size arteries with a predilection for arteries of the heart, mediastinum, meninges, and cervical spinal cord. The vessels first show intimal thickening due to a mononuclear cell infiltrate that progresses eventually to involve all layers in the arterial wall (Fig. 18.2). Subsequently, the artery becomes surrounded by a mixed inflammatory infiltrate. The intima and media develop fibrinoid necrosis that eventually results in thrombosis. Immunoglobulins are deposited in the walls of these arteries. During remissions, the vascular lesions consist of intimal and medial fibrosis and a mild perivasculitis, the residue of previous acute vasculitis episodes. Chronically affected dogs may eventually develop generalized amyloidosis.

It is of interest to note that canine juvenile polyarteritis syndrome is very similar to Kawasaki disease of children. In this disease, it is believed that autoantibodies directed against vascular endothelial cells initiate the inflammatory process and trigger a platelet-driven immunothrombosis. Epidemiologic studies on this disease in a commercial Beagle kennel have shown a remarkable peak in the disease prevalence occurring approximately every 5 years. (Kawasaki disease shows a similar cyclic effect, with each cycle lasting about 4 years.) This suggests that an infectious agent may be the trigger, but none has been detected yet. Cases may resolve rapidly following administration of high doses of prednisone.

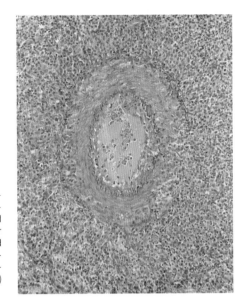

Fig. 18.2 An extramural coronary artery from a Beagle suffering from juvenile polyarteritis. The medium-sized muscular artery is characterized by medial necrosis, rupture elastic laminae, and perivascular accumulations of neutrophils, lymphocytes, and macrophages. H&E stain. (Snyder PW et al., Pathologic Features of Naturally Occurring Juvenile Polyarteritis in Beagle Dogs. Vet Pathol 1995; 32:337–345.) (Tizard IR, Vet Immunology, 10 Ed, 2016, Elsevier.)

POLYARTERITIS NODOSA

Polyarteritis nodosa occurs in dogs, cats, humans, and pigs. It is characterized by a widespread focal necrosis of the media of small and medium-size muscular arteries. The lesions are found in many organs, especially in the kidney.

On occasion, focal vascular lesions characterized by neutrophil infiltration may develop in small blood vessels throughout the body but especially in the skin. Affected dogs may develop mucocutaneous ulcers, bullae, edema, polyarthropathy, myopathy, anorexia, intermittent fever, and lethargy. Although called hypersensitivity vasculitis, a foreign antigen can be found in only a small proportion of cases. The cause or causes of polyarteritis nodosa and hypersensitivity vasculitis are unknown. Their histopathology suggests that they are a form of type III hypersensitivity reaction, perhaps triggered by an infectious agent. Immunosuppression with glucocorticoids, together with cyclophosphamide, has given encouraging results in treating canine hypersensitivity vasculitis. Polyarteritis nodosa is usually detected as an incidental finding on necropsy, although ocular defects may present clinically if the arteries of the eye are involved.

Nasal Philtrum Arteritis

An arteritis involving the nasal philtrum has been described in some large dog breeds such as St. Bernards, Giant Schnauzers, Newfoundlands, and Basset Hounds. Its cause is unknown.

Small Blood Vessel Diseases

CANINE VASCULITIS

Small vessel vasculitides predominantly affect arterioles, venules, and capillaries. These vasculitides may be primary diseases, perhaps triggered by antiendothelial cell autoantibodies or ANCA, although they are much more commonly a secondary response to the deposition of immune complexes originating in concurrent diseases. Many triggering factors resulting in secondary vasculitis have been identified. For example, vasculitis is a common consequence of many bacterial, fungal, protozoal, and viral infections. It is a feature of rickettsial infections and bartonellosis;

tick-transmitted infections such as leishmaniasis, anaplasmosis, or babesiosis; or virus infections due to feline immunodeficiency virus and feline coronavirus. In some of these cases, the infectious agents penetrate the blood vessel walls. When the animal mounts an innate immune response, the resulting inflammation can result in local thrombosis or hemorrhage. Likewise, localized infections or even a septicemia can trigger generalized vasculitis. It may be associated with an underlying food allergy, a drug reaction, or metabolic diseases such as diabetes mellitus. A unique form may also develop in dogs with cold agglutinin disease (see Chapter 11). Paraneoplastic vasculitis secondary to malignant disease also occurs. It may develop before the cancer itself becomes clinically apparent.

General Features of Vasculitis

Vasculitis may develop in any breed of dog. However, certain breeds, including Dachshunds, Rottweilers, Collies, Shetland Sheepdogs, and Jack Russell Terriers, appear to be predisposed. Vaccine-induced vasculitis tends to occur in small-breed dogs.

In acute cutaneous vasculitis, body extremities are commonly affected. These include the legs and feet, pinnae, nose and ears, tail tip, and scrotum. This is because these sites generally have limited collateral circulation. Other affected sites may include the oral cavity and mucous membranes. As a result of local tissue ischemia, cutaneous vasculitis presents with erythema, ecchymoses, purpura, hemorrhagic bullae, areas of necrosis, and consequent ulceration with exudation and crusting. The erythema and purpura are due to erythrocytes escaping into tissues (i.e., bruising). Subcutaneous vasculitis is less obvious and presents as palpable firm nodular lesions and swellings. Some affected dogs may be in considerable pain.

Systemic vasculitis presents with signs that are determined by the organ systems and the degree of tissue necrosis involved. These include depression, fever, lethargy, anorexia, generalized myalgia and arthralgia, and lymphadenopathy. Dogs may show edema of the extremities. If the vasculitis is sufficiently severe, it may progress to intravascular coagulation and shock. Chronic vasculitis may develop slowly, resulting in low-grade ischemia, patchy alopecia, scaling, erythema, and hyperpigmentation. These too tend to develop at sites with limited collateral circulation. Some animals may have concurrent polyarthropathy, myopathy, and neuropathy.

It is generally assumed that most cases of vasculitis are a result of a type III hypersensitivity response to immune complexes deposited in small or medium-size blood vessel walls. Consequent complement activation results in an influx of neutrophils with the release of tissue-degrading enzymes and oxidants. In some cases, a type IV hypersensitivity reaction mediated by cytotoxic T cells may have a similar effect.

In addition to secondary changes in surrounding tissues as a result of inadequate blood flow and consequent hypoxia, acute inflammation develops within the vessel walls. Depending on the severity of the vasculitis, these walls tend to be thickened and edematous. Areas of hyalinization and necrosis may develop. Endothelial cells are also damaged, resulting in swelling, hemorrhage, and necrosis. The vessel walls are infiltrated with inflammatory cells. If many of these cells are degenerating neutrophils (leucocytoclasia) and debris accumulates around the blood vessels (nuclear dust), then these are pathognomonic for the leukocytoclastic form of the disease. This is the most common form observed in dogs. While a neutrophil infiltration is most common, there are variations in cell state and the composition of the cellular infiltrate. Thus in lymphocytic vasculitis, cuffs of CD8$^+$ T cells tend to surround small arterioles. It should also be pointed out that the composition of the cellular infiltrate will vary over time. A granulomatous vasculitis probably reflects a subacute or chronic stage of the neutrophilic reaction.

Concomitant pathologic findings may include anemia, thrombocytopenia, lymphopenia, a neutrophil left shift, and often moderately raised liver enzymes. In addition, if the vasculitis is immune mediated, then immune complexes may be present in the bloodstream. Plasma analysis may show a hypergammaglobulinemia and reduced complement levels.

Immune Complex–Mediated Vasculitis

Leukocytoclastic Vasculitis. Leukocytoclastic vasculitis is a necrotizing inflammatory reaction involving the walls of small blood vessels. Both cutaneous and systemic forms occur as a result of impaired small blood vessel function. It is believed to result from a type III hypersensitivity response mediated by immune complexes deposited in or on blood vessel walls. Here, they interact with platelets and neutrophils. The resulting inflammation and thrombus formation can lead to edema, hemorrhage, and immunothrombosis.

IgG-containing immune complexes bind and activate Fc receptors on neutrophils. This can trigger the release of neutrophil extracellular traps (NETs). The activated neutrophils also release cytokines, proteases, peptides, and oxidants such as H_2O_2 and OCl^- as well as antimicrobial cathelicidins. The released NETs interact with von Willebrand factor (vWF) through electrostatic forces and bind to nearby blood vessel walls. Among the clotting factors found within neutrophil NETs is tissue factor (TF). TF can trigger thrombotic activity. NETs are also potent activators of the alternate complement pathway. The histones and DNA in the NETs are also proinflammatory.

Immune complexes interact with the Fc receptors on blood platelets to cause their activation and aggregation. This aggregation, together with their release of clotting factors such as vWF, platelet-activating factor, platelet factor-1, and HMGB-1, can trigger further neutrophil NET release. Platelets express CD40L that can bind to neutrophil CD40, triggering the respiratory burst that drives NET formation. These aggregated platelets can then bind to neutrophils to form neutrophil-platelet complexes.

Thus the NETs provide a scaffold to which vWF, platelets, fibronectin, and TF can attach. The interaction of these NETs, together with platelets and components of the coagulation pathway, results in intravascular thrombus formation (immunothrombosis) and the development of an associated vasculitis.

Numerous triggers of leukocytoclastic vasculitis have been identified, and a careful history, including recent drug treatments, is needed if the trigger is to be identified. The most common cause of these vasculitides in small animals is a type III hypersensitivity reaction, but the offending antigens may be difficult to identify, and at least half of canine vasculitis cases are idiopathic.

Clinical Disease. Dogs suffering from vasculitis present with anorexia, depression, malaise, and fever. Ulcers may form on the pinnae, oral mucosa, and lips. The skin overlying the extremities, including pinnae, feet, and over the hocks, is most commonly affected. Lesions may develop on the apical margin and then spread across the concave surface of the pinnae. Affected skin may be very painful, especially during the initial phase of the disease. These dogs can develop necrotic ulcers, bullae, edema, polyarthropathy, myopathy, anorexia, intermittent fever, and lethargy. These lesions may evolve over time so that ulcers may develop several days after the first appearance of lesions. If necrosis and ulcerations are extensive, then secondary bacterial and fungal infections may invade the raw, damaged skin areas. Untreated ulcers on the pinnae may result in deformities and notching of the pinnal margin (Fig. 18.3). Epidermal lesions include exudation, crusting, and ulceration. Many animals develop purpuric plaques and hemorrhage as well as papules and edema (Fig. 18.4). The purpuric lesions darken over time. The vasculitis is often associated with anemia, thrombocytopenia, or neutropenia, as well as a protein-losing nephropathy and musculoskeletal lesions. Vasculitis-associated disseminated intravascular coagulation may cause the thrombocytopenia.

Diagnosis and Treatment. Histologic examination of skin biopsies is required to identify the presence of a vasculitis. Damage to small and medium-size blood vessels leads to hemorrhage and edema. The neutrophilic vasculitis is usually leukocytoclastic. Thus the fragmentation of the nuclei of infiltrating pyknotic or karyorrhexic neutrophils will result in the accumulation of fragments of nuclear material around blood vessels. This is called leukocytoclasia (or nuclear dust). This nuclear dust is often the only evidence of a vascular lesion. Other lesions that may be present include

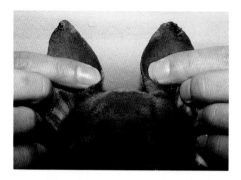

Fig. 18.3 An idiopathic pinnal vasculitis showing the resulting ear margin deformities. (Courtesy of Dr Robert Kennis.)

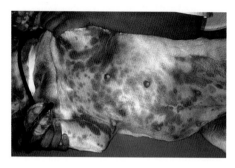

Fig. 18.4 An erythematous vasculitis in a dog with a recent history of tick bites. The lesions were multifocal coalescing erythematous macules. The dog recovered promptly on treatment with doxycycline. (Courtesy of Dr Robert Kennis.)

intramural inflammation and endothelial cell swelling, as well as hemorrhage and fibrinous necrosis in the blood vessel walls. Hypoxic changes will result in pale collagen and faded hair follicles.

Once a vasculitis is diagnosed, the cause must be identified. Underlying causes of vasculitis may include drug allergies, insect and tick bites, infections, adverse food reactions, and some autoimmune diseases. In reviewing the animal's history, care should be taken to obtain a history of all drugs and vaccines administered, as well as diet or any dietary supplements. If an infectious cause is suspected, then blood cultures are required.

The first step in treatment is to remove and avoid subsequent exposure to any offending drug or antigen if at all possible. Once a diagnosis of vasculitis is confirmed by histology, treatment and follow-up should be tailored to the specific animal. In general, patients should receive glucocorticoid therapy or cyclosporine. Immunosuppressive doses are required to induce remission, and relapses are not uncommon. Immunosuppression with corticosteroids, together with cyclophosphamide, has given encouraging results in treating canine hypersensitivity vasculitis. Pentoxifylline, a phosphodiesterase inhibitor, is also effective in the treatment of cutaneous vasculitis. It has antiinflammatory effects and reduces neutrophil adherence to vascular endothelium. In dogs, combined treatment with glucocorticoids and pentoxifylline appears to produce the best results. Pentoxifylline is, however, slow to act, and patience is required.

Vaccine-Induced Vasculopathy

On rare occasions, a lymphoplasmacytic vasculitis may develop at the injection site following rabies vaccination in dogs and cats. It results in the development of an ischemic dermatitis (Fig. 18.5). The viral antigen can be demonstrated in the walls of cutaneous blood vessels at the injection site. It may also be detected in the epithelium of nearby hair follicles.

This response to vaccines is most frequently diagnosed in small-breed dogs such as Toy or Miniature Poodles, Shih Tzu, Shetland Sheepdogs, Lhasa Apsos, Bichons Frises, and Yorkshire and Silky Terriers. It is rarely reported in large-breed dogs. There are no apparent age or sex

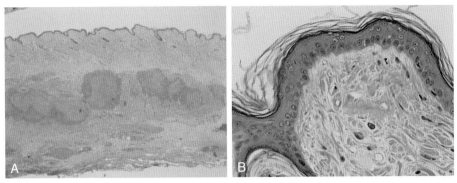

Fig. 18.5 A case of ischemic vasculopathy in a dog following rabies vaccination. (A) Lymphocytic panniculitis, follicular atrophy, and edema (× 10). (Courtesy of Dr. Karen Russell.) (B) Vasculopathy with loss of endothelial cells and hyalinization of vessel walls (× 40). (Courtesy of Dr Dominique Wiener.)

predilections. The lesion develops between 1 and 4 months after vaccination. It usually develops slowly as an area of alopecia with irregular margins. The site eventually becomes scaly, indurated, and pigmented, but visible inflammation is minimal. Smaller satellite lesions may develop nearby. Erosion and ulceration of the skin may occur in severe cases. A subgroup of these dogs may go on to develop a generalized vaccine-induced ischemic dermatopathy. However, these dogs will usually have a focal lesion at the injection site. Local muscle atrophy may be significant. Dogs may also show systemic signs such as lethargy, depression, and fever. Hair regrowth may eventually occur, but this may take up to 1 year and may be associated with changes in skin pigmentation. Similar reactions have been observed in response to leptospirosis vaccination.

The lesion should be biopsied. Histopathology reveals evidence of long-term deoxygenation, including dermal pallor, smudging, and prominent follicular atrophy in the superficial dermis, with perivascular accumulations of lymphocytes, monocytes, and occasional plasma cells in the deep dermis and panniculus. There may be evidence of vasculitis and some hemorrhage. Secondary dermal and epidermal vesiculation may also develop. There are few eosinophils seen in these reactions.

Treatment consists of appropriate antiinflammatory and immunosuppressive therapy. Administration of prednisolone supplemented by pentoxifylline has been reported to be effective. Topical glucocorticoids may also be useful. Animals should not be revaccinated.

Drug-Induced Vasculitis

Adverse responses to some drugs may trigger an immune-mediated vasculitis. Neutrophilic vasculitis may develop should a drug induce high-titered antibodies and generate large quantities of immune complexes. These complexes are often deposited in vessel walls within the skin. The immune complexes may contain antigens derived from the parent drug or its metabolites bound by host antibodies. The resulting vasculitis can range in severity from mild to life-threatening.

A temporal relationship with drug administration can often be identified, although it may be difficult to determine which specific drug is the cause, especially in patients receiving multiple medications. Three commonly used drugs that are known to trigger cutaneous vasculitis in dogs and cats include itraconazole, fenbendazole, and meloxicam. Antineutrophil antibodies have been detected in dogs with sulfonamide allergy. Fixed drug eruptions are circumscribed erythematous lesions that develop into local edema that eventually develops into bullae, which may then ulcerate.

ANCA-Associated Vasculitis

Antineutrophil cytoplasmic antibodies cause three distinct diseases in humans: granulomatosis with polyangiitis, microscopic polyangiitis, and eosinophilic granulomatosis. They do so by

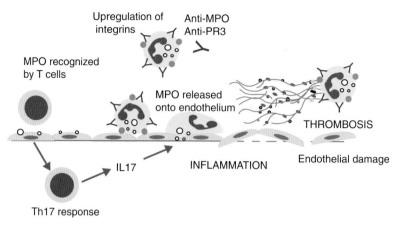

Fig. 18.6 The pathogenesis of antineutrophil cytoplasmic antibody-mediated vasculitis. Neutrophil enzymes such as myeloperoxidase (*MPO*), together with the enzymes associated with neutrophil extracellular trap release, cause damage to vascular endothelial cells and trigger blood clotting and immunothrombosis. A helper T type 17 (*Th17*) response also contributes to the inflammatory process. *IL17*, Interleukin-17.

triggering a vasculitis that affects small blood vessels, especially those in the skin, lungs, and kidneys. Their clinical presentation depends on the organs and tissues affected. The neutrophil cytoplasmic antigens myeloperoxidase and proteinase 3 are targeted by ANCA. These antineutrophil cytoplasmic antibodies are produced in many different autoimmune diseases (see Chapter 11). They can bind directly to neutrophil granules within or on blood vessel walls, release neutrophil enzymes and reactive oxygen species, and as a result cause local inflammation. ANCA can also trigger the release of NETs onto the vascular surface (Fig. 18.6). Activated neutrophils may bind and penetrate the vascular endothelium at these sites and trigger additional cell damage and inflammation. Released proteases can activate the alternate complement pathway and generate large quantities of C5a. This peptide in turn attracts more neutrophils and generates a self-amplifying inflammatory loop. Serum ANCA have been shown to be increased in some cases of juvenile polyarteritis in Beagles as well as in some dogs with chronic enteropathies.

Canine Dermatomyositis

As described in Chapter 12, an immune-mediated vasculopathy is the central lesion of canine dermatomyositis. These lesions lead to muscle ischemia and eventually result in muscle atrophy.

Breed-Specific Vasculitides

Racing Greyhounds. A systemic form of cutaneous and renal glomerular vasculopathy has been identified in racing Greyhounds. It is known colloquially as Alabama rot since the first cases were identified in that state in the 1980s. The etiology is unknown, and no infectious agents have yet been identified nor have immune complexes been detected in the vascular lesions. The disease is certainly genetically influenced, being restricted to certain litters of Greyhounds. However, it is widely believed that the disease trigger is an infectious or environmental factor that has yet to be identified since disease outbreaks occur in clusters, have the highest incidence from November to May, and appear to be associated with forested areas. A similar disease has been identified in Great Danes.

Affected animals develop multiple edematous, tender, and erythematous skin swellings. They form mainly on the hind legs (tarsus, stifle, and inner thigh) but occasionally on the forelimbs. The head and dorsum are usually spared. The lesions progress to sharply demarcated deep ulcers that discharge a serosanguinous fluid. Some dogs recover gradually as the ulcers heal. However, the lesions are predisposed to secondary infections. Some dogs may develop more severe disease with systemic signs such as fever and lethargy, icterus, anemia, and thrombocytopenia. Many of these dogs develop azotemia with acute renal failure and gastrointestinal symptoms. The dogs develop a microvascular thrombosis associated with endothelial damage and a consumptive thrombocytopenia.

Histopathology shows epidermal necrosis, subcutaneous hemorrhage, fibrinoid necrosis of small arterioles, a mixed inflammatory infiltrate, and sometimes thrombosis. The renal lesions consist of glomerular ischemia, congestion, and hemorrhage with intravascular coagulation—a thrombotic microangiopathy, tubular epithelial atrophy, and necrosis. Some glomeruli may contain deposits of IgG or IgM. Occasional cases may also have nonspecific lesions in the brain with focal necrosis, hemorrhage, and edema. The skin lesions heal with normal wound care, but recurrence is frequent. The prognosis is poor to guarded, especially in animals with renal disease.

Shar-Pei Fever. As pointed out in Chapter 14, Shar-Pei suffer from an inherited autoinflammatory disease called Shar-Pei fever as a result of a mutation in the gene encoding hyaluronan synthase 2. Some affected dogs may also develop multifocal areas of skin discoloration, with hemorrhagic papules and macules. They also develop extensive edema on the face and extremities. Many present with fever and malaise. Fluid-filled bullae may also develop. Over time, these lesions develop into areas of obvious deep and extensive ulceration and ischemic necrosis. Histologic examination shows a necrotizing neutrophilic vasculitis. Some affected dogs have responded positively to glucocorticosteroid therapy and cyclophosphamide.

Jack Russell Terriers. An idiopathic vasculitis that is probably familial has been reported in Jack Russell Terriers. In these cases, ulcers form over bony prominences and on the face. Dapsone has been reported to be an effective treatment, possibly supplemented with dexamethasone.

German Shepherd Dogs. A vaccine-proximate vasculitis has been reported in German Shepherd Dog puppies 4 to 7 weeks of age. It develops 7 to 10 days after receiving their first dose of vaccines (distemper, hepatitis, parvovirus, and parainfluenza viruses). However, some animals may develop the disease prior to vaccination or without a vaccination challenge. Genetic studies suggest that it is inherited as an autosomal recessive trait; however, its pathogenesis remains unknown.

The puppies present with transient lameness, anorexia, and fever. They go on to develop footpad swelling and depigmentation. There are areas of focal depigmentation, crusting, exudation, and eventually ulceration of the nose and the footpads as well as the nasal planum, tail, and ear tips. Many of the animals suffer severe discomfort and pain. Hematology and serum biochemistry are normal. Immunoglobulin levels and lymphocyte numbers also lie within normal ranges, and they possess neither ANA nor a positive Coombs test. Histopathology shows a multifocal nodular dermatitis where foci of mononuclear leukocytes and neutrophils surround foci of dermal collagen lysis and degenerate blood vessels. Depigmented areas have a mild interface dermatitis with limited destruction of basal cells.

Scottish Terriers. A familial vasculitis has been reported to occur in Scottish Terriers between 3 and 6 months of age. Animals developed severe but nonpainful ulceration of the nasal planum that also affected the nasal cartilage. This resulted from a leukocytoclastic vasculitis and pyogranulomatous inflammation. The cause is unknown.

EQUINE VASCULITIS

Purpura Hemorrhagica

The most common form of cutaneous vascular disease in horses is purpura hemorrhagica, a necrotizing vasculitis that develops after an acute *Streptococcus equi* infection. Preexisting high serum antibody levels to *S. equi* predispose horses to this condition. Other triggers can include infections with *Corynebacterium pseudotuberculosis*, *Prescottella (Rhodococcus) equi*, equine influenza virus, and equine herpesvirus type 1. In some cases, purpura may develop in the absence of any known prior bacterial or viral infection.

There are great variations in disease severity and clinical course, ranging from a mild transient reaction to fatal disease. Classically, clinical signs develop within 2 to 4 weeks following natural or vaccinal exposure to streptococcal antigens (Fig. 18.7). Horses develop urticaria, followed by severe, well-demarcated subcutaneous edema, especially involving the distal limbs and ventral abdomen, and the development of petechial or ecchymotic hemorrhages in the mucosa and subcutaneous tissues. Other signs may include depression and reluctance to move, fever, anorexia, tachycardia and tachypnea, colic, epistaxis, and weight loss. The edema may result in skin exudation, ulceration, crusting, and sloughing. Severe edema of the head may compromise breathing and feeding. Other abnormalities include anemia, neutrophilia, hyperglobulinemia, elevated muscle enzymes (due to rhabdomyolysis), and hyperproteinemia. Affected horses may have unusually high blood IgA levels.

The vasculitis may also affect the gastrointestinal tract, lungs, and muscle. In severe cases, some horses may develop a generalized leukocytoclastic vasculitis, resulting in thrombosis and infarction. Small intestine intussusception may complicate the disease, as does muscle infarction. There may be hemorrhage and necrosis of skeletal muscle. Infarctive purpura hemorrhagica is a rare and highly fatal form of the disease.

Immune complexes are found in the serum of affected horses and consist of streptococcal M or R proteins complexed with IgM or IgA. These immune complexes are deposited in blood vessel walls, resulting in vasculitis, edema, and hemorrhage. Complement components may also be deposited in association with the immune complexes. Skin biopsies show the presence of a severe leukocytoclastic vasculitis with a marked neutrophilic infiltration around affected blood vessels. This vasculitis may be associated with necrosis of the infarcted muscle. Immune complex deposition can also cause an membranoproliferative glomerulonephritis with resulting proteinuria and azoturia.

Immediate medical attention should be sought for affected horses. Any associated infections must be treated. Inflammation should be suppressed through the use of systemic glucocorticosteroids (dexamethasone and/or prednisolone). Horses may also be given nonsteroidal

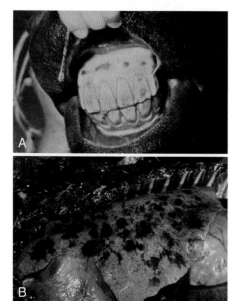

Fig. 18.7 (A) Petechial hemorrhages of oral mucous membranes in a horse with purpura hemorrhagica. (B) Hemorrhages on the surface of the lungs in a horse with purpura hemorrhagica. (Sellon DC, Long MT. Equine Infectious Diseases.1e, Saunders, 2007.)

antiinflammatory drugs (phenylbutazone or flunixin meglumine) and antibiotics to limit secondary infections.

Equine Pastern Vasculitis

This is a disease pattern primarily encountered in adult draft horses. Lesions appear on the nonpigmented caudal aspects of the pasterns but may extend as far as the cannon bone (Fig. 18.8). They are often bilateral. The hindlimbs are most commonly affected. The lesions are red and swollen. They may develop into ulcers or fissures with exudation and crusting. The lesions vary in severity from mild to an exudative form to a chronic proliferative form, and probably reflect several distinct causes. Secondary bacterial and fungal infections are common. The predisposing lesion appears to be a vasculitis. Biopsies of affected skin show a deep dermal neutrophil leukocytoclastic arteritis with nuclear dust, thickening, and edema of the blood vessel walls, with microhemorrhages. The etiology of the lesion is unknown, although photoactivation appears to be a trigger factor, and the prognosis is guarded.

Other Equine Vasculitides

Horses have been reported to develop other forms of vasculitis. About half are of unknown etiology. Of the others, these may be secondary to a photoaggravated dermatitis (confined to the nonpigmented areas of the skin) or to drug (penicillin, acepromazine) reactions. The most frequent findings in equine cutaneous vasculitis are crusts and scales and to a lesser extent, edema of the lower limbs (fore and hind), face, and head. Other signs may include alopecia, urticaria, edema, ulcers, and skin nodules. The usual lesion is a leukocytoclastic vasculitis. These may be accompanied by depression, fever, and anorexia as well as anemia, neutrophilia, hyperglycemia, and hyperglobulinemia. The vascular lesions are either cell poor or lymphohistiocytic. Treatment options include corticosteroids and pentoxifylline.

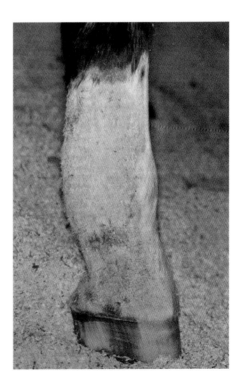

Fig. 18.8 Pastern vasculitis. Erythema, crusts, and hypotrichosis in the hind leg of an affected horse. (Psalla D, Rüfenacht S, Stoffel MH, et al. Equine pastern vasculitis: a clinical and histopathological study. *Vet J.* 2013;198:524–530.)

PORCINE VASCULITIS

Pigs suffer from sporadic cases of an immune complex–mediated thrombocytopenic purpura. This has been a specific problem in Gottingen minipigs, a line of small pigs used for experimental studies. The animals develop severe thrombocytopenia, anemia, excessive bleeding, and membranoproliferative lesions in their glomeruli. Some animals have a necrotizing vasculitis. The cause is unknown, although it is assumed to be due to a type III hypersensitivity to an unknown antigen. This same line of pigs may also develop a spontaneous polyarteritis. Its cause is unknown but is also probably immune mediated.

Sources of Additional Information

Carpenter JL, Andelman NC, Moore FM, et al. Idiopathic cutaneous and renal glomerular vasculopathy of greyhounds. *Vet Pathol*. 1988;25:401–407.

Dincer Z, Piccicuto V, Walker UJ, et al. Spontaneous and drug-induced arteritis/polyarteritis in the Göttingen Minipig—review. *Toxicol Pathol*. 2018;46:121–130.

Holm LP, Stevens KB, Walker DJ. Pathology and epidemiology of cutaneous and renal glomerular vasculopathy in dogs. *J Comp Path*. 2020;176:156–161.

Innerå M. Cutaneous vasculitis in small animals. *Vet Clin Small Anim*. 2013;43:113–134.

Malik R, Foster SF, Martin P, et al. Acute febrile neutrophilic vasculitis of the skin in young Shar-Pei dogs. *Aust Vet J*. 2002;80:200–206.

Misra DP, Agarwal V. Innate immune cells in the pathogenesis of primary systemic vasculitis. *Rheumatol Int*. 2016;36:169–182.

Nichols PR, Morris DO, Beale KM. A retrospective study of canine and feline cutaneous vasculitis. *Vet Dermatol*. 2001;12:255–264.

Psalla D, Rüfenacht S, Stoffel MH, et al. Equine pastern vasculitis: a clinical and histopathological study. *Vet J*. 2013;198:524–530.

Scott-Moncrieff JCR, Snyder PW, Glickman LT, et al. Systemic necrotizing vasculitis in nine young beagles. *J Amer Vet Med Assoc*. 1992;201:1553–1558.

Shochet L, Holdsworth S. Kitching AR. Animal models of ANCA associated vasculitis. *Front Immunol*. 2020. doi:10.3389/fimmu.2020.00525

Swann JW, Priestnall SL, Dawson C, et al. Histologic and clinical features of primary and secondary vasculitis: a retrospective study of 42 dogs (2004-2011). *J Vet Diagn Invest*. 2015;27:489–496.

Thibault S, Drolet R, Germain M-C, et al. Cutaneous and systemic necrotizing vasculitis in swine. *Vet Pathol*. 1998;35:108–116.

Weir JAM, Yager JA, Caswell JL, et al. Familial cutaneous vasculopathy of German Shepherds: clinical, genetic and preliminary pathological and immunological studies. *Can Vet J*. 1994;35:763–769.

White SD, Affolter VK, Dewey J, et al. Cutaneous vasculitis in equines: a retrospective study of 72 cases. *Vet Dermatol*. 2009;20:600–606.

Immune-Mediated Enteropathies

The gastrointestinal tract has a special role to play in the relationship between the body's immune responses, the commensal microbiota, and invading pathogens. Not only does it contain about 75% of the body's lymphoid tissues, but these also come into constant contact with the enormous diversity of foreign antigens originating in the microbiota as well as in foods. The immune system has to be discriminating—it cannot react very strongly to everything foreign that it encounters, especially if it does not pose a threat. As a result, the gastrointestinal tract is home to many regulatory and tolerance-inducing mechanisms that ensure that immune-mediated responses to all these antigens are either totally suppressed, as in the responses to foods, or at the very least are carefully regulated, as in the responses to the microbiota. Regulatory T (Treg) cells are essential for maintaining this intestinal homeostasis. For example, they must suppress any CD4+ effector T cells that become excessively activated by antigens originating in the normal microbiota. It is no surprise therefore that autoimmune responses directed against cellular antigens in the gut wall are almost unheard of (<50 cases of autoimmune enteropathy have been described in adult humans). On the other hand, if one considers the intestinal microbiota to be a constituent part of the animal body—the so-called superorganism—then inappropriate immune responses against the microbiota can be considered akin to autoimmunity. Similarly, food allergies can be considered to reflect a failure in immune regulation. As a result, the autoinflammatory diseases that affect the intestine, including inflammatory bowel disease (IBD) and other enteropathies, represent yet another consequence of a loss of peripheral tolerance. IBD develops as a result of inappropriate immune responses to either foods or the microbiota. Irrespective of the cause, these responses damage mucosal surfaces so that they share clinical features and even histopathology, and it may be difficult to distinguish between the two.

In humans, the two chronic IBDs are ulcerative colitis and Crohn disease. Neither have exact equivalents in domestic animals. Practically speaking, IBD (otherwise known as chronic inflammatory enteropathies) in domestic species can be subdivided into (1) food-responsive enteropathies if a change in diet will improve their clinical status, (2) steroid/immunosuppressive-responsive enteropathies if steroids or other immunosuppressive drugs can cause clinical improvement, and (3) unresponsive enteropathies if nothing works. Histologically, there is no apparent difference among the three. It may be assumed that the food-responsive disease probably reflects a food allergy, toxicity, or a dietary imbalance, whereas the immunosuppression-responsive group probably reflects immune-mediated responses to the commensal microbiota.

Genetic Predispositions

Over 240 genetic susceptibility loci for IBD have been identified in humans, yet they explain less than 15% of the disease variance. Five variants have been identified in the *NOD2* gene alone. This gene encodes the protein NOD2 (nucleotide-binding oligomerization domain-containing protein-2), a cytoplasmic pattern-recognition receptor (PRR) that recognizes certain bacterial molecules, including muramyl dipeptide. Two of these gene variants affect the translocation of NOD2 to the cell membrane or impair the body's NF-κB responses. Other implicated genes include those influencing autophagy and epithelial barrier function, as well as innate and adaptive immune responses.

Certain canine major histocompatibility complex (MHC) class II genes have been associated with the development of chronic enteropathies in French Bulldogs and Miniature Dachshunds. One haplotype, DLA-DRB1*002.01/DQA1*009.01/DQB1*001.01, appears to be protective against chronic enteropathy in French Bulldogs but not in Dachshunds. This same haplotype, DLA-DQA1/DQB1, is also protective against Doberman hepatitis. Conversely, DLA-DRB1*006.01 is overrepresented in French Bulldogs with chronic enteropathy as well as in cases of Doberman hepatitis.

Intestinal Immune Tolerance

FOOD ANTIGENS

The intestinal epithelium consists of a single layer of epithelial cells bound together by tight junctions. Scattered between these epithelial cells are numerous lymphocytes, dendritic cells (DCs), and secretory cells such as mucin-producing goblet cells. Treg cells are abundant in the intestinal mucosa, where they regulate responses to both the microbiota and food antigens. As a result, normal animals are highly tolerant of ingested protein antigens. Dietary proteins that succeed in penetrating the intestinal epithelium intact usually generate a strong Treg response. These Treg cells suppress Th2 cell activities, decrease B-cell immunoglobulin E (IgE) production, suppress effector T-cell emigration into tissues, induce interleukin-10 (IL10) and indoleamine 2,3-dioxygenase (IDO) production by DCs, and inhibit the activation of mast cells, eosinophils, and basophils. A population of intestinal DCs regulates this Treg cell activity and hence is ultimately responsible for oral tolerance (Fig. 19.1).

Specialized antigen-capturing cells in the intestinal epithelium, called microfold (M) cells, capture food proteins and deliver samples to DCs. Intestinal DCs can also extend their dendrites between the epithelial cells and sample food proteins from within the gut lumen. Once these proteins are captured, they are carried by the DCs to draining mesenteric lymph nodes or to Peyer patches. The DCs produce suppressive molecules such as IDO, IL10, and retinoic acid that cause any responding T cells to differentiate into Treg cells. The Treg cells in the mesenteric lymph nodes of orally tolerant animals in turn secrete the suppressive cytokines transforming growth factor-beta (TGFβ) and IL10; as a result, immune responses against food antigens are effectively blocked. Intraepithelial lymphocytes, predominantly T cells, are also tolerant of food and commensal antigens and play an important role in preventing allergic and inflammatory responses in the healthy gut. A second mechanism by which oral tolerance is induced is through the production of tolerosomes. These are exosomes shed by enterocytes. They carry MHC class II molecules

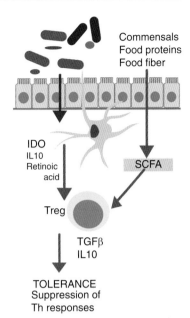

Fig. 19.1 The induction of oral tolerance. This tolerance must be directed not only against food allergens but also against the great diversity of antigens and pathogen-associated molecular pattern molecules generated by the commensal microbiota. It is important that tolerance affects all three populations of helper T *(Th)* cells. Failure to do so results in food allergies and inflammatory bowel disease. This tolerance is largely dependent on the production of effective regulatory T *(Treg)* cell populations. *IDO,* Indoleamine 2,3-dioxygenase; *IL,* interleukin; *SCFA,* short-chain fatty acids; *TGFβ,* transforming growth factor-beta.

on their surface and so can bind peptides sampled from the gut lumen. Purified tolerosomes fed to experimental animals induce tolerance. It is suggested that presentation of food antigens by tolerosomes selectively induces Treg formation.

Like other T cells, however, the Treg cell phenotypes are plastic. Tolerance is a flexible process, and should the intestine be invaded by pathogens, these cells can switch phenotypes, become effector cells, and play their part in the defense of the body. This may well result in the development of immune-mediated inflammatory disease. Provided the invaders are promtly destroyed, this inflammation should be short lived. If, however, the challenge persists, then so too will the inflammatory tissue response.

THE MICROBIOTA

One probable cause of chronic IBD is the development of inflammatory responses to antigens and metabolites produced by the intestinal microbiota. This loss of regulation may be triggered by disruption of the intestinal mucosal barrier that results in increased antigen access to the intestinal lymphoid tissues. This breach in the barrier is likely a result of dysbiosis, local mucosal infection, and a breakdown in tight junctions between epithelial cells. For example, inflammation in human ulcerative colitis is associated with greatly increased levels of anticommensal IgG in serum. If the integrity of the epithelial barrier is compromised, then normally innocuous members of the microbiota may penetrate the intestinal wall, bypass local tolerance mechanisms, activate inflammasomes, and as a result, generate both innate and adaptive immune responses.

Dysbiosis that triggers IBD can take many forms. These include decreases in microbial diversity or increases in the abundance of proinflammatory taxa. In many cases, it is not known whether these changes are the causes of disease or the results of chronic inflammation. It has been proposed that some pathogenic members of the microbiota (pathobionts) may directly drive the development of IBD by provoking local inflammation. It is possible that these pathobionts are normally controlled by intestinal IgA responses that block their invasion. Failure of these responses may then permit invasion, inflammation, and disease development. It is also of interest to note that IgA appears to selectively target a subset of the microbiota: those organisms that appear to be the most proinflammatory. In cases of IBD, the composition of this IgA-coated subset changes.

Other IBD cases may result from a local immunodeficiency such as a deficiency of IgA in German Shepherd Dogs. IgA normally serves to bind to many commensals and hence block their access to the mucosa. This process of immune exclusion normally serves to keep intestinal pathogens well away from the mucosal surface. In its absence, however, microbial antigens can gain access to intestinal tissues and so provoke defensive inflammatory responses.

Loss of Food Tolerance

GLUTEN-INDUCED ENTEROPATHY

Food hypersensitivities are well described in humans and are common in companion animals. They include several different syndromes, of which one of the most important is gluten-induced enteropathy (celiac disease) (Fig. 19.2). This enteropathy is characterized by chronic inflammation of the small intestine. It is triggered by ingestion of the cereal protein gluten, derived from wheat, barley, or rye, in genetically predisposed individuals. As a result, affected individuals mount a B-cell and cytotoxic T-cell response that attacks and destroys intestinal epithelial cells. Gluten contains two major proteins, glutenin and gliadin. It is the gliadin that causes the problems. Gliadin is a proline-rich protein that is resistant to intestinal digestion. When exposed to gliadin, the intestinal epithelial cells produce zonulin (a form of haptoglobin). As described previously, zonulin triggers disassembly of the intercellular tight junctions. As a result, intestinal permeability increases, and macromolecules can therefore penetrate to the submucosa. Once absorbed, the intact gliadin molecules trigger an innate immune response that increases the permeability of the intestinal epithelial barrier. As a result, the gliadin then gains access to the lamina propria. Because the gliadin is not digested, it can also trigger an antibody response. The responding B cells not only make IgA and IgG antibodies directed against gliadin, but they inadvertently also make antibodies against an intestinal enzyme, transglutaminase 2. (The transglutaminase complexes with the gliadin so that it too is processed and presented to B cells, an example of bystander activation.) The resulting attack on the transglutaminase causes activation of cytotoxic T cells. This in turn results in a loss of extracellular matrix and the destruction of intestinal epithelial cells. In effect,

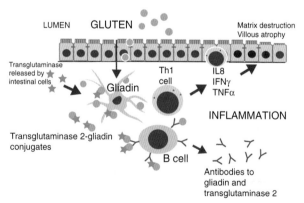

Fig. 19.2 The pathogenesis of gluten intolerance. Affected animals mount an autoimmune attack on the protein gliadin, a component of gluten. Transglutaminase 2 *(star)* binds to the gliadin *(circle)* and as a result, affected animals also mount an autoimmune attack on it. The combined immune attacks result in tissue destruction and villous atrophy. *IFNγ*, Interferon-gamma; *IL*, interleukin; *Th1*, helper T type 1; *TNFα*, tumor necrosis factor-alpha.

therefore, gluten sensitivity shares features of both food allergy and autoimmune diseases. The inflammatory response progressively increases in severity, eventually resulting in villous atrophy. Unlike typical allergies, the symptoms of gluten enteropathy may be delayed from hours to weeks after ingestion of the offending food. Diagnosis is often difficult owing to a lack of noninvasive diagnostic tests.

Gluten enteropathy in humans has also been linked to the development of a highly pruritic skin disease called dermatitis herpetiformis. IgA deposits are often found associated with the skin lesions in the human disease. A similar rare skin disease (not linked to gluten enteropathy) has been reported to occur in dogs. It presents as an intensely pruritic symmetric skin eruption with the development of groups of vesicles, papules, pustules, and urticaria. Canine dermatitis herpetiformis is probably immune mediated, but its pathogenesis is unclear.

Gluten-induced enteropathy is an inherited trait in some Irish Setters. This is an autosomal recessive disease under the control of a single gene locus. Unlike the situation in humans, this canine gene is not linked to the MHC. Affected animals usually present with vomiting, dehydration, abnormal or bloody stools, and protracted diarrhea. Pathologic changes include partial villus atrophy in the jejunum and increased intestinal permeability. This results in anorexia, poor growth, and weight loss. The disease can be managed by strict avoidance of the offending gluten.

Gluten exposure is also associated with paroxysmal gluten-sensitive dyskinesia in Border Terriers. Affected dogs present with neurologic signs such as difficulty walking, tremors, and dystonia of the limbs, head, and neck; evidence of pruritus such as scratching or licking the skin; the presence of autoantibodies against transglutaminase 2 and antigliadin antibodies; and gastrointestinal diseases such as vomiting, diarrhea, and abdominal cramping. Some dogs show only a few transient episodes, whereas others may suffer lifelong recurrent disease. Affected dogs must be placed on a gluten-free diet. (Box 19.1)

Canine Inflammatory Bowel Disease

DYSREGULATION OF INNATE IMMUNITY

Animals possess a diverse range of PRRs that can bind conserved microbial molecules such as lipopolysaccharides, flagellin, and nucleic acids. These PRRs can also bind and trigger responses to cell breakdown products and thus respond to tissue damage. Evidence suggests that excessive PRR signaling—especially of the toll-like receptors TLR2, TLR4, TLR5, and TLR9; NOD2; and the receptor for advanced glycation end products (RAGE)—is associated with the development of IBD (Fig. 19.3).

One PRR that contributes significantly to the pathogenesis of IBD is TLR5. Single nucleotide polymorphisms (SNPs) in the human *TLR5* gene are associated with the development of IBD. Likewise, three nonsynonymous SNPs in the *TLR5* gene and two in the *TLR4* gene are associated with IBD in German Shepherd Dogs. When the appropriate PRR genes were transfected into human embryonic kidney cells and exposed to their specific ligand—in this case, bacterial flagellin—it was found that genes from the susceptible dogs were hyperresponsive to the flagellin and greatly upregulated the NF-κB pathway. As a result the transfected cells produced much more tumor necrosis factor-alpha (TNFα) than cells containing the normal dog gene. Two other SNPs in *TLR 5* have been associated with the development of IBD in other dog breeds.

The expression of TLR2 is also significantly upregulated in the duodenal and colonic mucosa of dogs with IBD as compared to controls. This increase correlates generally with clinical disease severity. TLR2 binds microbial lipoproteins, molecules that are generated in large amounts by the intestinal microbiota. Although TLR2 is expressed at low levels on normal intestinal epithelial cells, if this expression should increase significantly, then it would be anticipated that increased signaling would result in excessive inflammasome activation and the production of increased quantities of proinflammatory cytokines.

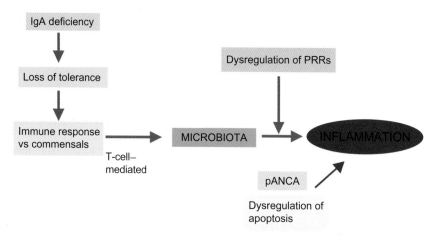

Fig. 19.3 A very simple view of the pathways involved in the breakdown of tolerance to the microbiota resulting in inflammatory bowel disease. *Ig,* Immunoglobulin; *pANCA,* antineutrophil cytoplasmic antibodies; *PRR,* pattern-recognition receptor.

It has also been reported that both TLR4 and TLR9 are upregulated in the duodenum and colon of dogs with IBD. TLR4 is of course the receptor for bacterial lipopolysaccharide that is also plentiful in the intestinal tract. TLR9 is the receptor for microbial DNA. As with TLR2, excessive signaling by these receptors may accentuate the intensity, duration, and severity of local inflammation.

NOD2 receptors are also PRRs. On examination of the SNPs within the *NOD2* gene, four of them have been found to be significantly associated with the development of IBD in German Shepherd Dogs. They are not associated with the disease in other breeds.

Genome-wide association studies (GWAS) on humans with IBD have also identified a variant in the antibody receptor gene *(FCGR2A)* as a predisposing factor. Commensal-IgG immune complexes crosslink their receptor FcγR on colonic macrophages and so induce IL1β production. Human ulcerative colitis patients make unusually high levels of anticommensal IgG. In response, their macrophages produce large amounts of IL1β as well as neutrophil-recruiting chemokines. These in turn increase the magnitude of IL1β-dependent helper T type 17 (Th17) responses.

RAGE, too, is a PRR. Its ligands include proteins of the S100 family (intracellular calcium-binding proteins that can act as alarmins). Cell-bound RAGE is a proinflammatory receptor. Cellular RAGE expression in the duodenum and colon of dogs with IBD is significantly increased when compared to normal control animals. On the other hand, soluble RAGE (sRAGE) acts as a decoy receptor and so suppresses inflammation. Serum sRAGE has been found to be significantly lower in dogs with IBD compared to healthy dogs. Its levels were not, however, correlated with the severity of histopathologic lesions or the clinical score. However, sRAGE did return to normal levels once animals were in complete remission.

Trefoil factors are small antimicrobial peptides produced by goblet cells that play an important role in epithelial healing. For example, they are upregulated in humans with IBD as a result of the body's repair efforts. Trefoil factor expression is significantly upregulated in the duodenum from IBD dogs but significantly lower in the colon. This latter finding may point to defective protective or repair mechanisms in the colon.

As expected, with all this upregulation of their PRRs, affected dogs also demonstrate upregulation of the NF-κB pathway in their duodenal mucosa. There are many more NF-κB–positive macrophages in the lamina propria of dogs with chronic enteropathy compared to control dogs. There are also more NF-κB–positive enterocytes in dogs with food-responsive diarrhea than in dogs with IBD. Resolution of these diseases is associated with decreased NF-κB activation in the macrophages of the lamina propria.

DYSREGULATION OF ADAPTIVE IMMUNITY

GWAS have demonstrated multiple gene loci associated with IBD development, especially in German Shepherd Dogs. One piece of supporting evidence is the association of SNPs in some MHC class II haplotypes with resistance to developing IBD. For example, the haplotype DLA-DRB1*01502/ DQA1*00601/ DQB1*02301 is associated with resistance to the disease. Conversely, the haplotype DLA-DRB1*01501/DQA1*00601/DQB1*00301 is associated with increased susceptibility.

B-Cell Changes

The major protective antibody produced by B cells in the healthy intestine is IgA. IgA acts by immune exclusion and so prevents potential microbial invaders from binding to and then penetrating the intestinal epithelial cell barrier. In human IBD and probably in animals as well, IgA production is decreased, while IgG production increases. This predominance of IgG, an immunoglobulin that activates complement, may provoke inflammation within the mucosa. This is especially the case if IgG binding results in macrophage activation, neutrophil recruitment, and triggering of Th17 responses.

Antineutrophil cytoplasmic antibodies (pANCA) have been detected in both humans and dogs with chronic intestinal inflammation. In dogs with food-responsive enteropathy, about two-thirds possess pANCA. In dogs with IBD, only about 25% are positive. Interestingly, after treatment, the number of IBD dogs with pANCA increased. pANCA titers do not correlate with clinical activity scores in dogs, and there is no evidence that pANCAs are pathogenic in the dog.

T-Cell Changes

One way by which T-cell functions are regulated is by carefully applied apoptosis. Unwanted T cells are killed, whereas required cells are protected. It is this regulation that accounts in part for peripheral tolerance. Examination of the lesions in IBD in dogs suggests that their apoptosis pathway may be dysregulated. Two genes are key to this regulation: caspase genes that participate in apoptosis and genes encoding proteins of the Bcl-2 family that protect against apoptosis. When the expression of these two gene families is examined in human IBD cases, it is found that caspases are downregulated and Bcl-2 genes are upregulated. Thus there is a significant association between Bcl-2 expression and the disease severity score. This of course implies that T-cell survival is enhanced. It is not far-fetched to suggest that this may be a mechanism behind the loss of tolerance and the persistence of inflammation within the intestinal wall. IL13 and IL33 are underexpressed in the duodenal mucosa of German Shepherd Dogs with chronic enteropathy. Both of these are Th2 cytokines, and their loss implies perhaps an imbalanced Th1:Th2 ratio. This suppression may also influence local production of IgA as well as altering the local microbial environment. Excessive type 1 and Th17 immune responses have also been implicated in human IBD.

Studies on cytokine gene expression in German Shepherd Dogs with IBD indicate, however, that duodenal IL17A gene expression is significantly lower in IBD dogs than in healthy controls! Likewise, there is no significant difference in duodenal interferon-gamma (IFNγ), IL10, IL22, and TGFβ expression between IBD dogs and healthy controls.

It is important to remind the reader at this stage that, while CD4+ T cells have been classified into discrete subtypes based on the cytokine mixture they secrete, this is an oversimplification. Studies on individual T cells in the intestinal wall have indicated that these phenotypes actually form a continuum. Mixed phenotypes are common, and single precursor cells may give rise to distinctly different helper cell types. These T cells will readily switch phenotypes as a result of exposure to different cytokines and environmental and microbial signals.

Dendritic Cell Changes

IBD-affected dogs have reduced numbers of DCs and macrophages in the mucosa of their duo-denum, ileum, and colon when compared to healthy controls. Given that some DC subpopu-lations have immunoregulatory functions, it is possible that this too may contribute to disease pathogenesis.

CLINICAL DISEASE

IBD is the commonest cause of chronic relapsing diarrhea in dogs. As a general rule, it is des-ignated as IBD if the diarrhea lasts more than 3 weeks. There should also be histologic demon-stration of mucosal inflammation. Animals develop persistent/recurrent vomiting and diarrhea. Associated with these are secondary consequences such as weight loss, ascites, and anemia.

Canine IBD is almost certainly not a single disease but a syndrome resulting from excessive intestinal inflammatory processes. Variations do occur in the histopathologic features, and these may be used to classify these diseases, but they rarely provide a definitive identification of its cause. Four syndromes appear to constitute IBD in dogs: lymphoplasmacytic colitis, eosinophilic coli-tis, histiocytic ulcerative colitis, and regional granulomatous colitis. These diseases are not always restricted to the large intestine but may affect the small intestine or in some cases, even extend to the stomach. Food-responsive diarrhea may also be included in the syndrome. There is no obvious gender predilection for canine IBD, although certain breeds are clearly predisposed. For example, lymphoproliferative enteropathy occurs in Basenjis, protein-losing enteropathy and nephropathy occur in Soft-Coated Wheaten Terriers, and histiocytic ulcerative colitis occurs in Boxers.

IBD generally develops in middle-aged animals and is rarely seen in animals under 1 year of age. The cellular infiltrate in the intestinal wall is usually mixed. Two of the most obvious types are lymphoplasmacytic enteritis and eosinophilic enteritis or gastroenteritis. Circumstantial evidence such as a lymphoplasmacytic infiltrate, relatively common both in dogs and cats, suggests that an immune-mediated process is involved. However, it is totally unclear whether an immune response is directed against the microbiota, certain foods, or even against unknown autoantigens.

It is common practice to assess the severity of these diseases using a clinical scoring system, either the Clinical Inflammatory Bowel Disease Activity Index (CIBDAI) or the Canine Chronic Enteropathy Clinical Activity Index (CCECAI). These provide an objective assessment of the animal's status but are of limited prognostic usefulness.

DIAGNOSIS

The diagnosis of idiopathic bowel disease is primarily based on the histology of the lesions. When analyzing cases of IBD, it is essential to exclude all other causes of enteritis such as infectious agents, poisons, food allergies, or parasites such as Giardia. Intestinal workup should include a biopsy as well as an appropriate range of blood and other laboratory tests (Fig. 19.4). Blood tests should include both leukocyte and thrombocyte counts as well as C-reactive protein levels. (CRP may be upregulated as much as 1000-fold in canine IBD.) Serum albumin levels may also be use-ful, since a significant number of affected dogs lose protein and may develop hypoalbuminemia. Fecal markers such as the neutrophil-derived proteins calprotectin, the S100 protein A12, and lactoferrin may also provide useful data. All three proteins are normally found within neutrophils and thus measure inflammatory cell escape into the intestinal contents. Radiology, ultrasonogra-phy, and endoscopy may provide more information such as evidence of changes in the thickness of the intestinal wall. The confirmatory evidence is an inflammatory infiltration of the mucosa of the large and small intestines as determined by biopsy.

In humans, serologic markers are often employed, and serologic tests used to determine etiology are being increasingly employed in dogs. Thus in humans with ulcerative colitis, high titers of pANCA

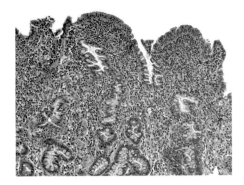

Fig. 19.4 An endoscopic biopsy from the duodenum of a 7-year-old spayed female Boxer with a 1-month history of vomiting, diarrhea, and weight loss. The lamina propria contains large numbers of lymphocytes, plasma cells, and few eosinophils. The villi are also blunted. 20 × . H&E stain. (Courtesy of Dr. Aline Rodrigues Hoffman.)

are 90% specific (although not very sensitive). In dogs, enzyme-linked immunosorbent assays have been used to test for antibodies to neutrophils (anticanine polymorphonuclear granulocyte antibodies [APMNA]), canine calprotectin, gliadins, and *Escherichia coli* outer membrane porin C (ompC). The detection of pANCAs in dogs is also a useful diagnostic test if available. Thus in a series of studies conducted in dogs with IBD, 39% to 76% of affected dogs had antibodies against ompC versus 0% to 13% in non-IBD controls. A combination of two serologic tests, ompC and APMNA, had a specificity of 93% to 99% and a sensitivity of 76% to 97% when compared to normal dogs.

TREATMENT

Since the etiology of these diseases remains largely unknown, treatment strategies are centered on reducing the intestinal inflammation. Many cases may be successfully managed by dietary manipulation such as increasing fiber levels, the use of probiotics, or antibiotic treatment. Some cases may respond positively to immunosuppressive and antiinflammatory therapies, thus providing circumstantial evidence of an immune pathogenesis. Therapeutic protocols depend on disease severity. In general, they involve initial dietary changes and possible use of pre- and probiotics. If no response is seen with a dietary trial, then this may be followed by immunosuppressive steroid treatment.

LYMPHOPLASMACYTIC ENTERITIS

While an inappropriate immune response to the microbiota may drive the local inflammatory processes in the intestinal wall, there is also likely to be a concomitant loss of tolerance in these tissues. For example, studies on steroid-responsive diarrhea in dogs have shown a major influx of CD4+ T cells, macrophages, and plasma cells producing IgG into the mucosa. Likewise, it has been demonstrated that many proinflammatory cytokines such as IL1, IL5, IL12p40, IFNγ, TNFα, and TGFβ may all be upregulated in affected tissues. There is also evidence that the NF-κB pathway is activated in cells located in the intestinal lamina propria of affected dogs.

This activation clearly points to a type 1 immune pathway, but there is also activation of some parts of the Th2 pathway as well. (In humans, IBD typically is associated with activation of the Th1 pathway only.) Of course it is possible that the two different pathways are activated in different disease types (e.g., Th1 cells in the lymphoplasmacytic pathway and Th2 responses in the eosinophilic pathways).

ANAL FURUNCULOSIS

Anal furunculosis is a chronic progressive inflammatory disease of the perineum that closely resembles perianal Crohn disease in humans. Sinus tracts develop in the perianal skin (Fig. 19.5).

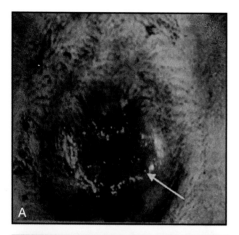

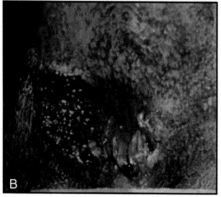

Fig. 19.5 Two distinct clinical presentations of anal furunculosis. (A) A discrete 2- to 4-mm wide, deep sinus or fistula *(white arrow)* within the perianal skin or mucocutaneous junction. (B) Extensive ulceration of the perianal skin and mucocutaneous junction with coalescence of lesions around the anal circumference. (House AK, Catchpole B. Gregory SP. Matrix metalloproteinase mRNA expression in canine anal furunculosis lesions. Vet Immunol Immunopathol 2007; 115:68-75.)

It most frequently affects middle-aged or old German Shepherd Dogs. In fact, German Shepherds account for 80% of cases, indicating that this is an inherited disease. There is a highly significant association with the MHC allele DLA-DRB1*00101. Homozygous animals develop the disease earlier in life. While its pathogenesis is unclear, anal furunculosis appears to be immune mediated. Affected tissues are infiltrated with T cells, plasma cells, and eosinophils. There may be local formation of ectopic lymphoid follicles. Cytokine profiles are consistent with an upregulated Th1 response; thus both IL2 and IFNγ levels are elevated. Likewise inflammatory cytokines IL1β, IL6, TNFα, IL8, IL10, and TGFβ are increased relative to control tissues. Biopsies of affected tissues show elevated levels of metalloproteases 9 and 13. These are produced by macrophages, so this is also consistent with macrophage activation due to an excessive Th1 response. Clinical signs are fecal tenesmus, straining, and bleeding. Treated animals respond well to prednisolone or cyclosporine. Anal furunculosis is also associated with the presence of colitis, suggesting that it and some forms of IBD may have a similar pathogenesis.

Equine Inflammatory Bowel Disease

IBD occurs in horses. As in dogs, there are probably diverse innate and adaptive immune mechanisms involved. Thus the intestinal cellular infiltrates may be eosinophilic, lymphoplasmacytic, or granulomatous. These diseases primarily involve the small intestine but in severe cases, may extend to the large intestine.

Clinical signs range widely from mild digestive disturbances to severe, unremitting colic and chronic diarrhea. They usually reflect malabsorption problems as evidenced by inappetence, weight loss with edema, and hypoalbuminemia. Standardbreds and Thoroughbreds appear predisposed to these diseases. Eosinophilic enteritis reflecting a local type 2 immune response is commonly attributed to parasites and related allergic responses. Lymphoplasmacytic enteritis is similar to that seen in dogs; its etiology is unknown (Fig. 19.6).

Limited attempts have been made to determine the etiology of equine IBD. One study, however, investigated whether affected horses have antibodies directed against the gluten derivative gliadin and the autoantigen transglutaminase 2. It was found that some horses did indeed possess antibodies directed against transglutaminase 2. These positive horses included both IBD horses and horses on a high-gluten diet. There was, however, no significant difference in antibody titers between the IBD horses and the gluten-fed control animals. Interestingly, a single IBD horse had high levels of autoantibodies against not only transglutaminase 2 but also against deamidated gluten peptides and equine endomysium. After 6 months on a gluten-free diet, this horse recovered clinically and had significantly improved duodenal histopathology.

Granulomatous enteritis may be focal or systemic and may preferentially occur in Standardbreds. In many cases, it reflects chronic infections with *Mycobacteria, Listeria,* or *Salmonella.* Animals usually have diffuse lesions in the small intestine. They suffer from villous atrophy, and the lesions consist of macrophage and epithelioid cell aggregates. Occasional giant cells may be present. In many respects, this resembles Johne disease in cattle.

A rare equine disease has been associated with a lymphoplasmacytic infiltrate in the lamina propria of the intestine. It results in a chronic enterocolitis and segmental or diffuse thickening of the small intestine. Villous atrophy is usually present. There is no apparent breed or sex predisposition, and horses of all ages appear susceptible. Affected horses are thin, lethargic, depressed, and suffer from chronic diarrhea. They are commonly hypoproteinemic and hypoalbuminemic.

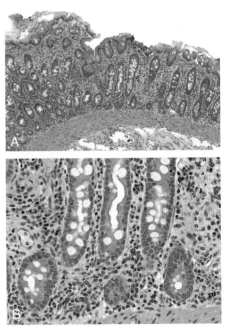

Fig. 19.6 Equine eosinophilic enteric disease showing an eosinophilic and lymphoplasmacytic colitis. H&E, A. 10× magnification. B. 40× magnification. (Courtesy of Dr. Dominique Wiener.)

Diagnosis requires a biopsy, but it is difficult to diagnose antemortem. It has been suggested that this disease may in fact be the early developmental stages of an intestinal lymphosarcoma.

A multisystemic eosinophilic epitheliotropic disease has been reported in young Standardbreds. They develop an eosinophilic infiltration of multiple organs, including the skin, oral cavity, esophagus, salivary glands, liver, lung, and mesenteric lymph nodes, in addition to the intestinal tract. The lesions may also contain lymphocytes and macrophages. Animals may also suffer from an exudative dermatitis affecting the face, limbs, and ventral abdomen that resembles pemphigus foliaceus. The hepatobiliary system may also be affected. Diagnosis is by biopsy of affected organs.

Eosinophilic diseases may affect many locations along the gastrointestinal tract. Eosinophils are normally present in small numbers and vary greatly between sites. Some horses may develop an eosinophilic enterocolitis. This involves massive infiltration of the mucosa with eosinophils plus lymphocytes and macrophages. Depending on the mucosal layer involved, it can result in recurrent colic rather than diarrhea. The infiltrates may be diffuse or segmental. Circumferential mural bands may also develop and so result in intestinal blockage. The lesions in these cases are usually restricted to the gastrointestinal tract, and affected animals do not necessarily develop an eosinophilia.

DIAGNOSIS AND TREATMENT

Diagnosis of equine IBD is one of exclusion. It therefore requires hematology, fecal egg counts, and bacterial cultures looking especially for *Salmonella*. Hypoproteinemia is a common finding. Rectal palpation may be useful in detecting a thickened bowel wall. Likewise, transabdominal ultrasound may identify thickened walls or lymphadenopathy. A rectal biopsy is diagnostic in about a third of patients.

Diverse drugs have been used to treat these diseases, although this is often unrewarding. These include steroids (dexamethasone or prednisolone), antibiotics, hydroxychloroquine, metronidazole, and sulfasalazine. Prolonged treatment is required. Anthelmintics may be used if the eosinophilic disease is attributed to parasites. Some horses may respond positively to dietary changes.

BOX 19.1 ■ Reoviruses and Celiac Disease

Gluten enteropathy occurs in about 1 in 133 persons in the United States. About 30% to 45% of the population also carry the risk alleles (HLA-DQ2) for celiac disease. Clearly, there must be other significant risk factors. Infectious agents, especially viruses, may serve as disease triggers. Among the viruses that do this are reoviruses, double-stranded RNA viruses that infect the intestine, trigger a strong type 1 interferon response, inhibit the production of Treg cells, and so can break oral tolerance. If gluten is fed at this time, then in the absence of tolerance the recipient will make the autoantibodies associated with gluten enteropathy. Epidemiologic studies have demonstrated that human celiac disease patients have significantly higher levels of antireovirus antibodies than healthy controls.

Bouziat R, Hinterleitner R, Brown JJ, et al. Reovirus infection triggers inflammatory responses to dietary antigens and development of celiac disease. *Science.* 2017;356:44–50.

Sources of Additional Information

Canine Inflammatory Bowel Disease

Allenspach K. Clinical immunology and immunopathology of the canine and feline intestine. *Vet Clin Small Anim.* 2011;41:345–360.

Burgener IA, König A, Allenspach K, et al. Upregulation of toll-like receptors in chronic enteropathies in dogs. *J Vet Intern Med.* 2008;22:553–560.

Cabrera-García AI, Protschka M, Alber G, et al. Dysregulation of gastrointestinal RAGE (receptor for advanced glycation end products) expression in dogs with chronic inflammatory enteropathy. *Vet Immunol Immunopathol.* 2021. doi:10.1016/j.vetimm .2021.110216.

Estruch JJ, Barken D, Bennett N, et al. Evaluation of novel serologic markers and autoantibodies in dogs with inflammatory bowel disease. *J Vet Intern Med.* 2020;34:1177–1186.

Heillman RM, Allenspach K. Pattern-recognition receptors: signaling pathways and dysregulation in canine chronic enteropathies—brief review. *J Vet Diag Invest.* 2017;29:781–787.

Heillman RM, Suchodolski JS. Is inflammatory bowel disease in dogs and cats associated with a Th1 or Th2 polarization?. *Vet Immunol Immunopathol.* 2015;168:131–134.

Kalck KA. Inflammatory bowel diseases in horses. *Vet Clin Equine.* 2009;25:303–315.

Kathrani A, Holder A, Catchpole B, et al. TLR5 risk-associated haplotype for canine inflammatory bowel disease confers hyper-responsiveness to flagellin. *PlosOne.* 2012. doi:10.1371/journal.pone.0030117.

Kathrani A, House A, Catchpole B, et al. Polymorphisms of the Tlr4 and Tlr5 gene are significantly associated with inflammatory bowel disease in German Shepherd dogs. *PlosOne.* 2010. doi:10.1371/journal. pone.0015740.

Kathrani A, Lee H, White C, et al. Association between nucleotide oligomerization domain two (Nod2) gene polymorphisms and canine inflammatory bowel disease. *Vet Immunol Immunopathol.* 2014;161:32–41.

Luckschander N, Allenspach K, Hall J, et al. Perinuclear antineutrophilic cytoplasmic antibody and response to treatment of diarrheic dogs with food responsive disease or inflammatory bowel disease. *J Vet Intern Med.* 2006;20:221–227.

McMahon LA, House AK, Catchpole B, et al. Expression of toll-like receptor 2 in duodenal biopsies from dogs with inflammatory bowel disease is associated with severity of disease. *Vet Immunol Immunopathol.* 2010;135:158–163.

Peiravan A, Bertolini F, Rothschild MF, et al. Genome-wide association studies of inflammatory bowel disease in German Shepherd dogs. *PlosOne.* 2018. doi:10.1371/journal.pone.0200685.

Equine Inflammatory Bowel Disease

Kemper DL, Perkins GA, Schumacher J, et al. Equine lymphocytic plasmacytic enterocolitis: a retrospective study of 14 cases. *Equine Vet J.* 2000;32:S108–S112.

Schmitz S, Garden OA, Werling D, et al. Gene expression of selected signature cytokines in T cell subsets in duodenal tissues of dogs with and without inflammatory bowel disease. *Vet Immunol Immunopathol.* 2012;146:87–91.

Schumacher J, Edwards JF, Cohen ND. Chronic idiopathic inflammatory bowel disease of the horse. *J Vet Intern Med.* 2000;14:258–265.

van der Kolk JH, van Putten LA, Mulder CJ, et al. Gluten-dependent antibodies in horses with inflammatory small bowel disease (ISBD). *Vet Quart.* 2012;32:3–11.

CHAPTER 20

Diagnostic Tests for Autoimmune Diseases

CHAPTER OUTLINE

Primary Binding Tests
Immunofluorescence Assays
    Antinuclear Antibodies
    ANCA Assays
Immunohistochemistry
Enzyme-Linked Immunosorbent Assays
Chemiluminescence Assays
Disposable Immunoassay Devices
Secondary Binding Tests
Antiglobulin Tests

Direct Antiglobulin Tests
Indirect Antiglobulin Tests
Rheumatoid Factor Tests
Passive Agglutination Tests
    C-Reactive Protein Levels
Cytotoxicity Tests
Flow Cytometry
Multiplex Immunoassays

By detecting specific autoantibodies in serum, it is possible to determine if an animal has mounted an autoimmune response. It is essential to point out, however, that the presence of autoantibodies in a diseased animal does not prove they are the cause of the disease in question. These tests may, however, be critical in establishing a diagnosis, providing an estimate of the severity of any autoimmune response, or even determining response to treatment. Serologic techniques used for the diagnosis of autoimmune diseases can be classified into two broad categories: primary binding tests that directly detect and measure the binding of antigen to antibody and secondary binding tests that detect the results of antigen-antibody interaction in vitro. Secondary tests are usually less sensitive than primary binding tests, but they may be simpler to perform in the clinic or require less complex technology.

Primary Binding Tests

Primary binding tests are performed by allowing antigen and autoantibody to combine and then detecting and measuring any immune complexes formed. To analyze these reactions, one of the reactants must first be labeled. Radioisotopes, fluorescent dyes, plastic beads, colloidal metals, reactive chemicals, and enzymes have all been used as labels in these tests.

Although radioisotopes have been used as labels for some primary binding tests such as drug testing, they have major disadvantages. Thus isotopes have a short half-life, are potentially hazardous, require expensive detection devices, and their use is accompanied by complex mandatory environmental regulations. As a result, isotope-based assays have largely been replaced by newer, highly sensitive chemiluminescence assays. Enzyme assays involving the production of luminescent products, such as luciferase, may be many times more sensitive than conventional dye-based enzyme assays but require sophisticated instruments to measure the luminescence produced.

Colored dyes linked to antibodies have been used in dipstick assays. Colloidal gold and colloidal selenium nanoparticles are colored and are commonly used as labels in simple immunochromatography tests such as lateral-flow assays.

IMMUNOFLUORESCENCE ASSAYS

Fluorescent dyes are widely employed as labels in primary binding tests. The most important of these is fluorescein isothiocyanate (FITC). FITC is a yellow dye that can be chemically linked to antibodies without affecting their reactivity. When radiated with invisible ultraviolet or blue light at 290 and 145 nm, FITC reemits visible green light at 525 nm. This green light can be readily seen under a fluorescent microscope or detected by a fluorometer. FITC-labeled antibodies are used in direct and indirect fluorescent antibody tests (Fig. 20.1). These are sensitive assays that permit the direct visualization of the reactants and their location within tissues.

While conventional histopathology is of critical importance in the diagnosis of autoimmune diseases, direct immunofluorescence assays are often required to confirm the presence and location of any immune reactants. Thus biopsy tissue sections may be stained using specific fluorescent antibodies to detect the presence of immunoglobulins, complement components, or specific antigens. This may be done either directly or indirectly. In the direct tests, a fluorescent-labeled antibody is used to detect the presence and location of a specific antigen in a smear or tissue

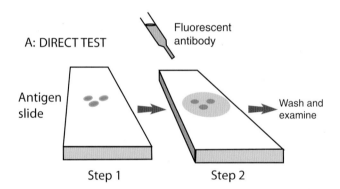

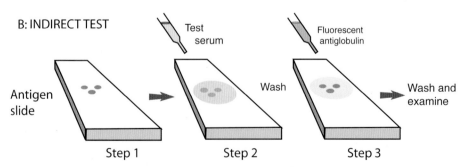

Fig. 20.1 Principles of immunofluorescence assays. (A) The direct fluorescent antibody assay. This technique is used to detect antigen by means of fluorescein isothiocyanate (FITC)-labeled antibody. (B) The indirect fluorescent antibody test may be used to detect either antigen or antibody. The antigen, in a section smear or culture, will bind antibody from the test serum. After washing, this antibody may be detected by binding to the FITC-labeled antiglobulin.

section. After incubation, unbound antibody is removed by washing and the slide examined under a fluorescent microscope to see if antigen is present and ascertain its location.

Indirect fluorescent antibody tests, in contrast, are used to measure antibodies in serum or other body fluids. In these tests, a known antigen is employed as a tissue smear, section, or cell culture on a slide or coverslip. This is incubated in the serum suspected of containing antibodies to that antigen. The serum is then washed off, leaving any specific antibodies bound to the antigen. These bound antibodies can then be visualized by incubating the smear with an FITC-labeled antiglobulin. After any unbound labeled antiglobulin is removed by washing, the presence of fluorescence indicates that antibodies were present in the test serum. The amount of these antibodies in the test serum may be estimated by testing increasing dilutions of serum on different antigen preparations.

To diagnose autoimmune skin diseases in dogs, direct immunofluorescence assays can be performed on skin tissue sections from the patient. In these cases, frozen or formalin fixed skin biopsy tissue sections are incubated with a fluorescent-labeled antiglobulin. The antiglobulin will bind to any autoantibodies present in the skin section. In the pemphigus group of diseases, for example, this will show a chicken wire–like staining pattern as the autoantibody is deposited on the intercellular desmosomes (see Fig. 10.3). Likewise, direct immunofluorescence of affected lupus skin lesions using an appropriately labeled antiglobulin will show a distinctive staining of the epidermal basement membrane (i.e., a lupus band) (see Fig. 15.5).

Indirect immunofluorescence assays on normal skin sections may be used to detect the presence of autoantibodies to desmosomes in the serum of pemphigus patients. However, this test varies in its sensitivity, depending on the target cells used and the specificity of the antiglobulin serum. Neonatal mouse skin appears to be most satisfactory, but not all pemphigus dogs may have detectable antiskin autoantibodies in their serum.

Direct immunofluorescence assays can also be used when diagnosing canine autoimmune thyroiditis. Thus a fluorescent anticanine immunoglobulin applied to a section of the affected thyroid gland will reveal not only the presence of any bound autoantibodies, but the staining pattern may also provide an indication as to the nature of the thyroid autoantigen involved.

Direct immunofluorescence assays are also used on frozen kidney sections to determine both the presence and distribution of immunoglobulin deposits within glomeruli. Thus the specific staining pattern obtained can demonstrate whether the antibodies are directed against the glomerular basement membrane (smooth pattern) or immune complexes have been deposited in or on the basement membrane to yield a granular pattern.

Antinuclear Antibodies

Antinuclear antibodies (ANA), as described in Chapter 15, are a mixture of different antibodies against diverse antigens located within the cell nuclei. They are the most sensitive biologic markers for analyzing the status of animals with diseases such as the systemic lupus erythematosus complex. Several different methods may be used to detect and measure these ANA. In humans, it is usual to first use a nonspecific screening test that measures ANA in general without reference to their specificity. If this is positive, then additional tests may be run to determine which specific antibodies are present. The three methods that are commonly used in humans are indirect immunofluorescence assays, enzyme-linked immunosorbent assays (ELISAs), and multiplex bead immunoassays.

ANA are normally demonstrated by immunofluorescence. Cultured cells or frozen sections of mouse or rat liver are used as the source of nuclear antigens. Dilutions of the patient's serum are applied to the section on a microscope slide. After incubation, the unbound material is washed off. Binding of ANA to the cell nuclei is revealed by incubating the tissue in an appropriate fluorescein-labeled antiglobulin and then rewashing. Several different nuclear staining patterns have been described for humans and their clinical correlations identified. In animals, staining patterns have been less thoroughly investigated so their significance is less clear.

An even staining pattern or staining of the nuclear rim is considered indicative of systemic lupus. A diffuse staining pattern is associated with autoantibodies to histones. Nucleolar fluorescence indicates the presence of autoantibodies directed against ribonucleoproteins (see Fig. 15.8). Serum from dogs that gives a speckled fluorescence pattern is associated with specific nuclear antigens such as Sm and suggests that the animal may have an autoimmune disease other than lupus.

Immunofluorescence assays on cells or tissues are only semiquantitative since the result depends in large part on the visual acuity of the test reader. This means in practice that, for consistency, one individual in a diagnostic laboratory is usually tasked with reading all these tests. Recent advances in imaging and image analysis have considerably simplified this task but not completely replaced human judgment. ANA test results must therefore be read with caution.

ANCA Assays

The detection of antineutrophil cytoplasmic antibodies (ANCA) is a diagnostic marker for many autoimmune diseases in humans such as the vasculitides. The most specific assays are indirect immunofluorescence assays used to measure antibodies directed against the major neutrophil antigens, myeloperoxidase (MPO) and proteinase 3 (PR3).

ANCA were first detected using indirect immunofluorescence assays using ethanol-fixed blood leukocytes as the cellular substrates. Two main fluorescence patterns are recognized: a diffuse granular cytoplasmic staining (cANCA) and perinuclear staining (pANCA) (see Fig. 11.3). It is now known that cANCA staining is due to antibodies directed against PR3, while pANCA staining is due to antibodies against the neutrophil MPO. While these can be read manually, automated fluorescent microscope systems have been developed to acquire and store high-resolution digital images and have the ability to assist in pattern interpretation and decision making. They are still being developed.

Once the specific neutrophil antigens were identified, it then became possible to develop antigen-specific ELISAs. Initially, these were simple direct ELISAs that used neutrophil antigens bound to polystyrene plates. These, however, lacked sensitivity, so second-generation methods have been developed. These include capture ELISAs, where the plate is coated with specific antibody, and competitive ELISAs. A more recent test has used a chemiluminescence assay in which beads are coated with either MPO or PR3. They are mixed and incubated with the patient's serum. After washing, they are mixed with antiimmunoglobulin G (anti-IgG) conjugated to luminol. When sodium hydroxide and peroxide solutions are added, they emit a flash of light that can be measured.

IMMUNOHISTOCHEMISTRY

Enzyme-labeled antibodies or antiglobulins can also be used to locate specific antigens in tissue sections. Horseradish peroxidase is the most widely employed enzyme label. The tests are performed in a manner similar to the immunofluorescence tests. In a direct immunoperoxidase test used to detect and locate antigen, the tissue section is treated with the enzyme-labeled antibody. After washing the slide, the tissue is incubated in a solution of the appropriate enzyme substrate. In the case of peroxidase-labeled antibodies, the bound antibody is detected by the development of a brown or black color at the site of antigen binding. In the indirect test, the presence of bound antibody can be detected by means of an enzyme-labeled antiglobulin. The use of these enzyme labels has an advantage over immunofluorescence techniques in that the tissue can be examined by conventional light microscopy and can be counterstained so that structural relationships are easier to see.

ENZYME-LINKED IMMUNOSORBENT ASSAYS

Among the most widely employed immunoassays in the diagnosis of autoimmune diseases are the ELISAs. As with other primary binding tests, ELISAs can be used to detect and measure either antibodies or antigens. They have good sensitivity and specificity and are technically simple. They are employed in many different formats, ranging from individual animal testing to automated high throughput screening of large numbers of samples. Depending on the nature of the enzyme label, they may or may not require specialized equipment to read. The most popular enzyme labels used in ELISAs include alkaline phosphatase, horseradish peroxidase, and β-galactosidase.

Different types of ELISAs are routinely used to test serum, plasma, cell culture fluid, cell lysates, saliva, and even urine. There are four main types of ELISAs: indirect, direct, sandwich, and competitive. To perform these assays, it is usual to use microwells in polystyrene plates (the commonly used plate uses 96 wells) (Fig. 20.2).

The simplest assay is the indirect ELISA used to detect antibodies to a specific antigen. In this test, the microwells are first coated with the antigen. Proteins bind firmly to polystyrene so that after any unbound antigen is removed by vigorous washing, the wells remain coated with a thin layer of antigen. These coated plates can be stored until required. When conducting the test, the test serum is first added to the wells. Any antibodies in the serum will bind to the antigen layer. After incubation and washing to remove unbound antibody, the presence of bound antibodies can be detected by adding a solution containing an enzyme-labeled antiglobulin. The labeled antiglobulin binds to any antibody present and, following incubation and washing, can be detected

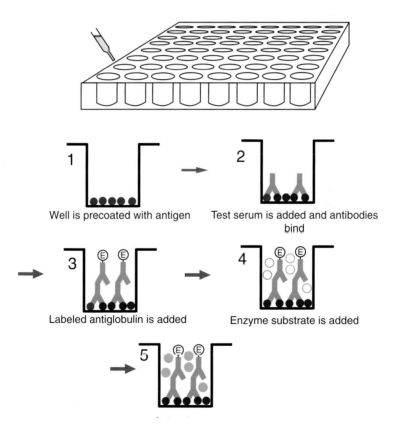

Fig. 20.2 The principle of the indirect enzyme-linked immunosorbent assay (ELISA) technique. Step 1: Antigen is bound to the wells in a styrene plate. Step 2: The test serum is added. Step 3: After washing, the presence of bound antibody is detected by means of an enzyme-labeled antiglobulin. Step 4: Addition of the enzyme substrate leads to a color change proportional to the amount of bound antibody. Step 5: This color change can be estimated visually or read in an ELISA reader (a specially adapted spectrophotometer).

and measured by adding a solution containing the enzyme substrate. The enzyme and substrate are selected so that a colored product develops in the well. The intensity of the color is proportional to the amount of enzyme-linked antiglobulin that is bound, which in turn is proportional to the amount of antibody present in the serum under test. The color intensity may be estimated visually or read in a specialized ELISA reader.

In a direct ELISA, a crude antigen solution is immobilized directly in a well and a labeled detection antibody added. After removing unbound antibody, enzyme substrate is added. The amount of color detected is proportional to the amount of specific antigen present on the plate.

A modification of this technique is the sandwich ELISA, which can also be used to detect and measure a specific antigen. (These tests get their name since they involve the formation of antibody-antigen-antibody layers.) In this case, the wells in polystyrene plates are first coated with a capture antibody. The antigen solution to be tested is then added to each well so that the capture antibody will bind any antigen present in the test solution. This step is followed, after washing, by another specific antibody, which also binds the antigen (the detection antibody). After washing to remove unbound detection antibody, enzyme-labeled antiglobulin and substrate, as described for the indirect technique, are added and the color change measured.

Antiglobulins are species specific. When performing sandwich ELISAs, it is important that the capture antibody and the detection antibody are from a different species and that a species-specific antiglobulin is used for visualization of the detection antibody. These are known as matched antibody pairs. This avoids false-positive results caused by binding of the antiglobulin to the capture antibody. In this assay, the intensity of the color generated is related directly to the amount of bound antigen.

Competitive ELISAs are often used to measure protein antigens such as thyroglobulin. In this technique, each microwell is first coated with specific capture antibody. In a single reaction, a mixture of the test sample and a standard amount of enzyme-labeled antigen are added to the well. The two antigens compete for the antibody-binding sites. As a result, the amount of labeled antigen that can be captured is inversely related to the concentration of antigen in the test sample. This technique is faster than other ELISA techniques. It can be made very sensitive if the sample antigen is permitted to react with the capture antibody before the labeled antigen is added. The result can be quantitated by reference to a standard curve.

CHEMILUMINESCENCE ASSAYS

Chemiluminescence is the emission of visible light in response to a chemical reaction. This phenomenon can be used in ELISAs to measure the concentration of the labeled reactants. These assays have a very high sensitivity, good specificity, a much wider dynamic range than simple colorimetric ELISAs, and are easy to measure. As a result, they are used in a wide range of diagnostic applications.

Two different types of chemical reaction are commonly employed in chemiluminescence assays. In the direct methods, the reactant, such as antigen, antibody, or antiglobulin, is labeled with a chemical that can emit light. Examples include acridinium or ruthenium esters, which when exposed to sodium hydroxide, emit a flash of light. Acridinium sulfonamide esters can be triggered by alkaline hydrogen peroxide. The light emitted by these reactants is of significantly greater intensity than those emitted by other reactions.

A second, indirect method uses enzymes as reactant labels. Reactions can be measured by using a substrate that emits light when acted on by the enzyme. For example, luminol (3-aminophthal hydrazide) emits a flash of light when it reacts with oxidized horseradish peroxidase. Luminol reduces the peroxidase and in doing so, generates two luminol radicals to form an electronically excited 3-aminophthalate dianion. The dianion releases light when it returns to the ground state. Thus the peroxidase is used as the label, and the luminol substrate is added later. The reaction results in the emission of light flashes at a wavelength of 425 nm. Luminol, when used with the correct enhancers (substituted phenols, naphthols, or aromatic amines), gives bright and stable light emission.

Another, similar system uses alkaline phosphatase as the enzyme and adamantane-1,2-dioxetane aryl phosphate (known to its friends as AMPPD) as the substrate. When the phosphate is cleaved off the AMPPD molecule, a flash of light is emitted at a wavelength of 470 nm. Enhancers such as ferrocyanide or metallic ions may be added to boost light emission. These assays are incredibly sensitive and can detect up to mol^{-16}/L of the label.

Chemiluminescence assays are employed in competitive ELISA tests (Fig. 20.3). For example, when measuring the thyroid hormone T4, microplate wells are coated with anti-T4. A measured amount of the patient's serum plus a constant amount of peroxidase-labeled T4 are then added to each well. The patient's T4 and the conjugated T4 compete for the bound antibody. After incubation for 60 minutes at 37°C, the wells are washed out and luminol substrate added. The plates are placed into the detecting chamber of a luminometer. The luminometer uses a fiberoptic light cable to transmit the light to a photomultiplier tube detector. This detects the photons from the labeled sample and converts them to electrical pulses and then to quantitative counts. The response is measured in relative light units (RLU). This may then be converted into absolute units (mg/dL) by comparison to a standard curve. One advantage of chemiluminescent assays over colorimetric assays is that they can measure a much wider range of light intensities compared simply to optical density. Chemiluminescence assays are good alternatives to radioimmunoassays and have largely replaced them in many diagnostic laboratories.

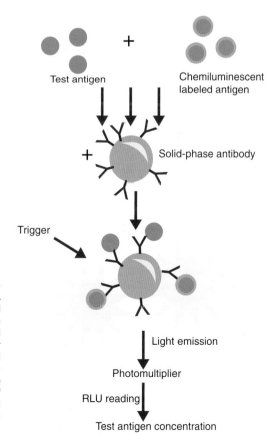

Fig. 20.3 The principle of a competitive binding assay using a chemiluminescent label. A fixed amount of labeled antigen is first mixed with the test sample. To the mixture is then added specific antibody bound to a solid substrate, in this case latex particles. After the reaction, the particles are washed and exposed to the exciting chemicals. The emitted light is detected and measured by relative light units (RLU). The greater the amount of antigen in the test sample, the less labeled antigen will bind. The test may be quantitated by reference to a standard curve.

DISPOSABLE IMMUNOASSAY DEVICES

Recent years have seen the development of simple immunoassay devices that can be employed in the clinic and provide results within a few minutes. These assays use a series of sequential reactions that are similar to ELISAs. They provide all the necessary reagents (antigens, antiglobulins, substrate, etc.) in excess so that the sample being tested becomes the limiting factor. Most disposable devices use this form of assay because the use of excess reagents makes the accurate metering of the sample unnecessary. The most popular of these are lateral-flow immunoassays that are increasingly employed in the diagnosis of infectious diseases but are only beginning to be used for the diagnosis of autoimmunity. One such use is the measurement of blood cytokine levels.

Secondary Binding Tests

The binding of antigens and antibodies is often followed by a secondary reaction. For example, if antibodies combine with soluble antigens, the resulting large immune complexes may precipitate out of solution. If antibodies bind to particulate antigens such as antigen-coated latex particles or red blood cells, then the particles will clump or agglutinate. These reactions can be employed in many different serological assays. Unfortunately, precipitation tests require large amounts of high-titered antibodies to produce a visible precipitate and as a result, are very insensitive. They are rarely used for the diagnosis of autoimmune diseases where sensitivity is important.

Agglutination tests in contrast are very sensitive and relatively easy to perform. For example, a slide agglutination test is widely used for the diagnosis of immune-mediated hemolytic anemia (IMHA) in dogs. A drop of blood from the patient is mixed on a microscope slide with saline, covered with a coverslip, and examined under the microscope. If the red cells remain clumped after dilution, this is considered evidence that the red cells are agglutinated rather than simply stuck together by normal rouleaux formation. The test, however, is prone to yield false-positive result, especially if the blood is insufficiently diluted in saline. While it has been traditional to use a saline-to-blood ratio of 1:1 or 4:1, evidence now suggests that a much greater dilution, 49:1, is more specific and much less prone to yielding false-positive results.

ANTIGLOBULIN TESTS

Because antibodies are bivalent, they normally crosslink particulate antigens such as bacteria or foreign red cells, which results in their clumping or agglutination. Antibody classes, however, differ in their ability to cause agglutination (e.g., IgM antibodies with 10 antigen-binding sites are more efficient than IgG antibodies with only 2). However, agglutination does not always happen because some antibodies cannot cause agglutination. These nonagglutinating antibodies are also called incomplete antibodies. The reason for their lack of agglutinating activity is not completely understood. (They are not incomplete!) One possibility is that the specific antigens with which they react lie deep within the surface coat of the particle, so deep that crosslinking cannot occur. Alternatively, some IgG antibodies may be unable to overcome the particle's negative surface charge. An additional suggestion is these antibodies are capable of only restricted movement in their hinge region, causing them to be functionally monovalent.

If it is necessary to detect nonagglutinating antibodies on the surface of particles such as bacteria or red cells, a direct antiglobulin test can be used. In this test, the washed particles are simply mixed with an antiglobulin. If antibodies are present on their surface, then they will be crosslinked by the antiglobulin, and agglutination will occur. This assay is sometimes called the Coombs test after Robin Coombs, the veterinarian who invented it.

Direct Antiglobulin Tests

The direct antiglobulin test is used to detect immunoglobulins on the surface of a patient's erythrocytes. Thus red cells are taken from the patient in EDTA/ACD anticoagulant, washed to remove all unbound immunoglobulin, and resuspended at 5% in buffered saline. Increasing dilutions of the antiglobulin solution in buffered saline are distributed across the rows in a 96-well plate, and an equal volume of the red cell suspension is added to each well. As the erythrocytes settle out of the suspension, they can be seen to either form a pellet (a negative result) or agglutinate. If immunoglobulins are present on the red cell surfaces, the antiglobulin will crosslink them and so cause agglutination (Fig. 20.4). For practical purposes, the best antiglobulin reagent used when testing dogs should have a broad specificity so that it will detect both canine IgM and complement C3 in addition to IgG. Since cell-bound IgM activates the classical complement system, detection of C3 on the target cell surface generally implies the presence of IgM. (As pointed out in Chapter 11, in some animals with IMHA, the IgM may elute from the red cells, leaving the C3 behind.)

Instead of using 96-well plates for direct agglutination tests, it is possible to use gel-based antiglobulin tests. These use whole blood samples rather than washed and resuspended red cells. The blood sample is layered into a tube containing a gel matrix impregnated with a rabbit antiglobulin specific

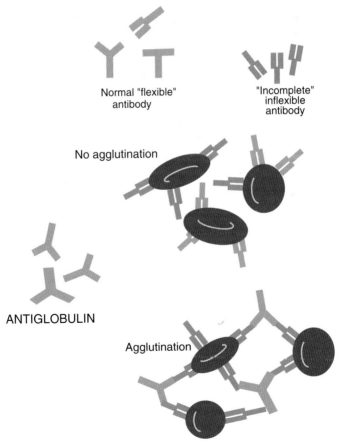

Normal "flexible" antibody

"Incomplete" inflexible antibody

No agglutination

ANTIGLOBULIN

Agglutination

Fig. 20.4 The direct antiglobulin test. The presence of the antiglobulin is required to agglutinate particles coated with nonagglutinating, incomplete antibodies.

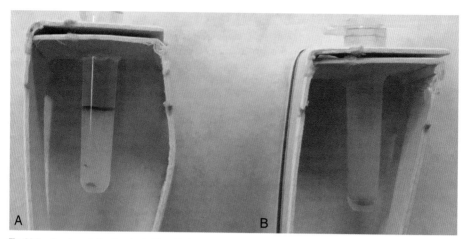

Fig. 20.5 A gel agglutination test. Blood is layered on top of a gel that contains anticanine immunoglobulin antibodies, and the tube is gently centrifuged. If the cells are coated in antierythrocyte antibodies, they cannot penetrate the gel (A) and remain on top. Nonantibody-coated control cells (B), in contrast, can pass through the gel. (Courtesy of Dr. Unity Jeffery.)

for the species to be tested. The tubes are gently centrifuged for a defined time. In a positive test, the clumped red cells will not penetrate the gel and hence layer at the top of the tube. If the test is negative, the individual red cells can pass through the gel and pellet at the bottom of the tube (Fig. 20.5).

Polyclonal antiglobulins directed against canine immunoglobulins are commercially available. They are usually produced by appropriate immunization of rabbits, sheep, or goats. Once these animals are fully immunized and their serum isolated, it must be absorbed by washed normal canine erythrocytes to ensure that false-positive reactions are not a result of natural antibodies directed against dog red cells themselves. Depending on the purity of the immunizing immunoglobulin, it is possible to make nonspecific antiglobulins against immunoglobulins of all classes or very specific antiglobulins directed against a single class. Antiglobulins are essential reagents in many immunologic tests.

Experience has shown, however, that somewhat different results may be obtained with the use of a polyvalent antiglobulin directed against multiple immunoglobulins as well as complement C3 when compared to a panel of monovalent reagents. It is also clear that different results may be obtained when the test is conducted at 4°C rather than at 37°C. Some of these differences appear to correlate with whether the IMHA is of the primary idiopathic type or secondary to some other concurrent disease.

Indirect Antiglobulin Tests

An indirect antiglobulin test may be used to detect and measure any autoantibodies circulating in the patient's bloodstream. The patient's serum is first exposed to a panel of normal canine erythrocytes. If autoantibodies are present, they will bind to the red cells. These can then be detected after washing by exposure to the antiglobulin. (Bear in mind, however, that the patient's blood may also contain antibodies directed against foreign blood groups on the donor erythrocytes, so this must be appropriately controlled.) Generally, only a very high titer of autoantibodies is considered clinically significant, and as a result, this test is not routinely used for diagnostic purposes in dogs.

RHEUMATOID FACTOR TESTS

Rheumatoid factors (RF) are autoantibodies directed against an animal's own IgG. In 1940, Erik Waaler discovered that antibodies in the serum of rheumatoid arthritis patients agglutinated antibody-coated sheep red cells. In 1949, Harry Rose rediscovered the phenomenon and developed it into a practical assay. Thus RF may be detected by the Rose-Waaler test. In this test, IgG is chemically or immunologically bound to carrier particles such as sheep red cells or latex beads. In the presence of rheumatoid factor (a natural antiglobulin), these particles are crosslinked and will visibly agglutinate.

Sensitized sheep erythrocytes are commonly used for the canine test and can be sensitized in several ways. One is to expose them to dilute tannic acid so that the cells become sticky and then coat them with purified canine IgG. Alternatively, sheep red cells may be exposed to subagglutinating dilutions of canine antisheep red blood cells and gently washed. When these IgG-coated red cells are mixed with RF-positive test serum on a microscope slide, any RF present will cause the red cells to agglutinate. More modern tests are now available, including nephelometry or ELISAs to detect RF and identify their immunoglobulin isotypes. Alternatively, canine IgG can be chemically bound to the surface of latex particles. A RF-positive serum will crosslink the latex particles so that they can be seen to agglutinate. Remember, however, this is a species-specific test, and human kits will not work with dog serum.

PASSIVE AGGLUTINATION TESTS

Since agglutination is a much more sensitive technique than precipitation, it is sometimes useful to convert a precipitating system to an agglutinating one. This may be done by chemically linking soluble antigen to inert particles such as red blood cells or latex beads. Erythrocytes are among the best particles for this purpose, and tests that employ coated erythrocytes are called passive hemagglutination tests.

Sensitized microspheres of polystyrene or latex are also commonly used in qualitative agglutination tests because of their uniformity and stability. Recent advances have developed particles with polystyrene cores covered by thin shells of reactive chemicals. The cores have a well-defined size that can be colored so they can be used in nephelometric assays (e.g., the shells may consist of polystyrene/polymethacrylate/polymethacrylamidoacetaldehyde dipentylacetal copolymer that allows covalent protein binding).

Latex agglutination may be used in direct agglutination tests to detect an antigen in a biologic sample. Thus antibodies are bound to latex particles. If these are mixed in an antigen solution, the antigen will bridge the particles, causing them to agglutinate (Fig. 20.6). Alternatively, latex agglutination can be used to detect the presence of antibodies in serum or plasma. This uses antigen-coated beads that will agglutinate when crosslinked by antibodies. As a result, the particle suspension clumps, and the aggregated particles settle out of suspension.

A reliable automated method of reading microparticle agglutination is nephelometry. This is based on the principle that a suspension of small particles will scatter light passing through, rather than just absorbing it. The amount of light scatter can be quantitated by collecting the light at an angle (30–90 degrees). The amount of scatter can be compared with a standard curve to arrive at a quantitative result. For example, these are used to assay C-reactive protein (CRP).

C-Reactive Protein Levels

CRP is an acute-phase reactant that is significantly elevated in animals with inflammatory lesions. Thus it is often a useful assay to measure disease severity. CRP can be measured by ELISA, nephelometry, or passive agglutination. Nephelometry, as described earlier, is a form of agglutination test. Thus monoclonal anti-CRP antibodies are covalently bound to latex particles. When mixed with positive serum, the particles will clump. Nephelometry measures the opacity of a particle suspension. In a positive case, the clumped latex particles will scatter the light. This scatter can be quantitated and calibrated by using a standard curve.

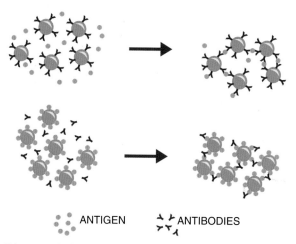

ANTIGEN   ANTIBODIES

Fig. 20.6 Latex particles coated with antigen are employed in several diagnostic tests for autoantibodies. Thus antibody-coated particles will be agglutinated by the presence of antigen in solution. Conversely, antigen-coated particles may be agglutinated by the presence of antibodies in solution, thus they can be employed for the detection of either antigen or antibodies as required.

CYTOTOXICITY TESTS

Complement may cause membrane damage not only to erythrocytes but also to nucleated cells. Antibodies against cell surface antigens may therefore be measured by reacting target cells with antibody and then adding a source of complement such as fresh guinea pig serum. The complement will be activated by the classical pathway, resulting in cell lysis (or hemolysis if red blood cells are used). The resulting loss of cell viability can be measured by the use of vital stains. A form of cytotoxic assay has been employed to detect antiplatelet antibodies.

There are two tests commonly used for the detection of antibodies to blood platelets: the direct fluorescent antibody test and the platelet factor 3 (PF3) test. In the former, the direct immunofluorescent assay is used to examine a bone marrow aspirate from the patient for the presence of antibody-coated megakaryocytes. If positive, the megakaryocytes will stain with labeled antidog immunoglobulin.

The PF3 test is a cytotoxic test that involves mixing the patient's plasma with normal platelet-rich plasma. Any autoantibodies present will bind to the platelets and damage them. This results in the release of PF3 (a phospholipid called thromboplastin) into the medium. The thromboplastin activates factor X. In the presence of factors XI and XII plus calcium, a fibrin clot will rapidly form. The time taken for this clot to form is noted. A positive result occurs when the time needed for the clot to form is significantly less in the presence of test serum than with control serum. False-positive responses may be obtained due to injury to the platelets by clotting factors in the patient's serum; hence it is important to use plasma. False-negative responses may also result from damage to the normal platelets so that the factor 3 escapes prematurely.

FLOW CYTOMETRY

Flow cytometry is an automated technique that rapidly scans single cells and is able to count and sort them by means of sets of cell surface markers. Thus cells are labeled with specific antibodies conjugated to fluorescent dyes. These labeled antibodies bind to specific cell surface antigens and even to intracellular proteins. The cell suspension is then passed through a capillary tube in single file. The labeled cells pass one by one through a laser beam that excites the dye molecules.

The emission spectra of these dyes are recorded and the markers on each individual cell identified. Flow cytometry can be used to quantify the numbers and size of each specific cell type in the mixture. It can also be used to sort specific cell populations for future studies. (The cells are not harmed by passage through the laser beam.) Flow cytometry can even be used to measure cell activation by using labels that specifically bind the phosphorylated state of the target protein. The main limitation of flow cytometry is that even the most sophisticated machines are limited to measuring fewer than 20 markers at any one time.

MULTIPLEX IMMUNOASSAYS

ELISA assays, as described previously, can conventionally measure only a single analyte, whereas the use of colored bead-based substrates permits many different immunoassays to be performed and analyzed simultaneously on a single sample. These multiplex immunoassays are available in several different formats depending on the manufacturer and whether they are designed to detect antibodies, antigens, oligonucleotides, enzyme substrates, or specific receptors.

Multiple sets of beads are internally colored with a specific mixture of two different fluorescent dyes. These mixtures are designed so that each set of beads can be readily differentiated. Then each set is coated with a different specific antibody, and the beads are mixed together (Fig. 20.7). The bead mixture is first added to the solution under test, such as serum. As a result, some of the beads in the mixture will capture the specific antigen being assayed. The bead mixture is then washed and mixed with fluorescent-labeled, antigen-specific reporter antibodies. These form a labeled antibody-antigen-antibody sandwich on the bead surface. A commonly used label is the fluorescent dye phycoerythrin conjugated to streptavidin, which binds specifically to biotinylated antibodies. (Avidin and biotin bind each other strongly and specifically.) After washing, the bead suspension is then passed through a dual laser flow-based detection instrument—essentially a specialized flow cytometer. One laser identifies the color of the bead (and thus which antigen is being detected), while the other measures the intensity of the reporter fluorescence (and hence the amount of bound antigen). High-speed digital processors can record the signals from each bead and with appropriate software, translate the results into usable data.

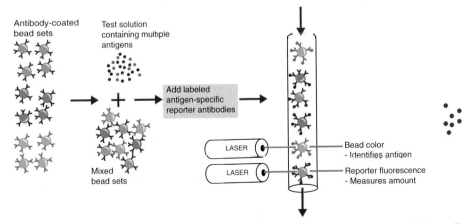

Fig. 20.7 The principle of multiplex particle-based immunoassays. Colored beads are coated with specific antibody. The beads are then mixed with the test solution so that specific antigens, if present, will bind to the colored beads. The antigens on the beads are next labeled with fluorescent antibodies. Finally, the bead suspension is passed through a flow cytometer, where lasers illuminate them and detect both the bead color and the labeled antibody. This identifies both the presence and amount of specific antigen in the test solution.

In an alternative to flow-based assays, labeled magnetic beads can be employed. After reacting with their specific reagents, the beads can be captured in such a way that they form a monolayer on a metal surface. When the layer of beads is illuminated with two sources of light of specific wavelengths, they will fluoresce. Light of one wavelength can identify the antigen on each bead, while the other can determine its amount. These automated assays can simultaneously and rapidly detect and quantitate many different analytes from a single biologic sample. They will inevitably grow in importance and sophistication as time passes.

Sources of Additional Information

Baslund B, Segelmark M, Wilk A, et al. Screening for antineutrophil cytoplasmic antibodies (ANCA): is indirect immunofluorescence the method of choice. *Clin Exp Immunol.* 1995;99:486–492.

Cinquanta L, Fontana DE, Bizzaro N. Chemiluminescent antibody technology: what does it change in auto-antibody detection? *Autoimmun Highlights.* 2017. doi:10.1007/s13317-017-0097-2.

Kapmeyer WH, Pauly H-E, Tuengler P. Automated nephelometric immunoassays with novel shell/core particles. *J Clin Lab Analysis.* 1988;2:76–83.

Molina-Bolivar JA, Galisteo-Gonzalez F. Latex immunoagglutination assays. *J Macromolecular Sci.* 2005. doi:10.1081/MC.200045819.

Pieck CJ, Teske E, van Leeuwen MW, et al. Good agreement of conventional and gel-based direct agglutination test in immune-mediated hemolytic anemia. *Acta Vet Scand.* 2012. doi:10.1186/1751-0147-54-10.

Schmidt T, Mauracher S, Bender L, et al. A novel lateral flow immunoassay for the rapid detection of anti-Dsg3 serum antibodies in pemphigus vulgaris. *Exp Dermatol.* 2018;27:233–237.

Siddiqui J, Remick DG. Improved sensitivity of colorimetric compared to chemiluminescence ELISAs for cytokine assays. *J Immunoassay Immunochem.* 2003;24:273–283.

Sun PL, Jeffrey U. Effect of dilution of canine blood samples on the specificity of saline agglutination tests for immune-mediated hemolysis. *J Vet Intern Med.* 2020;34:2374–2383.

Tamamoto T, Nagao A, Sugano M. Detection of anti-neutrophil cytoplasmic antibodies in dogs with immune-mediated inflammatory diseases. *Vet Immunol Immunopathol.* 2018;203:47–51.

Warman SM, Murray JK, Ridyard A, et al. Pattern of Coombs' test reactivity has diagnostic significance in dogs with immune-mediated hemolytic anemia. *J Small Anim Pract.* 2008;49:525–530.

The Treatment of Immune-Mediated Diseases

Immune-mediated diseases encompass diverse syndromes with a multitude of clinical presentations, but in general they all involve the development of excessive or inappropriate inflammatory and immune responses. Thus treatment usually involves the administration of immunosuppressive and antiinflammatory medication. In general, glucocorticoids are employed as the first-line treatment, but these may be supplemented with a second immunosuppressive drug such as cyclosporine if necessary. It is not recommended that three such drugs be used at the same time. They are rarely required, and they significantly increase the risks of adverse side effects. Some drug combinations are also recognized as provoking severe side effects and significantly increasing the risks of developing opportunistic infections. Should the use of three or more drugs be deemed necessary, the veterinarian should ensure that they each use different suppressive pathways so that they complement each other.

Glucocorticosteroids

Until recently, the only medications proven to ameliorate severe immune-mediated inflammatory diseases were the glucocorticosteroids—powerful, broad-spectrum antiinflammatory drugs. As a result they are the most widely employed antiinflammatory agents, and their prolonged use is often necessary for the treatment of autoimmune diseases. Corticosteroids are able to suppress both immunologic and inflammatory responses. They also work rapidly. Unfortunately, their use is complicated by their diverse and serious adverse effects.

Corticosteroids affect many different cell types. They are lipid soluble and as a result, can pass through cell membranes directly into cells, where they bind to receptors in the cytosol. The natural corticosteroid, cortisol (hydrocortisone), binds to two different receptors, a glucocorticoid receptor and a mineralocorticoid receptor. Most therapeutic corticosteroids, however, are designed so that they do not bind the mineralocorticoid receptor. The glucocorticoid receptor is found in most body cells and mediates the antiinflammatory responses. Some therapeutic glucocorticoids do not bind directly to glucocorticoid receptors but when given orally, are converted to active derivatives. Thus cortisone is converted to cortisol and prednisone is converted to prednisolone.

Unbound glucocorticoid receptors are found free in the cytoplasm but once they bind a glucocorticoid, the complexes are rapidly transported to the cell nucleus, where they bind to DNA and regulate gene transcription. There are at least eight different forms of the glucocorticoid receptor, and it is likely that each has a slightly different biologic function. Once they bind to DNA, the glucocorticoid receptor complexes trigger two different gene transcription processes: transactivation and transrepression.

TRANSACTIVATION

In transactivation, the steroid-receptor complex binds to specific DNA sequences called glucocorticoid response elements (GREs) and activates gene transcription. To add complexity to the process, the complexes may bind to different GREs in different cell types or at different stages in cell development. Among the most important targets of glucocorticoids is the NF-κB pathway. As a result, they stimulate the synthesis of IκB, the inhibitor of the key regulator of gene transcription, NF-κB (Fig. 21.1; see also Fig. 2.5). In a resting cell, NF-κB is inactive since its nuclear binding site is masked by IκB. When a lymphocyte is stimulated by antigens or cytokines, signals from its receptors cause the two molecules to dissociate and the IκB is degraded, while the released

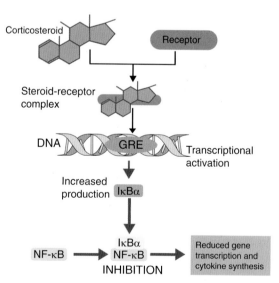

Fig. 21.1   Glucocorticosteroids can cross the plasma membrane and bind to receptors in the cytosol. The steroid-receptor complex can then bind to glucocorticoid response elements (GRE) on the nuclear DNA to increase the synthesis of IκBα. IκBα binds to NF-κB and prevents it from translocating to the cell nucleus. This effectively blocks all the many pathways mediated by NF-κB.

NF-κB can then move into the nucleus, where it activates the genes involved in inflammation and immunity. Glucocorticosteroids, however, stimulate the synthesis of excess IκB. As a result, its levels remain high and so IκB continues to suppress NF-κB–mediated processes, including cytokine synthesis and T-cell responses in activated cells.

TRANSREPRESSION

Steroid-receptor complexes may also bind to some specific gene enhancers and prevent them from binding to DNA. As a result, this will interfere with downstream proinflammatory signaling pathways. They may also bind to negative GREs that can inhibit gene transcription.

Corticosteroids suppress both the innate and adaptive immune systems. For example, they suppress leukocyte production and circulation and modulate the activities of inflammatory mediators, thus suppressing innate responses. They influence the effector mechanisms of lymphocytes and promote regulatory T (Treg) responses, and so suppress adaptive immunity as well.

EFFECTS ON LEUKOCYTES

The effects of corticosteroids on blood leukocytes vary among species. In horses, the number of circulating eosinophils, basophils, and lymphocytes declines within a few hours of corticosteroid administration as a result of increased sequestration in the bone marrow. Blood neutrophil counts, on the other hand, increase as a result of decreased adherence to vascular endothelium and reduced emigration into inflamed tissues. Neutrophil, monocyte, and eosinophil chemotaxis are suppressed by corticosteroids. Corticosteroids suppress the cytotoxic and phagocytic abilities of neutrophils in some species, but in others, such as the horse, they have no discernable effect. They may also block neutrophil nitric oxide synthase and so prevent the production of antibacterial nitric oxide. Macrophage production of prostaglandins and proinflammatory cytokines such as interleukin-1 (IL1), as well as antigen processing, are reduced in some species. Steroid-treated macrophages also tend to assume an M2 phenotype and release antiinflammatory cytokines. Glucocorticoids also decrease dendritic cell (DC) cytokine production and suppress antigen presentation.

EFFECTS ON LYMPHOCYTES

Glucocorticoid suppression of helper T type 1 (Th1) mediated inflammation is their most obvious therapeutic benefit. Corticosteroids inhibit the ability of Th1 cells to produce IL1, IL6, IL8, IL12, interferon-gamma (IFNγ), and tumor necrosis factor-alpha (TNFα). These are the major cytokines that promote type 1 immune responses and inflammation. Corticosteroids also upregulate the expression of the IL1 receptor CD121b. This is a decoy receptor that binds active IL1 but does not generate a signal, thus blocking IL1 functions. Conversely, glucocorticoids upregulate the production of IL4, IL10, and IL13 by Th2 cells. As a result, they force a change in the Th1/Th2 balance rather than a nonspecific immunosuppression. They also act on Th17 cells to suppress their differentiation and cytokine production. Steroids act on cytotoxic T cells to inhibit their effector functions and cytokine release while promoting their apoptosis.

In addition to suppressing Th1 responses, glucocorticoids increase Treg numbers. They do this in part by upregulating FoxP3 expression as well as by modulating the cytokine mixture within the T-cell environment. In the absence of FoxP3+ Treg cells, glucocorticoids are ineffective. Dexamethasone administered in the absence of Treg cells completely loses its ability to suppress inflammation. It appears that the dexamethasone acts on Tregs to induce a specific microRNA. This miRNA targets a protein called Rictor. Rictor controls cell growth and when its production is suppressed, this upregulates Treg cell functions.

The effects of corticosteroids on antibody responses are variable and depend on both timing and dose. In general, B cells tend to be corticosteroid resistant, and enormous doses are usually required to decrease B-cell receptor signaling and suppress antibody synthesis.

EFFECTS ON CYTOKINE PRODUCTION

Glucocorticoids act through JAK-STAT signaling pathways to reduce the production of IL5, IL9, and IL13 by innate lymphoid cells. IL10 production may be upregulated.

They enhance the production of lipocortin, which inhibits phospholipase A_2 and so interrupts arachidonic acid metabolism. This in turn inhibits leukotriene synthesis. They also inhibit cyclo-oxygenase (COX2) gene transcription and so block prostaglandin synthesis.

In humans, glucocorticoids inhibit eosinophil production of IL1, TNFα, and IL4 as well as IL3, IL5, and granulocyte macrophage colony-stimulating factor (GM-CSF). They reduce eosinophils' life span by promoting their apoptosis. This results in a rapid and profound fall in the numbers of circulating eosinophils and a decrease in the recruitment of eosinophils to sites of inflammation.

Synthetic corticosteroids act on small blood vessels to suppress acute inflammation by preventing increased vascular permeability and vasodilation and thus prevent edema formation and fibrin deposition. In the later stages of inflammation, they inhibit capillary and fibroblast proliferation and enhance collagen breakdown. As a result, corticosteroids also delay wound and fracture healing.

AVAILABLE GLUCOCORTICOIDS

Glucocorticoids are classified based on their biologic half-lives. Budesonide has a half-life of 2 hours in the dog, where it is used in the management of canine inflammatory bowel disease. Hydrocortisone is a short-acting molecule with a half-life of 8 to 12 hours. Prednisone, predniso-lone, and methylprednisolone have intermediate half-lives of 12 to 36 hours and have less sodium retention activity than hydrocortisone. (Prednisone is a prodrug that is converted in vivo to its active molecule, prednisolone.) Long-acting corticosteroids such as dexamethasone and triamcin-olone have half-lives of 24 to 54 hours. Cats achieve much higher plasma levels with oral predniso-lone than with prednisone, implying that they convert prednisone to prednisolone less efficiently.

ADVERSE EFFECTS

While highly effective, glucocorticoid treatment is not without significant risks. The wide distri-bution of glucocorticoid receptors in many different cell types makes adverse events inevitable. Most importantly, they have the potential to supply the body's corticosteroid needs, suppress the pituitary-adrenal axis, and induce Cushing syndrome (i.e., iatrogenic hyperadrenocorticism). Side effects include polyuria, increased thirst, and appetite leading to obesity. They also cause cutane-ous and muscle atrophy with alopecia and delayed wound healing. In addition, by suppressing inflammation and phagocytosis, corticosteroids can render animals susceptible to secondary infec-tions. For example, they predispose dogs to bacterial urinary tract and fungal infections as well as demodicosis and toxoplasmosis in cats.

Because these adverse events are generally a result of prolonged high doses, oral glucocorticoids are best used for short-term palliative treatments such as the suppression of acute disease. Once a satisfactory clinical response has been induced, the dose of corticosteroids should be gradually reduced to enable the adrenal cortex to resume its normal functions. This is generally achieved by lengthening the dose interval and then decreasing the amount given.

When systemic corticosteroid therapy is initiated, medium-acting oral prednisolone (2–4 mg/kg every 24 hours), dexamethasone (0.2–0.4 mg/kg orally), or triamcinolone (0.2–0.6 mg/kg orally) are usually the agents selected for companion animal treatment. They can be administered once daily or divided and given twice daily for 10 to 14 days. Thereafter the dose and frequency should be reduced in accordance with the patient's clinical state. If improvement is not noted by 2 weeks, consideration should be given to alternative diagnoses. If long-term treatment is determined to be necessary, the dose should be gradually reduced by first administering the second daily dose on alternate days and continuing to reduce it to the minimal dose that still controls the disease. Animals receiving long-term treatment should be examined regularly to monitor for adverse effects. Cats may require higher doses than dogs to achieve a significant clinical response, although an initial dose of 1 to 2 mg/kg daily of prednisolone is usually effective. As in other species, the dose should be tapered as soon as possible to the lowest dose that controls the disease.

Oral glucocorticoid pulse therapy may have significant benefits in animals that require long-term immunosuppressive treatment. In this procedure, dogs receive a therapeutic dose of prednisone or prednisolone at 10 mg/kg orally once daily for 3 days, followed by a daily low dose (<2 mg/kg). If the animal's response is unsatisfactory, the 3-day pulse may be repeated but no more frequently than once weekly. This technique has produced significantly faster remissions in dogs with pemphigus foliaceus than dogs that received conventional therapy (>2 mg/kg daily).

Calcineurin Inhibitors

CYCLOSPORINE

Cyclosporine (also called ciclosporin) is a cyclic peptide derived from a soil fungus, *Tolypocladium inflatum*. This fungus yields several natural forms of cyclosporine, of which the most important is cyclosporin A, a circular peptide of 11 amino acids. Cyclosporine acts as a molecular glue with two distinct surfaces that allow it to bind two proteins simultaneously. Cyclosporine interferes with the NF-AT signal transduction pathway (Fig. 21.2). When it enters the T cell, one surface of the peptide binds to an intracellular receptor called cyclophilin, whereas the other surface binds

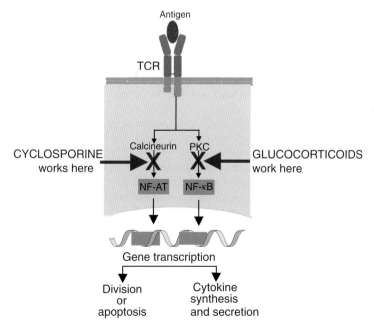

Fig. 21.2 While glucocorticoids block the NF-κB signal transduction pathway, cyclosporine blocks the NF-AT pathway. Both pathways are essential for an effective immune response. *PKC,* Protein kinase C; *TCR,* T-cell receptor.

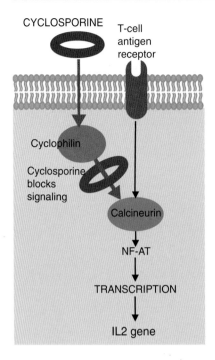

Fig. 21.3 The mechanism of action of calcineurin inhibitors. They essentially act as a molecular glue that binds calcineurin to cyclophilin and effectively blocks the NF-AT signal transduction pathway. *IL,* Interleukin.

to the intracellular transmitter calcineurin (Fig. 21.3). Cyclosporine therefore blocks cyclophilin-calcineurin interactions and as a result, interferes with many NF-AT–mediated T-cell functions such as the production of IL2, IL3, IL4, GM-CSF, TNFα, and IFNγ. The primary effect of cyclosporine treatment is therefore the blocking of Th cell responses.

Cyclosporine also has indirect suppressive effects on macrophages, B cells, and natural killer cells. It inhibits degranulation of neutrophils, eosinophils, and mast cells, and suppresses eicosanoid formation. It reduces eosinophil survival, granule release, and cytokine production. Thus cyclosporine prevents inflammation by inhibiting the functions of many of the participating cells. In many respects, it has similar effects to glucocorticoids. Cyclosporine simply interferes with different cell signaling pathways.

Oral cyclosporine therapy has proved very effective in treating immune-mediated diseases. When compared to systemic glucocorticoids, cyclosporine is equally effective but with significantly fewer and less severe side effects. It appears to have a wide safety margin in dogs. It is, however, slower to act, taking 2 to 3 weeks to show evidence of effectiveness. The major adverse effect reported in dogs is gastroenteritis (nausea, vomiting, and diarrhea). Other side effects may include anorexia leading to weight loss and gingival enlargement. Opportunistic infections are rare, and cyclosporine has no apparent effect on the skin microbiota. Once cyclosporine therapy is seen to be working, usually by 4 to 6 weeks, then the daily dose may be gradually reduced to a level that maintains the disease in remission.

Cyclosporine is the preferred first-line therapy for perianal furunculosis and keratoconjunctivitis sicca (in the form of eye drops or ointment). It is considered second-line therapy in many other autoimmune diseases.

Cyclosporine is a well-tolerated alternative to glucocorticoid therapy in cats. As in dogs, improvements will not be seen until 2 to 3 weeks after initiation of therapy. Vomiting and diarrhea may occur in some cats.

Cyclosporine is metabolized in the liver through cytochrome P450 enzymes. These actively transport it across hepatocytes to the bile, where it is excreted into the intestine. This metabolic pathway is inhibited by azole antifungal drugs such as ketoconazole. Thus concurrent administration of 2.5 to 5 mg/kg ketoconazole once daily reduces cyclosporine secretion and permits the dose (and cost) of cyclosporine to be reduced by 30% to 50%.

Cyclosporine is highly lipophilic and as a result, it was first introduced as a coarse suspension in vegetable oil. Unfortunately, as a result, the absorption of the drug into the body was erratic and unpredictable. This has now largely been replaced with modified cyclosporine, an ultramicronized suspension that forms microemulsions in aqueous solutions and the absorption of which is much more predictable. Modified cyclosporine should be used whenever possible.

The use of sustained-release cyclosporine delivery devices implanted close to affected organs has yielded encouraging results when treating chronic autoimmune diseases such as equine recurrent uveitis. These implants use several different biodegradable polymers and can be designed to release defined doses of cyclosporine into the tissues for up to several years.

Tacrolimus is a macrolide antibiotic produced by the fungus *Streptomyces tsukubaensis*. It also interferes with the NF-AT pathway by preventing an activating molecule, immunophilin, from binding to calcineurin in a manner similar to cyclosporine. It therefore inhibits the production of several key cytokines, including IL2, IL3, IL4, IL5, IFNγ, and TNFα. Tacrolimus is a much more potent immunosuppressant than cyclosporine. It downregulates cytokine production by mast cells, basophils, eosinophils, keratinocytes, and Langerhans cells. Given orally, it may cause severe intestinal toxicity in dogs, resulting in ulceration, vasculitis, anorexia, and vomiting. Topically, it has been used to treat cutaneous lupus erythematosus, pemphigus foliaceus, and pemphigus erythematosus. It has also been used to treat perianal furunculosis and keratoconjunctivitis sicca. A related macrolide antibiotic calcineurin inhibitor, pimecrolimus, has been shown to be safe and effective when used in the form of oil-based eye drops to treat keratoconjunctivitis sicca in dogs.

Phosphodiesterase Inhibitors

PENTOXIFYLLINE

Phosphodiesterases are enzymes with multiple functions. Most importantly, they stimulate cell signaling (Fig. 21.4). Pentoxifylline (PTX) is a widely employed, competitive phosphodiesterase inhibitor that can reverse this. It also inhibits the NF-κB pathway. As a result, PTX decreases the

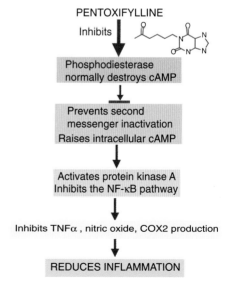

Fig. 21.4 Pentoxifylline is a phosphodiesterase inhibitor. As a result, it can block several signaling pathways, the most important of which is the NF-κB pathway; thus it effectively inhibits the production of many proinflammatory cytokines. *cAMP*, Cyclic adenosine monophosphate; *COX2*, cyclooxygenase; *TNFα*, tumor necrosis factor-alpha.

PENTOXIFYLLINE

Inhibits

Phosphodiesterase normally destroys cAMP

Prevents second messenger inactivation Raises intracellular cAMP

Activates protein kinase A Inhibits the NF-κB pathway

Inhibits TNFα, nitric oxide, COX2 production

REDUCES INFLAMMATION

production of inflammatory cytokines (IL1, IL6, and TNFα) and leukotrienes. It therefore acts as an antiinflammatory agent. PTX also facilitates blood flow by decreasing blood viscosity and the flexibility of red blood cells so that they suffer less damage when passing through small blood vessels. Given orally, it is safe and moderately effective in reducing the severity of some autoimmune diseases, especially those mediated by T cells. It is, however, slow to act, with a response time of 4 to 10 weeks. It is also recommended for the treatment of some forms of vasculitis, including rabies vaccine–induced alopecia. It has been used successfully to treat canine dermatomyositis and lupoid onychodystrophy. Side effects include vomiting, diarrhea, and anorexia. Given its vascular effects, it should not be given to animals with bleeding problems.

Antimetabolites

Cytotoxic drugs inhibit cell division by blocking nucleic acid synthesis and activity. The major cytotoxic drugs currently in use are alkylating agents, folic acid antagonists, and DNA synthesis inhibitors (Fig. 21.5).

CYCLOPHOSPHAMIDE

Alkylating agents crosslink DNA helices, preventing their separation and replication and so preventing mitosis. The most important of these is cyclophosphamide. It is toxic for dividing cells, especially for dividing lymphocytes. As a result, it is widely employed as an anticancer agent and as a powerful immunosuppressant. It inhibits B-cell activity, including antibody synthesis, by preventing B cells from renewing their antigen receptors. At high doses, it can also inhibit T-cell responses, especially primary immune responses. It blocks mitogen- and antigen-induced production of IFNγ. Early in therapy, cyclophosphamide tends to be more effective against B cells than T cells. In long-term therapy, it affects both cell populations. It also suppresses macrophage functions. Cyclophosphamide may be administered parenterally or orally and is inactive until biotransformed by hepatic microsomal enzymes to active metabolites in the liver. It is of interest to note that corticosteroids inhibit hepatic microsomal enzymes and so reduce its potency. The main toxic effect of cyclophosphamide is bone marrow suppression, leading to leukopenia and a predisposition to infection. It has a half-life of about 6 hours and is largely excreted through the kidneys. As a result it may cause a hemorrhagic cystitis. Other adverse effects may include thrombocytopenia

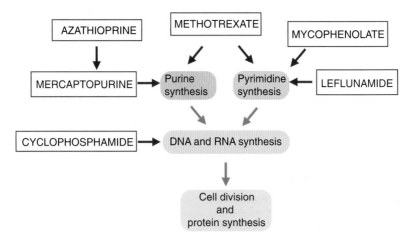

Fig. 21.5 Cytotoxic drugs act at many different points on the cell division pathways. They especially inhibit the production of the purines and pyrimidines that are essential for DNA and RNA synthesis.

and anemia. Cyclophosphamide may be of benefit in the treatment of immune-mediated skin diseases, although its toxicity suggests that other, less-toxic alternatives should be considered first. It should not be used for the treatment of immune-mediated hemolytic anemia (IMHA).

FOLIC ACID ANTAGONISTS

Methotrexate is a folic acid antagonist that has two mechanisms of action. Acting directly, it binds to dihydrofolate reductase and blocks the synthesis of tetrahydrofolate, inhibiting the synthesis of both pyrimidines and purines. As a result, it interferes with DNA synthesis. This blocks B-cell division so that it can also suppress antibody formation. Its side effects are similar to those of cyclophosphamide. Methotrexate also acts indirectly on the intestinal microbiota to alter its composition in such a way that Th1 and Th17 cell activation are minimized. Low doses of methotrexate are used for the treatment of systemic lupus, rheumatoid arthritis, vasculitis, and inflammatory bowel disease in humans. Much higher doses are used for cancer chemotherapy.

AZATHIOPRINE

Azathioprine is a nucleoside analog that suppresses purine synthesis and hence lymphocyte activation and mitosis. It is a prodrug that is oxidized by thiopurine methyltransferase in the liver to two active metabolites, 6-mercaptopurine and 6-thioinosinic acid. These metabolites inhibit both DNA and RNA synthesis. T and B cells are especially susceptible to this effect since they lack a salvage pathway that can repair purine biosynthesis. Thus azathioprine affects rapidly dividing cells such as T cells when they respond to an antigen. Azathioprine can suppress both primary and secondary antibody responses if given after antigen exposure. Azathioprine also has significant antiinflammatory activity since it inhibits the production of macrophages. It has no effect on the synthesis of cytokines or immunoglobulins but tends to suppress T-cell–mediated responses to a greater extent than B-cell responses. Its major toxic effects include bone marrow depression affecting leukocytes rather than platelets or red cells, acute pancreatitis, liver necrosis, and gastroenteritis. It is favored by many clinicians for the treatment of immune-mediated skin diseases because of its combination of antiinflammatory and immunosuppressive activity. It has also been reported to be of benefit in IMHA and myasthenia gravis. It is commonly used in association with corticosteroids; however, it may take up to 11 days before its effects can be seen. Myelosuppression, hepatotoxicity, and pancreatitis may develop in treated animals. As a result, marrow function should be monitored and the dose adjusted if necessary. There are breed-related variations in azathioprine metabolism in dogs that may also influence its effectiveness and toxicity. Long-term treatment may predispose to demodicosis, pyoderma, or fungal infections. Azathioprine should not be used in cats since they have low levels of the enzyme thiopurine methyltransferase that breaks down 6-mercaptopurine.

MYCOPHENOLATE MOFETIL

Mycophenolate mofetil is also a prodrug that is metabolized to mycophenolic acid. This inhibits inosine-5'- monophosphate dehydrogenase, found in activated but not resting lymphocytes. This causes the depletion of guanosine nucleotides and so prevents synthesis of DNA. It therefore blocks both B- and T-cell proliferation, T-cell differentiation, antibody formation, and DC maturation. It may also be antifibrotic. Oral mycophenolate has been reported to be effective in controlling canine diseases such as immune-mediated thrombocytopenia and hemolytic anemia, meningoencephalitis, polymyositis, acquired myasthenia gravis, and pemphigus foliaceus and pemphigus vulgaris, as well as systemic histiocytosis. It is well tolerated by dogs, but its most significant side effects are severe diarrhea, weight loss, and a leukocytosis. It should not be combined with azathioprine.

LEFLUNOMIDE

Leflunomide is a synthetic isoxazole derivative that is metabolized to its active metabolite malononitrilamide and selectively inhibits pyrimidine synthesis. As a result, it blocks DNA and RNA synthesis and inhibits lymphocyte division. Leflunomide suppresses T and B cells that lack a pyrimidine salvage pathway. It also inhibits several tyrosine kinases. Given orally, it is been used to treat several canine autoimmune and inflammatory diseases, especially in cases refractory to corticosteroid treatment or where corticosteroids are contraindicated. Examples include IMHA, immune-mediated thrombocytopenia, nonsuppurative encephalitis/meningitis, immune-mediated polymyositis, myasthenia gravis, immune-mediated polyarthritis, and pemphigus foliaceus. It also appears to be effective in cats with rheumatoid arthritis. Adverse events include gastrointestinal disturbances and bone marrow suppression.

VINCRISTINE

Vincristine is an alkaloid derived from the periwinkle plant and is normally used to treat leukemias. It prevents cell division and thus inhibits leukocyte production and maturation. Its use in autoimmune diseases is restricted to immune-mediated thrombocytopenia where paradoxically, it appears to stimulate thrombopoiesis by activating megakaryocytes while slowing platelet phagocytosis by macrophages. When administered with prednisolone, it is associated with a faster recovery of platelet numbers as compared to prednisolone alone. Unfortunately, it may also induce a neutropenia, especially in dogs that are also receiving cyclosporine.

CYTARABINE

Cytarabine, also called cytosine arabinoside, is an antimetabolite that acts by blocking the actions of DNA polymerase. It is therefore an effective inhibitor of lymphocyte division and a potent immunosuppressant, and is widely used for the treatment of leukemias. It can cross the blood-brain barrier and has been used successfully in combination with prednisolone to treat inflammatory nervous system diseases such as meningitis of unknown origin and steroid-responsive meningitis-arteritis in dogs. It appears to be especially effective when administered by constant rate infusion.

Antiinflammatory Drugs

SULFASALAZINE

Sulfasalazine is an aminosalicylate approved by the US Food and Drug Administration for the treatment of chronic inflammatory diseases. The sulfa component has antimicrobial properties and the salicylate has antiinflammatory effects. It is used in humans to treat rheumatoid arthritis, some types of inflammatory arthritis, ulcerative colitis, and Crohn disease. It also appears to be effective in treating neutrophilic cutaneous vasculitis. It is often used off-label for some immunologic skin diseases such as alopecia areata and pemphigus. It is unclear just how it works, but it reduces leukotriene production and inhibits the cellular release of IL1. In addition, sulfasalazine inhibits the chemotactic response to leukotriene B4, reduces the synthesis of platelet -activating factor, and inhibits the expression of adhesion molecules by leukocytes.

DAPSONE

Otherwise known as diaminodiphenyl sulfone, dapsone is primarily an antibacterial drug. It is also effective in treating humans with mild cutaneous lupus erythematosus, dermatitis herpetiformis, and thrombocytopenia. It appears to inhibit the respiratory burst system in neutrophils. It probably acts by specifically inhibiting neutrophil myeloperoxidase and hence reduces both inflammation and tissue damage.

MISOPROSTOL

Misoprostol is a synthetic prostaglandin E1 analog. It has been shown to elevate intracellular levels of cyclic adenosine monophosphate. This in turn reduces the production of the inflammatory cytokines IL1, TNFα, and leukotriene B4. It also reduces lymphocyte proliferation and granulocyte activation.

HYDROXYCHLOROQUINE

An antimalarial drug with some antiinflammatory properties, hydroxychloroquine is widely used to treat chronic inflammatory diseases such as rheumatoid arthritis and systemic lupus erythematosus. It increases lysosomal pH in antigen-presenting cells and blocks signaling by toll-like receptors, especially TLR7 and TLR9. These two TLRs are responsive to foreign nucleic acids. As a result, it reduces B-cell and DC production of the proinflammatory cytokines INFα, IL6, and TNFα. It has been used for the control of rheumatoid arthritis in humans.

TETRACYCLINE/NIACINAMIDE COMBINATIONS

Antibiotics of the tetracycline family such as tetracycline, doxycycline, and minocycline have both antiinflammatory and immune-modulating properties (Fig. 21.6). Their effects on inflammation and immunity are broad. They suppress lymphocyte proliferation and inhibit neutrophil migration and chemotaxis as well as the production of nitric oxide. They also inhibit T-cell migration, activation, and proliferation, and upregulate the suppressive cytokine IL10. It has been demonstrated recently that as a result of their bacterial evolutionary origins, mitochondrial protein synthesis is also inhibited by tetracycline antibiotics. This interferes with cellular electron transport and the generation of oxidants. As a result, tissue damage is reduced. Tetracyclines inhibit the production

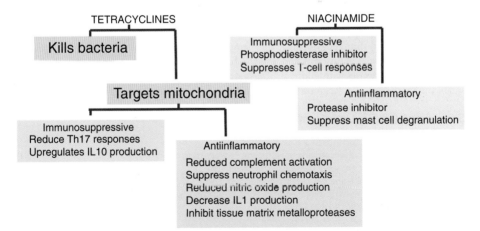

Fig. 21.6 While tetracyclines and niacinamide have many other functions, both have effects on the innate and adaptive immune systems. Thus tetracyclines kill bacteria and interfere with mitochondrial function. (Mitochondria have evolved from bacteria.) As a result, the mixture appears to be effective in treating many autoimmune diseases, especially of the skin, and helps avoid the excessive use of glucocorticosteroids. *IL,* Interleukin; *Th17,* helper T type 17 (cell).

of IL1β and IL17 by inflammatory T cells as well as matrix metalloprotease-13, thus reducing both inflammation and matrix destruction.

Niacinamide inhibits serum phosphodiesterase, increases mast cell stability, and inhibits the production of multiple cytokines and chemokines, including IL1β, IL6, IL8, TNFα, TGFβ. It reduces both neutrophil immigration and lymphocyte activation, and suppresses prostaglandin and cyclooxygenase production.

The combination of doxycycline and niacinamide appears to limit lymphocyte proliferation as well as neutrophil and eosinophil chemotaxis. This combination has been used to treat mild autoimmune skin diseases in dogs, such as cutaneous lupus erythematosus. The combination has been reported to be efficacious, with a 90% response rate when compared to corticosteroids in a double-blind, placebo-controlled trial. It generally takes 3 to 8 weeks before clinical effects may be noticed. It is considered to be a steroid-sparing agent. This is an important quality in diseases such as the pemphigus complexes, where treatment must be continued for years. Once an effect is achieved, some dogs may be maintained in remission on twice- or even once-daily dosing. Side effects include vomiting and diarrhea.

INTRAVENOUS IMMUNOGLOBULIN THERAPY

Although immunoglobulin replacement is appropriate for animals with antibody deficiencies, human intravenous immunoglobulin (IVIG) therapy is immunosuppressive and antiinflammatory. Human IVIG has been used to treat autoimmune and inflammatory diseases in domestic animals. This is a pooled IgG preparation derived from the plasma of a large number of healthy donors. Administered intravenously, its beneficial effects are probably mediated by IgG molecules with sialic acid on their Fc region. These stimulate IL33 production, which then promotes IL4 production, which in turn upregulates the inhibitory receptor FcγR2b on effector macrophages and DCs. In addition, administration of IVIG has been shown to increase production of TGFβ and IL10 by Treg cells and numerous other activities. In dogs, it may act by saturating Fc receptors such as CD16 and CD32 on monocytes. IVIG may also interfere with Fas-mediated apoptosis.

When administered to dogs, IVIG causes a mild thrombocytopenia, leukopenia, increased total plasma protein, and increases in fibrin degradation products, thrombin-antithrombin complexes, and C-reactive protein. In effect, it enhances blood coagulation and some inflammatory responses. It also binds to canine monocytes and lymphocytes (CD4+T, CD8+T, and B cells) and inhibits antibody-mediated phagocytosis by monocytes. IVIG has been used in dogs to treat successfully IMHA, thrombocytopenia, and pemphigus, as well as severe cutaneous drug reactions such as erythema multiforme and Stevens-Johnson syndrome. Most authors have reported positive clinical responses with minimal adverse reactions; however, the number of such reports is small, and more controlled trials of IVIG use in animal diseases are urgently required.

Sources of Additional Information

Glucocorticosteroids

Bizikova P, Olivry T. Oral glucocorticoid pulse therapy for induction of treatment of canine pemphigus foliaceus—a comparative study. *Vet Dermatol.* 2015;26:534 e77.

Elenkov EJ. Glucocorticoids and the Th1/Th2 balance. *Ann NY Acad Sci.* 2004;1024:138–146.

Hardy RS, Raza K, Cooper MS. Therapeutic glucocorticoids: mechanisms of action in rheumatic diseases. *Nature Rev Immunol.* 2020;16:133–144.

Rhen T, Cidlowski JA. Anti-inflammatory action of glucocorticoids: new mechanisms for old drugs. *N Engl J Med.* 2005;353:1711–1723.

Calcineurin Inhibitors

Archer TM, Boothe DM, Langston VC, et al. Oral cyclosporine treatment in dogs: a review of the literature. *J Vet Intern Med.* 2014;28:1–20.

Cummings FO, Rizzo SA. Treatment of presumptive primary immune-mediated thrombocytopenia with mycophenolate mofetil versus cyclosporine in dogs. *J Small Anim Pract*. 2017;58:96–102.

Fellman CL, Stokes JV, Archer TM, et al. Cyclosporine A affects the in vitro expression of T cell activation-related molecules and cytokines in dogs. *Vet Immunol Immunopathol*. 2011;140:175–180.

Janes MR, Fruman DA. Immune regulation by rapamycin: moving beyond T cells. *Sci Signl*. 2009;2:65–68.

Palmeiro BS. Cyclosporine in veterinary dermatology. *Vet Clin Small Anim*. 2013;43:153–171.

Suto T, Karonitsch T. The immunobiology of mTOR in autoimmunity. *J Autoimmunity*. 2020. doi:10.1016/j. jaut.2019.102373.

Antiinflammatory Drugs

Greenfield SM, Punchard NA, Teare JP, et al. The mode of action of the aminosalicylates in inflammatory bowel disease. *Aliment Pharmacol Ther*. 1993;7:369–383.

Ji Q, Zhang L, Jia H, et al. Pentoxifylline inhibits endotoxin-induced NF-kappa-B activation and associated production of proinflammatory cytokines. *Ann Clin Lab Sci*. 2004;34:427–436.

Mushtaq S, Sakar R. Sulfasalazine in dermatology: a lesser explored drug with broad therapeutic potential. *Int J Womens Derm*. 2020;6:191–198.

Nayak RR, Alexander M, Deshpande I, et al. Methotrexate impacts conserved pathways in diverse human gut bacteria leading to decreased host immune activation. *Cell Host Microbe*. 2021;29:362–377.

Sacre K, Criswell L, McCune M. Hydroxychloroquine is associated with impaired interferon-alpha and tumor necrosis factor-alpha production by plasmacytoid dendritic cells in systemic lupus erythematosus. *Arthritis Res Ther*. 2012. doi:10.1186/ar3895.

Sapadin AN, Fleischmajer R. Tetracyclines: nonantibiotic properties and their clinical implications. *J Am Acad Dermatol*. 2006;54:258–265.

Weinberg SE, Chandel NS. Targeting bacteria within us to diminish infections and autoimmunity. *Immunity*. 2021. doi:10.1016/j.immuni.2020.12.006.

Intravenous Immunoglobulin Therapy

Bianco D, Armstrong PJ, Washabau RJ. A prospective, randomized, double blinded, placebo-controlled study of human intravenous immunoglobulin for the acute management of presumptive primary immune-mediated thrombocytopenia in dogs. *J Vet Intern Med*. 2009;23:1071–1078.

Gelfand EW. Intravenous immune globulin in autoimmune and inflammatory diseases. *N Engl J Med*. 2012;367:2015–2025.

Hirschvogel K, Jurina K, Steinberg TA, et al. Clinical course of acute canine polyradiculoneuritis following treatment with human IV immunoglobulin. *J Am Anim Hosp Assn*. 2012;48:299–309.

Lowrie M, Thomson S, Smith P, et al. Effect of a constant rate infusion of cytosine arabinoside on mortality in dogs with meningoencephalitis of unknown origin. *Vet J*. 2016;213:1–5.

Sibley TA, Miller MM, Fogle JE. Human intravenous immunoglobulin (hIVIG) inhibits anti-CD32 antibody binding to canine DH82 cells and canine monocytes in vitro. *Vet Immunol Immunopathol*. 2013;151:229–234.

General

Archer TM, Mulligan C, Narayanan L, et al. Effects of oral administration of 5 immunosuppressive agents on activated T cell cytokine expression in healthy dogs. *J Vet Intern Med*. 2020;34:1206–1213.

Dinarello CA. Anti-inflammatory agents: present and future. *Cell*. 2010;140:935–950.

Tater KC, Gwaltney-Brant S, Wismer T. Dermatological topical products used in the US population and their toxicity to dogs and cats. *Vet Dermatol*. 2019;30:474–e140.

Thompson AW, Forrester JV. Therapeutic advances in immunosuppression. *Clin Exp Immunol*. 1994;98:351–357.

Viviano KR. Update on immunosuppressive therapies for dogs and cats. *Vet Clin Small Anim*. 2013;43:1149–1170.

Whitley NT, Day MJ. Immunomodulatory drugs and their application to the management of canine immune-mediated disease. *J Small Anim Pract*. 2011;52:70–85.

Experimental Autoimmune Disease Models

Laboratory animal models have proved enormously useful in elucidating the pathogenesis of many autoimmune diseases. Three types of models have been most widely used. These include (1) spontaneous disease models, in which specific strains of laboratory animals have been identified as suffering from an autoimmune disease; (2) induced models, in which the disease can be induced experimentally, usually by active immunization against a specific autoantigen or by passive transfer of antibodies or T cells; and (3) genetically engineered animal models, where manipulation of a known critical gene induces the disease. Genetically engineered models may be divided into transgenic models, where specific genes have been inserted, and knockout models, from which specific genes have been removed.

Examples of spontaneous models of autoimmunity include the obese strain (OS) of chickens that develop autoimmune thyroiditis, the nonobese diabetic (NOD) mouse that develops type

1 diabetes mellitus, and the New Zealand mouse hybrids (NZB x NZW) that develop a disease resembling systemic lupus erythematosus (SLE). Examples of induced autoimmune disease include many that can be triggered by injecting high doses of suspected autoantigens together with a powerful adjuvant such as experimental autoimmune encephalitis or experimental autoimmune thyroiditis. This technique can overcome peripheral tolerance and trigger an autoimmune response to many different autoantigens. More recently, methods have been developed to deliberately manipulate the mouse genome by either adding or subtracting specific genes. Thus knockout mice use reverse genetics to delete specific genes, such as the *lpr* gene, from mice of specific genotypes, enabling their effects to be explored in detail. All these models have provided useful and important information on disease etiology, pathogenesis, and potential treatments.

Endocrine Diseases

AUTOIMMUNE THYROIDITIS

An experimental autoimmune thyroiditis resembling the human disease Hashimoto thyroiditis can be induced in mice simply by immunization against mouse thyroglobulin. The thyroglobulin can be adjuvanted with either bacterial lipopolysaccharide or Freund's complete adjuvant. Immunized animals develop a lymphocytic thyroiditis. The susceptibility of different mouse strains to this experimental disease is directly related to their major histocompatibility complex (MHC) class II haplotypes—some haplotypes are susceptible, while others are resistant. This form of the disease is T-cell mediated since it can be passively transferred to normal syngeneic mice by adoptive transfer of T cells. In vitro T-cell proliferative responses to thyroglobulin correlate well with disease severity in these animals. A slightly different form of lymphocytic thyroiditis can be induced by immunizing susceptible mouse strains with a different autoantigen, recombinant murine thyroid peroxidase.

Obese Strain Chickens

OS chickens develop a spontaneous autoimmune thyroiditis in their first months of life. This strain was developed at Cornell University by R. K. Cole when he noticed that symptoms of hypothyroidism developed in a closed line of chickens he was developing. He went a step further and derived the OS by breeding hypothyroid hens with normal males. Eventually, over 90% of the birds of this strain developed the disease. Histopathology shows a severe lymphoplasmacytic infiltration of their thyroids. These lymphoid cells, primarily B cells, can form themselves into germinal centers, a feature also seen in humans with Hashimoto disease. These B cells make autoantibodies against thyroglobulin, although others may make autoantibodies against liver, kidney, pancreas, and red cell antigens without causing lesions in these other organs.

Neonatal bursectomy will prevent the development of these antithyroglobulin antibodies and thus decrease disease severity. Neonatal thymectomy, in contrast, results in more severe disease and very high antibody levels. This has been interpreted as indicating that the disease is caused by B cells as a result of a loss of regulatory T (Treg) cell functions. This is supported by the observation that OS chickens mount an exaggerated response to foreign antigens such as sheep red cells.

The antibodies to thyroglobulin may activate complement or alternatively cause thyroid cell destruction through antibody-dependent cell-mediated cytotoxicity. However, passive transfer of high titered antisera from OS birds alone does not induce disease in normal recipients. Conversely, the disease can be induced in bursectomized OS birds by transfer of bursal cells. The disease can also be triggered by passively administered antibodies if the thyroid is first surgically damaged.

Analysis of the infiltrating lymphocytes indicates that while these are mainly B cells, there are also large numbers of T cells present. Initially, cytotoxic T cells play a minor role in its pathogenesis, but their importance gradually increases so that they destroy thyroid cells later in the course of the disease. Evidence also suggests that there may be a primary defect within the thyroid itself since degenerative lesions develop in the thyroid early in life before the autoantibodies first appear. The development of the disease is controlled by three gene loci. One gene within the chicken MHC and one outside the MHC appear to control immune aggression against the thyroid cells. The third gene acts within the thyroid to predispose it to immunologic attack.

AUTOIMMUNE DIABETES

NOD Mice

The most widely used mouse model of spontaneous autoimmunity is the NOD mouse strain, which was developed in Japan. As a result of extensive outbreeding, there are many available NOD substrains. The prevalence of diabetes varies between individual substrains and laboratories. Thus housing, health status, and diet all have an effect on disease expression. Some NOD mice may also develop autoimmune hemolytic anemia (AIHA), Sjögren syndrome, or autoimmune thyroiditis. Other lines may also develop a spontaneous autoimmune neuropathy.

The disease first appears at weaning. Immature NOD mice develop a lymphocytic infiltration of the pancreatic islets that results in the loss of insulin-producing beta cells. When 90% of the beta cell mass is destroyed, then clinical signs of diabetes develop abruptly. Once all the beta cells are destroyed, the mice develop hyperglycemia, glucosuria, and insulin-dependent diabetes mellitus (IDDM). Their disease resembles human type 1 diabetes and is rapidly lethal in the absence of insulin treatment. It is especially severe in older female mice. Thus more than 90% of female mice develop the disease by 24 weeks, whereas fewer than 40% of male mice develop the disease by 40 weeks.

Development of clinical disease is preceded by an insulitis, resulting in disruption of the islet structure as well as development of a leukocyte infiltrate detectable at weaning. In the infiltrate, CD4+ T cells predominate. The initial lesions probably develop when macrophages infiltrate the islets. These act as antigen-presenting cells that activate T cells. T cells are the prime effector cells, and the disease can be transmitted between syngeneic mice by adoptive transfer of T cells. The triggering autoantigen is a secreted form of the enzyme glutamic acid decarboxylase (GAD). The T-cell response to GAD coincides with the development of insulinitis. There is also evidence of epitope spreading, since the initial responding cells first recognize its C-terminus but over time, they recognize other parts of the GAD molecule as well. NOD mice also have defects in natural killer (NK) and NKT-cell function.

At least 30 genes associated with the diabetic phenotype have been identified in NOD mice. The more of these genes an animal has, the greater its chances of developing the disease. Disease susceptibility also depends on their MHC haplotype. NOD mice have a regular class I region, a unique class II region, and they lack an I-E homolog. Within the MHC, there is a five-nucleotide substitution in the *I-Ab* gene that alters two amino acids. The modified gene is designated I-Ag7. However, other mouse strains that possess I-Ag7 are not diabetic, indicating that additional genes are certainly involved. Several of these other genes have been mapped to specific chromosomes. Thus the I-Ag7 gene (*Idd-1*) is located within the MHC on chromosome 17. A second predisposing gene, *Idd-2*, is found on chromosome 9. Other susceptibility genes, including *Idd-3* on chromosome 3 and *Idd-4* on chromosome 11, also play a role.

Checkpoint blockade of the programmed death 1 (PD-1) pathway in NOD mice will induce fulminating autoimmune diabetes. The PD-1 blockade results in activation of CD8+ T cells that respond by producing high levels of interferon-gamma (IFNγ). This in turn activates blood monocytes that are cytotoxic for islet beta cells through their production of nitric oxide.

The development of diabetes in NOD mice is also influenced by their microbiota. Thus conventional NOD mice that lack MyD88 (MyD88 is an adaptor molecule for the toll-like receptors) do not develop diabetes, whereas totally germ-free MyD88- NOD mice do. If commensal bacteria are fed to these germ-free NOD mice, their diabetes is less severe. The interaction of the intestinal microbiota with the immune system results in an immunosuppression that reduces the predisposition of these mice to develop diabetes. Experimental bacterial infections may also reduce the severity of the disease.

BB Rats

The spontaneous BioBreeding (BB) rat model of IDDM was discovered in a Wistar rat colony in Ottawa, Canada, and phenotypically selected. Insulinitis develops at puberty, and diabetes develops by 8 to 16 weeks. The onset of hyperglycemia is sudden, and insulin is needed if the animals are to survive. NK cells appear to be the major effector cells, but T cells are also critical, as determined by passive transfer experiments. BB rats, like NOD mice, may also develop thyroiditis and Sjögren syndrome. The critical gene implicated in this model appears to be the MHCII, RT1^{u} haplotype. Both susceptibility and the incidence of disease depend in part on the presence of viral infections within the colony. BB rats are also immunocompromised since they carry a recessive lymphopenia mutation.

Neurologic Diseases

EXPERIMENTAL AUTOIMMUNE ENCEPHALOMYELITIS

An autoimmune brain disease known as experimental autoimmune encephalomyelitis (EAE) can be induced by immunizing mice with brain tissue or purified neuronal components emulsified in Freund's complete adjuvant. This can be done in many different species, but most studies have involved mice and rats. Depending on their genetic background, rodents develop a focal encephalitis and myelitis. Their brain lesions consist of a vasculitis with mononuclear cell infiltration, perivascular demyelination, and axon damage. Antibodies to brain tissue can be detected in the serum of these animals, although the lesion itself is a result of a T-cell–mediated response. The major autoantigen is myelin basic protein, but other components such as proteolipid protein are also antigenic. Immunized rats generally develop a single, monophasic neurologic disease with paralysis, while certain strains of mice develop a relapsing-remitting form of disease that closely resembles multiple sclerosis (MS) in humans. Passive EAE can be transferred from affected to normal rats by syngeneic lymphocytes.

A similar encephalitis used to occur in humans following administration of rabies vaccines containing brain tissue. For this reason, the use of adult animal brain tissue vaccines was stopped, and suckling mouse brain tissue obtained prior to myelination was substituted (Chapter 7).

The microbiome is required to initiate EAE since germ-free animals or antibiotic-treated mice are resistant. It is also both interesting and relevant that in mice developing EAE, there is a progressive change in their intestinal microbiota over time following the induction of the disease. The change involves a drastic reduction in *Lactobacilli* and a corresponding increase in *Clostridia*. It has been suggested that this may be a result of progressive changes in immunoregulatory pathways.

Other animal models of MS include a chronic demyelinating disease caused in mice by infection with Theiler's murine encephalomyelitis virus and toxin-induced models caused by cuprizone, a copper-chelating agent.

EXPERIMENTAL AUTOIMMUNE NEURITIS

Experimental autoimmune neuritis (EAN) can be induced in animals such as rabbits, guinea pigs, mice, and especially rats by immunization with constituents from peripheral nerves. Initially, the procedure involved injecting crude homogenized sciatic nerve in Freund's complete adjuvant. Nowadays, purified peripheral nerve myelin proteins (P0, P2, or PMP22), gangliosides, or even synthetic peptides are used as immunogens. Acute demyelinating EAN generally presents as a self-limiting flaccid paralysis with ataxia beginning around 10 to 15 days after immunization.

Weakness begins in the tail and spreads forward. In severe cases, it may result in quadriplegia. After several days, the animal slowly recovers but may have some residual motor defects. Experimentally, the process can be modified to induce a chronic relapsing demyelinating neuropathy. The disease appears to be primarily T-cell mediated, involving both helper T type 1 (Th1) and Th17 immune responses. Perivascular T-cell infiltrates invade the nerves after 10 to 12 days and 2 to 3 days before myelin destruction and onset of paralysis. The main effector cells are, however, activated macrophages that produce reactive oxygen metabolites as well as nitric oxide that destroys the myelin sheaths. Autoantibodies to other nerve components such as glycolipids may contribute to subsequent nerve damage. As a result, affected nerves are infiltrated with CD4+ Th1 cells. These are followed by a wave of CD8+ cells. M2 macrophages and Th17 cells are also present in the lesions. Recovery is associated with increased interleukin-10 (IL10) levels and T-cell apoptosis. Tregs continue to accumulate during the recovery phase of the disease. Because it primarily affects peripheral nerves, EAN is used as an experimental model of diseases such as Guillain-Barré syndrome and other inflammatory neuropathies.

Depending on the immunizing antigen, different forms of EAN may be induced. Thus GN1 gangliosides from myelin sheaths can produce ataxic EAN. This is the form of disease that most closely resembles human Guillain-Barré syndrome. It is of interest to note that when administered to rats with EAN, the checkpoint molecule PD-L1 (see Chapter 2), an inhibitor of T-cell function, results in alleviation of the disease. It inhibits lymphocyte infiltration by decreasing both CD4+ and CD17+ T-cell numbers. A variant EAN may be also induced by immunization of rabbits against gangliosides and galactocerebrosides. It too is characterized by flaccid limb paralysis and high levels of antiganglioside antibodies but an absence of lymphocyte infiltration.

Eye Diseases

Several rodent models of Sjögren syndrome, autoimmune uveitis, and keratoconjunctivitis sicca exist. There are many published studies on adjuvant-induced sialoadenitis in all the laboratory animals in addition to cats. In the case of cats, four injections of cat parotid gland tissue in Freund's complete adjuvant eventually resulted in severe parotid inflammation.

Mild disease develops in NZB/NZW mice, but severe sialoadenitis develops in the MRL+ mouse. This strain develops a CD4+ T-cell infiltration of its lacrimal glands. The response appears to be primarily of the Th2 type. The lpr/lpr mouse has lost its ability to cause apoptosis through a defective fas gene so the MRL/lpr mouse also develops much more severe disease. Another model of this disease is the NOD mouse. Thus some NOD strains can develop lacrimal inflammatory disease. This is, however, primarily Th1 mediated. The NZB/W F1 mouse also develops a form of Sjögren syndrome in addition to other lupuslike lesions. These mice not only develop antinuclear antibodies (ANA) but also rheumatoid factors. It is unclear whether they develop antibodies to SSA or SSB autoantigens. They develop mononuclear cell infiltrates within their salivary and lacrimal glands.

Experimental autoimmune uveitis (EAU) can be induced in nonhuman primates, Lewis rats, or C57Bl/6 mice by the injection of many different retinal antigens. These include retinal S-protein or interphotoreceptor retinoid-binding protein (IRBP) incorporated in Freund's complete adjuvant. Other effective antigens include phosducin, recoverin, rhodopsin, and opsin. In Lewis rats, both IRBP and retinal S-protein induce the disease, whereas in mice, IRBP is more effective. The resulting disease closely resembles the natural uveitis seen in humans. It is also possible to induce an experimental disease with selected peptides from these antigens. These responses appear to be primarily T-cell mediated. Depending on the model, some trigger a Th17-mediated response and others promote a Th1 response. For example, the intense stimulation caused by Freund's complete adjuvant models tend to promote Th17-dominant responses, whereas a less intense signal provided by passive transfer of antigen-pulsed dendritic cells promotes Th1 responses. EAU can also be induced in mice by immunization with selected peptides from human IRBP, by muramyl dipeptide, or by proteoglycans injected systemically. Even Freund's complete adjuvant given without any antigen can induce a uveitis in retinal-binding protein- TCR transgenic mice. Like so many other autoimmune disease models, the severity of EAU is influenced by the intestinal microbiota. Germ-free mice are protected against the development of severe retinal inflammation. They have higher numbers of Treg cells and lower numbers of IFNγ and IL17-producing T cells.

Reproductive Diseases

As described in Chapter 9, vaccination of rabbits, horses, and pigs with zona pellucida glycopeptide ZP3 can induce ovarian inflammation, atrophy, and infertility. Experimental autoimmune orchitis can also be induced in many species, including monkeys, guinea pigs, rabbits, rats, and mice. This has generally been done by incorporating a testicular extract in Freund's complete adjuvant plus Bordetella pertussigens. The two adjuvants are considered necessary to break down tolerance. This results in a T-cell–mediated disruption of the seminal tubules and of spermatogenesis. In an alternative model, A/J and C3H/He mice given two subcutaneous injections of viable syngeneic testicular germ cells without an adjuvant will also develop an orchitis in which lymphocytes surround the tubules and block spermatogenesis.

Skin Diseases

Considerable efforts have gone into developing animal models of alopecia areata. Some mouse strains such as the C3H/HeJ strain develop a spontaneous alopecia areata-like disease. Like other mammals, they develop a mixed, T-cell–dominated infiltrate in and around the bulb region of the hair follicle. Likewise, the Dundee experimental bald rat (DEBR) also develops spontaneous adult-onset alopecia. Both are used to study possible treatments.

Experimental pemphigus-like disease has been induced by immunizing rabbits with an ethanol extract of esophageal mucosa in Freund's complete adjuvant. Autoantibodies are produced and the rabbits develop subepidermal bullae. A more sophisticated model has been developed in mice as a result of the adoptive transfer of lymphocytes from immunized or naïve desmoglein-3 (Dsg-3)$^{-/-}$ knockout mice into mice expressing Dsg-3. The donor lymphocytes, never having been exposed to Dsg-3, are not tolerant to it. As a result, they attack Dsg-3–positive keratinocytes in the skin of the recipient and cause epidermal acantholysis in the oral and esophageal mucosa. These mice also develop patchy hair loss. This "graft versus host" model is a useful tool to investigate potential immunosuppressive therapies. A similar technique has also been used to study pemphigus directed against desmocollin-3 either alone or in association with Dsg-3. As might be anticipated, mice that respond to both autoantigens develop a much more severe disease.

It is possible to induce a disease resembling bullous pemphigoid in neonatal mice by passively administering rabbit antiserum against mouse BP180. However, serum from human bullous pemphigoid patients will not cause blistering in mice since mouse and human type XVII collagens are structurally different. As a result, humanized mouse models have been developed where mice express human collagen in their basement membrane. Skin grafts from these mice placed on syngeneic normal mice induce a strong antibody response and subepidermal blistering. Passive transfer studies have shown that these lesions are induced by CD4$^+$ T cells.

Epidermolysis bullosa acquisita, in contrast, can be studied by administering specific antibodies against type VII collagen to wild-type (SJL/J) mice. After 4 to 8 weeks, the recipient mice begin to develop subepidermal blisters on the face and around the ears.

Blood Diseases

One of the first spontaneous models of immune-mediated hemolytic anemia (IMHA) to be characterized was the New Zealand black (NZB) mouse. These mice develop an autoimmune anemia by 6 months of age. This was first used to identify the genes that influence disease development. These include both susceptibility and protective genes. They were also used to identify the key red cell autoantigens such as band 3, band 4.1, and the Rh complex. These models have clarified the role of different immunoglobulin subclasses and complement in its pathogenesis and most recently have shown that oxidative stress is directly related to the severity of the anemia.

A widely used experimental model of AIHA is the Playfair and Marshall-Clarke model. In this model, AIHA is induced in mice by weekly intraperitoneal injections of rat red cells. Initially, the mice make antirat red cell antibodies, but this eventually changes. Autoantibodies to mouse red cells develop within 5 to 6 weeks and result in a shortened red cell lifespan and the development of anemia. This disease appears to result from dysregulation of Treg cell function. It possibly results as a consequence of epitope spreading from rat antigens to mouse autoantigens.

The HOD transgenic mouse model uses a triple fusion protein consisting of hen lysozyme, ovalbumin, and human Duffy blood group expressed together on the surface of its red cells. These mice are phenotypically normal. However, HOD mice can be crossed with other strains, and the F1 offspring develop clinical variants of hemolytic anemia such as age-related onset and female predominance, as well as a relapsing-remitting or sustained disease.

A drug-induced form of IMHA can be induced in strain A mice by repeated injections or feeding of levodopa. The injections induce IgM and IgG anti–red cell antibodies while oral administration induces IgA-mediated disease. Its pathogenesis is unclear.

Muscle Diseases

MYASTHENIA GRAVIS

Experimental autoimmune myasthenia gravis (EAMG) can be induced in rats and mice by immunization with purified acetylcholine receptors (AChRs) obtained from the electric ray eel, *Torpedo californica*. Some mouse strains such as C57Bl, SJL, and AKR are quite susceptible, and 50% to 70% of immunized animals will develop the disease. Conversely, resistant strains such as BALB/c will not develop the disease. Alternatively, EAMG can be induced in mice by the injection of purified mouse AChRs in Freund's complete adjuvant followed by two or three booster injections. Myasthenic symptoms develop 7 to 14 days after the last injection. In the Lewis rat, EAMG can be induced by a single injection of rat AChRs in complete Freund's adjuvant. IgM antibodies appear by about 7 days. Because they can activate the complement system, the antibodies attract neutrophils that attack and destroy the postsynaptic membrane. As a result, extrajunctional ACh production rises. Once the B cells switch classes to IgG, however, these antibodies are deposited on the postsynaptic membrane and cause a chronic progressive loss of AChRs.

EAMG can also be induced by immunization with a synthetic peptide that corresponds to an epitope occupying positions 97 to 116 of the rat AChR alpha subunit. This can break immunologic tolerance and so cause a slowly progressive myasthenic disease. The simplest method of inducing EAMG is, however, to passively transfer anti-AChR IgG from an affected individual to a normal animal. This may come from a human patient, an immunized donor animal, or a specifically derived monoclonal antibody.

An experimental autoimmune myocarditis can be initiated in susceptible strains of rats and mice by immunization with cardiac myosin. As in other such models, its MHC haplotype is the most important factor that controls disease development. The disease is characterized by infiltration of the myocardium with CD4$^+$ T cells.

Liver Diseases

An experimental autoimmune hepatitis can be induced in male C57BL/6 strain mice by immunizing them with a syngeneic liver homogenate incorporated with Freund's complete adjuvant. BALB/c and C3H mice strains are much less susceptible. This method does not work in Lewis rats. The hepatitis lasts for at least 6 months. It results in the development of perivascular inflammation within the liver. This can be transferred to normal mice by spleen cells or purified T cells.

As described in Chapter 13, repeated immunization of sheep with human glomerular basement membrane eventually results in the development of an acute glomerulonephritis in these animals. IgA nephropathy is a form of immune complex nephropathy that can be experimentally induced in rats. These rats are first given staphylococcal enterotoxin B intravenously while at the same time they are fed prolonged high doses of bovine serum albumin. They are then injected with carbon tetrachloride subcutaneously! The albumin induces high levels of IgA, while the enterotoxin permits it to enter the bloodstream, and the carbon tetrachloride causes a transient nephritis that triggers the IgA deposition. Another, more simple model involves mixing IgG from nephropathy patients with galactose-deficient IgA in vitro and then simply injecting the immune complexes intravenously into rats. The complexes get deposited in the rat kidneys and result in glomerular lesions identical to those found in human patients.

Systemic Lupus Erythematosus

SLE is very complex, so it is unsurprising that there are many different murine models of the disease. These include spontaneous models such as New Zealand and Scurfy mice, and induced models of lupus such as those induced by pristane and graft-versus-host responses.

SPONTANEOUS MOUSE MODELS

New Zealand Mice

Inbred NZB mice spontaneously develop a syndrome that bears a striking resemblance to SLE. The mice develop immune complex glomerulonephritis. They become hypergammaglobulinemic and hypocomplementemic, and they develop AIHA. Some may also develop lymphoid tumors. NZB mice produce autoantibodies against nuclear antigens, red blood cells, and T cells, and their B cells are polyclonally activated.

New Zealand white (NZW) mice, in contrast, are phenotypically normal, but the F1 cross between NZW and NZB mice develops an even more severe SLE-like syndrome. These animals develop lymphadenopathy, splenomegaly, elevated ANA, and an immune complex glomerulonephritis. Death results from kidney failure at 10 to 12 months. The disease susceptibility is strongly biased in favor of females. Studies on the inheritance of these traits in mice suggest that the onset of disease is linked to three susceptibility loci: Sle1 influences loss of tolerance to nuclear antigens, Sle2 affects B-cell hyperactivity, and Sle3 suppresses CD4$^+$ T-cell death.

Scurfy Mice

Scurfy (Sf) mice arose at the Oak Ridge National Laboratory in 1949 as a result of a spontaneous mutation. This was the first X-linked disease to be reported in mice. It was not until the late 1990s that the mutation was located in the gene encoding the Treg cell transcription factor Forkhead box protein 3 (FoxP3). As a result, Sf mice cannot make functional Treg cells. In the absence of Treg-mediated peripheral tolerance, Sf mice develop a generalized autoimmune disorder that resembles systemic lupus, including an interface dermatitis, glomerulonephritis, polymyositis, anemia, lymphopenia, and arthritis as well as autoantibodies against histones, Sm ribonucleoprotein, dsDNA, and many other antigens. They derive their name from a lupuslike hyperkeratosis that develops in their skin and tails as a result of uncontrolled T-cell activity. Sf mice develop splenomegaly and lymphadenopathy, and live for only 3 to 4 weeks.

Yaa Mice

Male BXSB mice develop an accelerated lupuslike syndrome. These males possess a Y chromosome containing a mutant gene called *Yaa* ("autoimmune accelerator"). This mutant gene is a result of a duplication of a 4-Mbp segment of DNA derived from the pseudoautosomal region of the X chromosome by translocation to the Y chromosome. The duplicated segment contains multiple genes, including those for TLR7. Affected males develop follicular T cells and germinal centers, are B-cell depleted, and have a monocytosis. The animals develop an enlarged spleen and a massive lymphadenopathy, hemolytic anemia, hypergammaglobulinemia, and ANA, as well as an immune complex–mediated glomerulonephritis. The disease is believed to result from the duplication of the *TLR7* gene. There is evidence clearly showing that an imbalance of the TLR7/TLR9 receptor functions may predispose to developing some forms of lupus in mice.

lpr and *gld* Mice

The cell surface molecule Fas, otherwise known as CD95, and its ligand Fas-L (CD95-L), play a key role in T-cell–mediated cytotoxicity. One function of cytotoxic T cells is to get rid of unwanted lymphocytes. For example, those lymphocytes that fail the negative selection test within the thymic medulla need to be eliminated. Likewise, anergic cells generated by peripheral tolerance need to be removed and recycled. Thus mutations that render Fas or its ligand defective so that apoptosis cannot occur result in the accumulation of unwanted and unneeded T cells. The mutation in the Fas-ligand gene is called *gld*. The mutation in the Fas gene is called *lpr*. The consequences of either mutation are very similar. Both *lpr*-and *gld*-mutated mice develop multiple autoimmune responses resembling lupus accompanied by lymphoproliferation. This lymphoproliferation results in massive lymphadenopathy and splenomegaly, known as autoimmune lymphoproliferative syndrome. The autoimmune diseases that develop in response to defects in the Fas pathway include immune cytopenias such as AIHA, neutropenias, and thrombocytopenias. These mutations have been recorded in humans. Affected individuals may develop SLE-like disease. Other manifestations may include Guillain-Barré syndrome, autoimmune intestinal diseases, and autoimmune glomerulonephritis. As many as 10% to 20% of affected individuals may develop lymphomas since malignant T cells cannot be killed.

FELINE AUTOIMMUNE LYMPHOPROLIFERATIVE SYNDROME

Feline autoimmune lymphoproliferative syndrome (FALPS) has been reported to occur in British Shorthair cats and their crosses. It is an inherited disease resulting from a *gld* mutation in the gene encoding Fas-ligand. The mutation involves the insertion of an adenine in the third exon of the gener resulting in a frameshift and the generation of a premature stop codon. This results in a severely truncated, nonfunctional Fas-L protein. Homozygous cats develop the disease, while heterozygotes are clinically normal but carry one copy of the gene and so act as carriers. Affected kittens appear normal at birth. Beginning around 6 to 12 weeks, they develop a generalized, rapidly progressive, nonpainful lymphadenopathy accompanied by abdominal distention (due to splenomegaly and hepatomegaly) and a regenerative anemia. All the lymph nodes in the body are enlarged as a result of a diffuse obliterating accumulation of T cells. Diagnosis may be based on lymph node cytology as well as postmortem histopathology. Genetic testing can reveal the defect. There is no treatment and the prognosis is bad. Affected kittens die by 4 months of age.

INDUCED MOUSE MODELS

Pristane-Induced Lupus

Pristane is a mineral oil used to induce ascitic fluid when injected into the peritoneal cavity of mice. (This is how hybridomas were originally grown.) It also induces ANA and the development of a glomerulonephritis. It is believed that pristane acts by inducing overproduction of type 1 IFN, IL6, and IL12. When injected into joints, pristane also induces arthritis by stimulating TNFα overproduction. It may also act by stimulating the pattern-recognition receptor TLR7.

Chronic Graft-Versus-Host Disease

An SLE-like disease can be induced in (C56Bl/10 x DBA/2) F1 mice by inducing chronic graft-versus-host disease. A single injection of donor lymphocytes into recipient mice can induce this disease. Autoantibodies to multiple autoantigens are detected in 10 to 14 days. Disease depends on the model used, but B6 cells administered to (B6 x DBA) F1 hybrid mice result in a massive host polyclonal B-cell activation accompanied by ANA, lupus-specific antibodies, and a glomerulonephritis.

CANINE MODELS

A lupuslike disease has been induced in dogs by immunization with the glycosaminoglycan heparan sulfate. The dogs developed a mild to moderate proteinuria. They also developed skin lesions, including alopecia, erythema, crusting, scaling, and seborrhea. Immunofluorescence assays showed deposition of IgM and complement at the dermal-epidermal junction. Three of eight immunized dogs developed lameness. All the immunized dogs developed ANA titers greater than 1:128.

Autoimmune Arthritis

As with the other diseases and models discussed in this chapter, laboratory animals contribute significantly to our knowledge of disease pathogenesis and provide a key resource for the testing of potential therapeutic processes, especially drugs. While the selected models usually mirror the human disease closely, they also tend to progress much faster than the human disease. For example, bone resorption and formation are more pronounced in rodent arthritis models than in humans. MRL-lpr/lpr mice spontaneously develop a form of arthritis that resembles human rheumatoid arthritis. These mice also produce high levels of IgG and IgM rheumatoid factors. Multiple experimental systems have also been developed that have some features in common with human rheumatoid arthritis. These include collagen-induced arthritis, immune complex arthritis, adjuvant arthritis, and streptococcal cell wall arthritis.

RAT TYPE II COLLAGEN ARTHRITIS

A model system has been established in which heterologous or homologous type II collagen, a major component of joint synovia, is injected together with Freund's incomplete adjuvant into female rats at the tail base and over the back on day 0 and 7 days later. Clinical arthritis develops between days 10 and 13. The animals develop a polyarthritis that resembles human rheumatoid arthritis insofar as it is characterized by significant pannus-associated cartilage destruction, the deposition of immune complexes on articular surfaces, bone resorption, periosteal proliferation, and synovitis. It is mediated by both antibodies and T cells.

MOUSE TYPE II COLLAGEN ARTHRITIS

Selected mouse strains such as the DBA/1 strain will also develop arthritis when immunized with bovine type II collagen. The arthritis is not symmetric, and one or more paws or joints may be affected. The lesions are similar to those that develop in rats with collagen arthritis.

ADJUVANT ARTHRITIS

Unlike most of the other disease models, an arthritis can be readily induced in susceptible male Lewis rats by injecting an oil-in-water emulsion containing killed *Mycobacteria* (i.e., Freund's complete adjuvant). The antigenic material is inoculated intradermally at the tail base or into one of the footpads. After 9 to 10 days, systemic illness (anorexia and weight loss) develops, with inflammation in the tarsal, carpal, phalangeal, and spinal joints. This may be accompanied by lesions in the eyes, nose, ears, and skin. Cartilage destruction tends to be minimal despite severe inflammation and bone loss. Animals usually develop a splenomegaly and hepatomegaly as well as an anterior uveitis. This is a purely T-cell–mediated disease, and antibodies apparently play no role. It is possible that the T cells may recognize cross-reacting proteoglycans or heat shock proteins from the tubercle bacillus. The disease is a relapsing-remitting one and may persist for several months. It may be modified by injecting the adjuvant around a specific joint or into a footpad.

The importance of the antiinflammatory effects of the microbiota is readily seen in this model. Germ-free F344 rats develop severe adjuvant arthritis, whereas specific pathogen-free and conventional rats develop a mild disease. The severity of the disease in germ-free animals can be reduced simply by infecting them with *Escherichia coli*.

IMMUNE COMPLEX ARTHRITIS

In principle, any animal can be immunized against a foreign antigen. Once immune, if this same antigen is then injected into a joint, local formation of immune complexes will result in the development of local inflammation and joint destruction. This is, in effect, a localized Arthus reaction within the joint. It can be induced not only in rats and mice but also in rabbits and guinea pigs.

STREPTOCOCCAL CELL WALL ARTHRITIS

Peptidoglycan-polysaccharide polymers derived from *Streptococcus pyogenes* or *Staphylococcus aureus* when injected into the joints of susceptible rodents (female Lewis rats) also generate a rheumatoid arthritis–like polyarthritis. There is massive immigration of macrophages and neutrophils into the joints that may result in cartilage and bone destruction. The process is mediated by the combined efforts of B cells, T cells, and macrophages. These polymers can also cause the formation of splenic, peritoneal, and liver granulomas.

TRANSGENIC MODELS

TNFα knockout mice that have been transfected with the gene for the membrane-bound form of TNFα that lacks its membrane cleavage site, overexpress membrane TNF and develop a severe arthritis in their paws at 3 weeks of age. Likewise, HLA-B27 transgenic and β2-microglobulin–deficient mice develop spondyloarthropathies.

Immune-Mediated Vasculitis

Multiple rodent models have been developed for both myeloperoxidase (MPO) and proteinase 3 (PR3) antineutrophil cytoplasmic antibody (ANCA)–associated vasculitides. There are few spontaneous disease models, but spontaneous crescentic glomerulitis/Kinjoh (SCG/Kinjoh) rats/mice make circulating MPO-ANCA; however, they make many other autoantibodies as well. Most experimental efforts have focused on the anti-MPO responses. Unfortunately, there are as yet no good models for organ damage other than the lungs and kidney.

Most of the earliest models have involved the passive administration of anti-MPO antibodies or T cells. These have proved to be useful in clarifying the mechanisms of acute vascular injury. Likewise, active immunization with MPO that triggers both B- and T-cell responses has proven useful. One important passive transfer model employs purified antibodies or spleen cells taken from MPO-deficient mice that have been immunized with MPO. These are then transferred into wild-type or recombination activating gene (RAG)–deficient recipients. Over about 6 to 13 days, the recipient mice develop a necrotizing glomerulonephritis and in some cases, they develop lesions in their pulmonary capillaries. Interestingly, the development of lesions is accentuated by administration of endotoxin to mimic the effects of an infection. As in so many of these animal models, the genetic background of the mice has a significant effect on the severity of the reaction. A modification of this model using passively transferred bone marrow cells has shown that MPO expression on hematopoietic cells is necessary for disease induction.

Another autoimmune model has been developed by immunizing mice with MPO in Freund's complete adjuvant. This model has shown that T cells and IL17 are also needed for disease induction. A similar active immunization model has been developed in the Wistar-Kyoto rat strain. These animals produce anti-MPO-ANCA antibodies and T cells, and develop a crescentic glomerulonephritis and pulmonary capillary disease. It should be noted that experimental immunization of rodents with PR3-ANCA has so far failed to generate any cases of glomerulonephritis or lung disease.

Inflammatory Intestinal Diseases

There are three general types of animal models that are used in research into inflammatory bowel disease (IBD): chemically induced models, models induced by adoptive transfer, and spontaneous models. In all these cases, animals develop a Th1 dominant autoimmune response.

Chemically induced models tend to be relatively easy to induce and provide reproducible results. Overall, they induce diseases that closely resemble the lesions observed in humans. They include the dextran sulfate model and the trinitrobenzene sulfonic acid–induced colitis model.

When ingested, dextran sulfate disrupts the colonic epithelial barrier and as a result, it exposes the lamina propria directly to the intestinal contents, including the microbiota. This leads to local tissue injury and the development of acute inflammation. This treatment may induce either an acute disease lasting 4 to 7 days or a chronic disease lasting several months. Affected animals lose weight and develop diarrhea. Gender affects the severity and duration of the colitis since males are more susceptible than females. Genetic background is also important, so that C3H mice are more susceptible than BALB/c. Interestingly, the development of acute colitis is suppressed by the presence of the intestinal microbiota, while germ-free mice develop a much more severe disease with intestinal hemorrhage.

The trinitrobenzene sulfonic acid–induced colitis model acts through a very different process. This molecule is a reactive hapten. As a result, it binds chemically to epithelial cell proteins, acts as a hapten, and triggers a type IV immune response (something like a poison ivy dermatitis on the skin). The animal develops an acute colitis that lasts 5 to 7 days with inflammation, diarrhea, and eventual weight loss. BALB/c mice are especially susceptible. This model does not work on germ-free mice. It appears to depend on a functioning *NOD2* gene. Another haptenating molecule, oxazolone, produces a somewhat similar disease following intrarectal application to mice.

ADOPTIVE TRANSFER MODELS

Models that employ T cells are especially relevant when investigating the immunologic aspects of IBD. Adoptive transfer of naïve T cells depleted of Tregs from healthy wild-type mice into immunodeficient syngeneic recipients induces severe colitis and small intestine inflammation.

The disease develops 5 to 10 weeks following the T-cell transfer. The lesions closely resemble those of human IBD. The severity of the disease is affected by the microbiota, especially the presence of segmented filamentous bacteria.

SPONTANEOUS MODELS

Naturally occurring IBD can occur in C3H/HeJBir and SAMP1/Yit mice as well as in cottontop tamarins and juvenile rhesus macaques. The C3H/HeJBir mice develop a colitis at 3 to 6 weeks of age, but it generally resolves by 10 to 12 weeks. The SAMP1/Yit mice, in contrast, develop disease in the terminal ileum and cecum by 20 weeks that gets progressively more severe.

GENETICALLY ENGINEERED MODELS

While many different proteins (and their genes) are implicated in the pathogenesis of IBD, several stand out because of the magnitude and nature of the consequences of knocking them out. For example, the *NOD2* gene encodes an intracellular pattern-recognition receptor for the bacterial pathogen-associated molecular pattern muramyl dipeptide. If this gene is knocked out or otherwise inactivated, the mice become highly susceptible to dextran sulfate–induced injury. This injury is exacerbated under germ-free conditions, suggesting that the *NOD2* gene plays a key role in the relationship between the animal and its microbiota. Some NOD2 mutants lack Paneth cells, resulting in decreased production of their antibacterial peptides. These mice also become very susceptible to dextran sulfate injury. None of these NOD2 mutants develop ileitis or colitis spontaneously.

Genes that control the autophagy process (the removal of unwanted proteins and organelles from cells) also play a critical role in the pathogenesis of IBD. An autophagy-related gene *(Atg)* appears to be a susceptibility gene for Crohn disease. Two different *Atg* knockouts have been developed. One reduces Paneth cell numbers; the other impairs the capture of bacteria such as *Salmonella* within the autophagosomes of epithelial cells. Mice engineered to lack the *Atg* gene in thymic epithelial cells spontaneously develop colitis.

As might be anticipated, cytokines that play a key role in inflammation are important players in IBD. Mice with deletions in genes encoding IL2, IL2Ra, IL10, and TNF overproduce Th1 cytokines and so develop IBD. Likewise, overexpression of IL7 or a deletion of the *TCR-α*gene results in a Th2-mediated form of IBD.

IL10-deficient mice lose Treg function but develop excessive Th1 and Th17 functions. These knockout mice develop a spontaneous chronic colitis at 2 to 3 months of age, depending on their microbiota and genetic background. BALB/c and C3H mice are susceptible. Germ-free mice do not develop the disease. The presence of *Helicobacter* appears to be essential.

In mice, deletion of the multiple drug-resistant gene *mdr1a* results in the development of chronic colitis around 3 months of age. This results from defect in the epithelial barrier and consequent activation of intestinal T cells. The microbiota are required to trigger this colitis. *mdr* polymorphisms are also associated with human ulcerative colitis. As a result, this is a widely used model in pharmaceutic research.

Sources of Additional Information

Endocrine Diseases

Chen Y-G, Mathews CE, Driver JP. The role of NOD mice in type 1 diabetes research: lessons from the past and recommendations for the future. *Front Endocrinol.* 2018. doi:10.3389/fendo.2018.00051.

Hu H, Zakharov PN, Peterson OJ, et al. Cytocidal macrophages in symbiosis with CD4 and CD8 T cells cause acute diabetes following checkpoint blockade of PD-1 in NOD mice. *Proc Natl Acad Sci.* 2020. doi:10.1073/pnas.2019743117.

Ng HP, Banga JP, Kung AWC. Development of a murine model of autoimmune thyroiditis induced with homologous mouse thyroid peroxidase. *Endocrinology*. 2004;145:809–816.

Wick G, Boyd R, Hála K, et al. Pathogenesis of spontaneous autoimmune thyroiditis in obese strain (OS) chickens. *Clin Exp Immunol*. 1982;47:1–18.

Neurologic Diseases

Yang M, Rainone A, Shi XQ, et al. A new animal model of spontaneous autoimmune peripheral neuropathy. Implications for Guillain-Barré syndrome. *Acta Neuropathol Comm*. 2014. doi:10.1186/2051-5960-2-5.

Eye Diseases

Bagavant H, Michroska A, Deshmukh US. The NZB/F1 mouse model for Sjogren's syndrome: a historical perspective and lessons learned. *Autoimm Rev*. 2020. doi:10.1016/j.autrev.2020.102686.

Dua HS, Abrams MS, Barrett JA, et al. The effect of retinal autoantigens and their peptides on the inhibition of experimental autoimmune uveitis. *Eye*. 1992;6:447–452.

Reproductive Diseases

Naito M, Terayama H, Hirai S, et al. Experimental autoimmune orchitis as a model of immunological male autoimmunity. *Med Mol Morphol*. 2012;45:185–189.

Skin Diseases

Michie HJ, Jahoda CAB, Oliver RF, et al. The DEBR rat: an animal model of human alopecia areata. *Brit J Dermatol*. 1991;125:94–100.

Takae Y, Nishikawa T, Amagai M. Pemphigus mouse model as a tool to evaluate various immunosuppressive therapies. *Exp Dermatol*. 2008;18:252–260.

Blood Diseases

Howie HL, Hudson KE. Murine models of autoimmune hemolytic anemia. *Curr Opin Hematol*. 2018;25:473–481.

Muscle Diseases

Mantegazza R, Cordiglieri C, Consonni A, et al. Animal models of myasthenia gravis: utility and limitations. *Int J Gen Med*. 2016;9:53–64.

Liver and Kidney Diseases

Bygren P, Wieslander J, Heinegard D. Glomerulonephritis induced in sheep by immunization with glomerular basement membrane. *Kidney Internatl*. 1987;31:25–31.

Lohse AW, Manns M, Dienes H-P, et al. Experimental autoimmune hepatitis: disease induction, time course and T-cell reactivity. *Hepatol*. 1990;11:24–30.

Moldoveanu Z, Suzuki H, Reily C, et al. Experimental evidence of pathogenic role of IgG autoantibodies in IgA nephropathy. *J Autoimmunity*. 2021. doi:10.1016/j.jaut.2021.102593.

Systemic Lupus Erythematosus

Aberdein D, Munday JS, Gandolfi B, et al. A FAS-ligand variant associated with autoimmune lymphoproliferative syndrome in cats. *Mamm Genome*. 2017;28:47–55.

Choi E, Shin I, Youn H, et al. Development of canine systemic lupus erythematosus model. *J Vet Med Assoc*. 2004;51:375–383.

Izui S, Twamoto M, Fossati L, et al. The Yaa gene model of systemic lupus erythematosus. *Immunol Rev*. 1995;144:137–155.

Moore E, Putterman C. Are lupus animal models useful for understanding and developing new therapies for human SLE?. *J Autoimm*. 2020. doi:10.1016/j.jaut.2020.102490.

Autoimmune Arthritis

Bendele AM. Animal models of rheumatoid arthritis. *J Musculoskel Neuron Interact*. 2001;1:377–385.

Immune-Mediated Vasculitis

Salama AD, Little MA. Animal models of ANCA associated vasculitis. *Curr Opin Rheumatol*. 2012;24:1–7.

Inflammatory Intestinal Diseases

Kiesler P, Fuss IJ, Strober W. Experimental models of inflammatory bowel disease. *Cell Mol Gastro Hepatol*. 2015. doi:10.1016/j.jcmgh.2015.01.006.

Misoguchi A, Misoguchi E. Animal models of IBD: linkage to human disease. *Curr Opin Pharmacol*. 2010;10:578–587.

Page numbers followed by "*f*" indicate figures, "*t*" indicate tables, and "*b*" indicate boxes